On Phlebotomy by Abū Bakr Muḥammad ibn Zakariyyāʾ al-Rāzī

Islamic Philosophy, Theology and Science

TEXTS AND STUDIES

Founding Editor

Hans Daiber

Edited by

Anna Akasoy
Emilie Savage-Smith
Ayman Shihadeh

VOLUME 136

The titles published in this series are listed at *brill.com/ipts*

On Phlebotomy by Abū Bakr Muḥammad ibn Zakariyyāʾ al-Rāzī

A Bilingual Edition of *Maqāla fī l-Faṣd* and *Maʿamar baHaqqaza*

Edited, translated and commented by

Juhan Björn

BRILL

ISSN 0169-8729
ISBN 978-90-04-76227-5
ISBN 978-90-04-76229-9 (PDF)
DOI https://doi.org/10.1163/9789004762299

Library of Congress Control Number: 2026940672

Brill and Koninklijke Brill BV are part of De Gruyter Brill.
www.degruyterbrill.com

Questions about General Product Safety Regulation: productsafety@degruyterbrill.com

Cover illustration: Seljuk Minai dish, first half of the 13th century. © Staatliche Museen zu Berlin, Museum für Islamische Kunst / Johannes Kramer

For my grandparents

Contents

Preface

The objective of this study is to present a revised text-critical edition, translation, and commentary, based on the unique copy of *Maqāla fī l-Faṣd* together with its anonymous Hebrew translation, *Ma'amar baHaqqaza le'al-Rāzī*, attributed to Abū Bakr Muḥammad ibn Zakariyyā' al-Rāzī. The Arabic edition was originally published as a doctoral dissertation in September 2023 and defended in October 2023 in Lund, Sweden.[1]

In this publication, the aim is to present a revised version of the previous publication, now including its hitherto unpublished Hebrew translation as a separate treatise. The inclusion of the Hebrew edition offers new findings and insights that have not previously been published. This approach aims to contribute to a comprehensive understanding of medieval medical knowledge and its transmission, emphasising the interconnectedness of diverse scholarly traditions and shedding light on scholarly and translation activities in medieval Europe. The dual structure of this volume thus serves Arabic and Hebrew readers independently, providing each with a self-contained analysis. Together, they form a comprehensive study, enhancing our understanding of *Maqāla fī l-Faṣd* and its historical significance, making one of al-Rāzī's lesser-known treatises accessible to readers.

Since the present publication is directly linked to my doctoral dissertation, I would like to extend my gratitude to my previous supervisors, Professor Emeritus Gerrit Bos and Professor Emerita Lena Ambjörn. Their guidance, mentorship, and encouragement have been valuable from the very beginning of my journey in the study of Arabic and Hebrew manuscripts. I am also grateful to Professor Peter E. Pormann for his valuable feedback at the defence of my doctoral dissertation. Finally, I would like to express my gratitude to Bengt Lindskogs stiftelse for the financial support received for working with the Hebrew edition.

---

1 Cf. Al-Rāzī, Muḥammad Ibn Zakarīyā, 865–925. *On Phlebotomy* / Abū Bakr Muḥammad ibn Zakariyyā' al-Rāzī; edition, translation and commentary by Juhan Björn, 2023.

The Arabic alphabet has been transliterated as follows:

k	ك	ḍ	ض	d	د	a, ʾ	أ ء
l	ل	ṭ	ط	ḏ	ذ	b	ب
m	م	ẓ	ظ	r	ر	t	ت
n	ن	ʿ	ع	z	ز	ṯ	ث
h	ه	ġ	غ	s	س	ǧ	ج
w, ū	و	f	ف	š	ش	ḥ	ح
y, ī	ي	q	ق	ṣ	ص	ḫ	خ

The Hebrew alphabet has been transliterated as follows:

s	שׂ	s	ס	ḥ	ח	a, ʾ	א
t	ת	ʿ	ע	ṭ	ט	b, v	ב
ǧ	ג׳	p, f	פ	i, y	י	g	ג
		ṣ	צ	k, ḵ	כ	d	ד
		q	ק	l	ל	h	ה
		r	ר	m	מ	v, w	ו
		š	שׁ	n	נ	z	ז

CHAPTER 1

The Medical Framework

This book presents a critical edition and translation of Abū Bakr Muḥammad ibn Zakariyyāʾ al-Rāzī's *Maqāla fī l-Faṣd* together with its Hebrew translation, *Maʾamar baHaqqaza leʾal-Rāzī*. Before introducing the author and the treatise itself, it is essential to briefly outline the medical framework that is reflected in this work. The foundations of this theory were laid in ancient Greece during the fourth century B.C., a time when both the profound value of health and the inherent human vulnerability to disease were acknowledged as fundamental aspects of life.[1] This early emphasis on health spurred the development of sophisticated medical thought, with Hippocrates emerging as the revered 'father of medicine,' whose fame and enduring influence extended across geographical, religious, and linguistic boundaries.[2] The extensive *Hippocratic Corpus*, compiled over several centuries, established foundational medical principles that were elaborated by subsequent generations.[3]

Building upon this early Greek foundation, the Hellenistic period (330–30 B.C.[4]) witnessed significant developments in medical knowledge and practice. As only a few original treatises from this era survive, most of our understanding of its medical advancements comes from fragments preserved by later authors.[5] This period also witnessed the emergence of pharmacology as a distinct field. With the conquest and growth of Alexandria as a central trading hub, herbs and spices from Africa and India became more widely available, contributing to the development of this area of investigation for authors like Theophrastus (c. 371–278). The investigation of new substances continued to expand, particularly in the botanical and medical writings advanced by the school of Herophilus. Moreover, the anatomical discoveries of Herophilus and Erasistratus further contributed to the development of new surgical techniques and instruments, with Alexandrian surgeons gaining particular fame for their skills in treating fractures and dislocations.[6]

1 Holmes, *Medicine*, pp. 554–555.
2 Pormann, *The Cambridge Companion to Hippocrates*, p. xiii.
3 Pormann, *The Cambridge Companion to Hippocrates*, p. 19.
4 Nutton, *Ancient Medicine*, p. 156.
5 Nutton, *Ancient Medicine*, p. 140.
6 Nutton, *Ancient Medicine*, pp. 141–142.

Grounded in the Aristotelian framework of four primary qualities and four elements, the *Hippocratic Corpus* offered a coherent system of medical theory and practice. According to this theory, disease was attributed to states of excess or deficiency; treatment aimed at restoring balance; and diet and exercise were viewed as crucial for enabling the body to counteract potentially harmful imbalances. The *Corpus* posited that the body's natural temperament made it continuously susceptible to imbalance, with each temperament associated with specific physical and psychological conditions. Furthermore, as noted in the Hippocratic treatises like *Epidemics* and *Airs, Waters and Places*, external factors affected the body.[7] Physicians had to be acquainted not only with the patient's individual constitution, but also with the season, winds, weather, geographical location, the sun's cycles, and the cosmos in general.[8]

Among the central aspects of Hellenistic medicine is humoral pathology, i.e., the doctrine of the four humours. The concept was introduced by Hippocrates of Cos (mid-fifth century B.C.) in his treatise *On the Nature of Man*, later adopted and further developed by Galen of Pergamon (129–c. 216 A.D.), who became the most influential of the Greek physicians[9]—as Temkin puts it, "no physician after Galen was comparable to him."[10] Even though the origins of the doctrine of the four humours can be traced back to the Hippocratic school of medicine, it was Galen who emphasised the four humours—yellow bile, blood, phlegm, and black bile—as *the* Hippocratic humours, together with their association with the Aristotelian qualities,[11] where fire was hot and dry, air was hot and moist, water was cold and moist, and earth was cold and dry.[12] There was also a fifth element among the celestial bodies, namely *aether*, which was considered more divine than the earthly elements, and which was believed to exist in all living creatures in the so-called innate heat and in the semen, credited with the power of generating life.[13]

To better understand how these fundamental substances were central to health, it is important to examine the nature and characteristics attributed

7 Nutton, *Ancient Medicine*, p. 145.

8 Nutton, *Ancient Medicine*, p. 75.

9 Pormann & Savage-Smith, *Medieval Islamic Medicine*, p. 9. According to Siegel, the notion of the four humours can be attributed to Pythagoras (530 B.C.) and his school, which are considered the originators of this concept. However, the Hippocratic treatises were not consistent regarding the number of the humours. Additionally, Praxagoras considered there to be nine or ten humours (Siegel, *Galen's System of Physiology and Medicine*, p. 216).

10 Temkin, *Galenism*, p. 125.

11 Brain, *Galen on Bloodletting*, p. 6.

12 Temkin, *Galenism*, p. 103.

13 Brain, *Galen on Bloodletting*, p. 6.

to each of the humours. The four humours each possessed a pair of primary qualities: yellow bile is hot and dry, blood hot and moist, phlegm cold and moist, and black bile cold and dry.[14] These qualities also defined the four elements with which the humours were associated: yellow bile with fire, blood with air, phlegm with water, and black bile with earth. Each humour was further linked to a specific temperament: yellow bile with the choleric, blood with the sanguine, phlegm with the phlegmatic, and black bile with the melancholic temperament. Finally, the humours were associated with the four seasons: yellow bile with summer and autumn, blood with summer and spring, phlegm with winter, and black bile with autumn.[15] Notably, yellow bile, blood, and phlegm are actual components of the body, whereas black bile was posited to complete the harmony of four.[16] The prevailing understanding was that the humours themselves were not inherently harmful, but that illness arose from their excess or deficiency. While a mere imbalance did not necessarily lead to illness, sickness occurred when an excessive amount of a humour settled in a specific area. Although health was generally considered the normal state of the body, the third book of the *Aphorisms* suggests that perfect health, not disease, was the rarity, highlighting the inherent fragility of human well-being. Some authors broadened the notion of health to include a permissible degree of imbalance—only when such imbalance became excessive did illness manifest.[17]

Among the humours, blood was considered the most well-tempered,[18] both as a humour of its own and a balanced mixture of all the humours.[19] Its primary task was to serve as nutrition for the body.[20] In Galen's physiological system, food from the stomach underwent digestion, or concoction, in the liver, transforming into nutritious blood that was then distributed via the veins to nourish the body.[21] Phlegm was recognised as a corrupt moisture, apparent in various body fluids. Yellow bile was understood as a foam generated during blood formation in the liver, with half of it flowing with the blood, and the other half settling in the gallbladder. Black bile was seen as a dark substance that, similarly to yellow bile, was produced during blood formation in the liver, half of

14 Brain, *Galen on Bloodletting*, pp. 6–7.
15 Siegel, *Galen's System of Physiology and Medicine*, p. 218.
16 Brain, *Galen on Bloodletting*, pp. 6–7.
17 Nutton, *Ancient Medicine*, pp. 80–81.
18 Brain, *Galen on Bloodletting*, p. 8.
19 Siegel, *Galen's System of Physiology and Medicine*, p. 217.
20 Brain, *Galen on Bloodletting*, p. 123.
21 Nutton, *Ancient Medicine*, p. 233.

it remaining in the blood, while the other half ended up in the spleen. Accordingly, the blood flowing in the veins was a mixture of blood, yellow bile, and black bile.[22]

According to Nutton (2004), early texts like *Nature of Man* refer to black bile as 'the so-called black bile,' suggesting that the concept was not initially widespread. Over time, diseases came to be attributed to black bile, and it gained status as a distinct humour rather than just a type of bile, despite never being observed in its pure form. Its existence was seemingly confirmed through empirical observations of the body, such as the dark colour of warts and moles, the appearance of dark blood in scars, and dark vomit, which were taken as evidence that the body contained a dark and mysterious substance, the antithesis of life-giving blood, which was seen as its complete opposite.[23] Nutton also suggests that bile and phlegm received more attention than other bodily fluids, likely due to their apparent visibility and straightforward association with illness. Their unappealing appearance often coincided with ailments such as a runny nose, coughing or spitting sputum, and cloudy urine—all conditions readily linked to disease. Consequently, it was logical to assume that a coarse substance could obstruct the flow of air throughout the body or cause arthritis by settling on a joint. Bile, being visibly present in vomit and diarrhoea, naturally led to the idea that it could damage internal surfaces and bodily processes, much like it disrupts digestion. Furthermore, both these substances were observed to occur seasonally.[24]

Underlying Galen's entire system was the fundamental belief that Nature was the creator and controller of all living things, and that health resided in maintaining a natural balance.[25] As Tallmadge May (1996) explains, 'Nature' was understood as "the primary essence which is the basis of all bodies that are generated and decay."[26] Through his anatomical experiments, Galen sought to demonstrate the wisdom of Nature, or the Creator. Echoing Plato and Aristotle, he believed that every part, from an insect's eye to any other component of a living being, was intentionally created for a specific purpose. Even the smallest structures were designed with their proper function in mind, along with a precise balance of elements, qualities, or humours that facilitated that specific function.[27] In Galen's view, disease was an unnatural state of the body, a dis-

22 Pormann & Savage-Smith, *Medieval Islamic Medicine*, p. 44.
23 Nutton, *Ancient Medicine*, p. 84.
24 Nutton, *Ancient Medicine*, p. 80.
25 Brain, *Galen on Bloodletting*, p. 7.
26 Galen, *UP*, May's introduction, p. 10.
27 Nutton, *Ancient Medicine*, pp. 234–235.

ruption of this harmonious equilibrium between the four humours and their associated qualities.[28] A too hot patient needed to be treated by cooling, a too dry patient by damping, and so on.[29] Consequently, the function of medicine, as he stated in *On Treatment by Venesection*, was "both to restore all the natural functions of the parts of the body when they have been corrupted, and to preserve them once they have been restored."[30]

As the humours flowed in the blood, phlebotomy became a central means to restore the balance between the humours. Even though it was Galen who became a pioneer in applying phlebotomy to treat a wide variety of diseases,[31] the procedure had been used for a long time by various civilisations. Garrison (1913) describes phlebotomy as one of the oldest and most common therapeutic devices, used by ancient Egyptians, Babylonians, and native Americans, who used fishbones, thorns, sharp stones, and horns as instruments for phlebotomy and cupping. Moreover, phlebotomy is even mentioned in the Talmud.[32] In other words, despite having been used for a long time by various civilisations, it was Galen who established the antique tradition of phlebotomy as a fashionable practice,[33] that he used to treat both physical and psychological conditions: illnesses in the parts, sciatica, rheumatism, insanity, melancholia,[34] hepatitis, angina, ophthalmia, and epilepsy, and according to his records, he successfully treated a patient suffering from *anorexia nervosa* as well.[35] Apart from phlebotomy, Galen used diet, cupping, and purging to rectify humoral imbalances.[36] He understood that different methods had different effects, with phlebotomy primarily emptying the veins, while fasting emptied the entire body. However, phlebotomy was faster to conduct and provided immediate results, while fasting took a long time and was more challenging for the patient.[37]

Galen also emphasised the importance of a proper diet. Yet, his understanding of diet extended beyond just food and drink, encompassing a person's entire lifestyle, including exercise, sleep, and environmental influences. He recog-

28 Brain, *Galen on Bloodletting*, p. 4.
29 Brain, *Galen on Bloodletting*, p. 7.
30 Galen, *Cur. Rat. Ven. Sect.*, p. 71.
31 Garrison, *The History of Bloodletting*, pp. 8–9, Brain, *Galen on Bloodletting*, p. 145.
32 Garrison, *The History of Bloodletting*, pp. 1–3.
33 Brain, *Galen on Bloodletting*, pp. 1–2.
34 Garrison, *The History of Bloodletting*, p. 10.
35 Brain, *Galen on Bloodletting*, p. 129; 133.
36 Pormann & Savage-Smith, *Medieval Islamic Medicine*, pp. 43–44.
37 Brain, *Galen on Bloodletting*, p. 122.

nised that consuming unsuitable foods could lead to illness, and a proper diet could maintain and restore health. In his works, he connected the properties of foodstuffs to the four humours and their associated qualities, categorising them as either heating, cooling, moistening, or drying, and noting their ability to thicken or thin the humours. Following the approach of his predecessors, Galen also classified foodstuffs based on their digestibility, strength, and suitability for human consumption.[38] He considered white meat, poultry, and fish to be more easily digestible than red meat, and believed that pork, due to its resemblance to human flesh, was the easiest meat to digest. For the sick, he recommended white wines, soups, barley broth, and gradually reintroducing their regular diet. Despite the enduring validity of much of his dietary advice, he almost entirely prohibited consuming fresh fruit, regarding them as a frequent source of illness.[39] Alongside a proper diet, Galen emphasised the importance of physical exercise and bathing in moderation.[40]

Regarding the balancing of humours, Savage-Smith (2013) argues that in practice, they were less central to therapy than the term 'humoral pathology' implies.[41] Firstly, therapy itself was not necessarily based on directly addressing humoral *imbalances*, but involved administering simple drugs based on their *qualities* (warm, cold, dry, moist) to counteract perceived symptoms; there was no direct 'humoral justification' for these therapies.[42] Secondly, the practical application of humoral theory in therapy was problematic because blood vessels, as mentioned above, carried a mixture of humours (blood, yellow bile, and black bile—and for some medical authorities even phlegm), implying that procedures like phlebotomy would remove multiple humours, making it impossible to selectively adjust the balance of a single humour.[43] However, when resorting to drugs, Galen aimed to correct imbalances by using a substance with a quality opposite to the nature of the disorder. He primarily studied simple drugs and observed how they affected the body through one of the primary qualities. He also recognised a category of drugs proven to be efficient by experience, even though it was difficult to assign any specific quality to their

38 Nutton, *Ancient Medicine*, pp. 240–241.

39 Nutton, *Ancient Medicine*, p. 241.

40 Nutton, *Ancient Medicine*, pp. 241–242.

41 Savage-Smith, *Were the Four Humours Fundamental to Medieval Islamic Medical Practice?*, p. 103.

42 Savage-Smith, *Were the Four Humours Fundamental to Medieval Islamic Medical Practice?*, p. 92.

43 Savage-Smith, *Were the Four Humours Fundamental to Medieval Islamic Medical Practice?*, p. 98. This inability to isolate and restore the balance of individual humours, according to Savage-Smith, is evident in the medical literature.

activity. These composite drugs could target specific *humours*: for instance, phlegmagogues could be used to draw out phlegm, and cholagogues to expel excess bile.[44]

In addition to the humoral theory, ancient physicians worked with other key physiological ideas. Another fundamental concept in the Greek medical theory was *pneuma*, of which Galen identifies three types: vital pneuma, that is generated in the heart and in the arteries, produced from the inhalation and vaporisation of the humours; psychic pneuma, generated from a further refinement of the vital pneuma in the retiform web through the carotid arteries, reaching the ventricles of the brain;[45] and natural pneuma, generated in the liver and distributed through the veins.[46] In addition to pneuma, Galen's physiological system, explained in his *De usu partium*, is based on the idea that each division of the soul has a special power or faculty. He assigned the psychic faculty to the brain, the vital faculty to the heart, and the natural faculty to the liver. Additionally, most of the other body parts had their faculties, such as the attractive faculty to attract nutriment, the retentive faculty to hold the nutriment, and the expulsive faculty to get rid of surplus material. Galen assigned these faculties to various parts of the body, such as the uterus, the arteries, the muscles, and the veins, while being aware that assigning these faculties did not actually explain much, but rather served as a label until the true essence of the cause behind actions could be understood.[47] The faculties of attraction, assimilation, excretion, and growth, found in every living organism, allowed each part of the body to absorb what it needed to function properly. Ultimately, Galen viewed the body as a self-regulating microcosm that responds to changes and actively seeks what it requires to function and survive.[48]

In summary, health was viewed as a vulnerable state, influenced by numerous factors including air, lifestyle, diet, sleep, and exercise. Moreover, it was in a constant state of flux due to climate, seasonal shifts, and ageing. This perspective emphasised individual constitution, each person having their own ideal balance, perpetually at risk of disruption from external changes. However, many of these changes were predictable and thus preventable. For instance, knowing that fevers could result from excess bile, which was prevalent in summer and autumn, one could take dietary precautions to limit bile production. Sim-

---

44 Nutton, *Ancient Medicine*, pp. 242–243.

45 Galen, *PHP* VII 3, pp. 444–445. For an explanation how this works, see Galen, *PHP* VII 3–4, pp. 442–453.

46 Galen, *UP*, p. 48.

47 Galen, *UP*, pp. 49–50.

48 Nutton, *Ancient Medicine*, p. 233.

ilarly, understanding that blood increased in spring and early summer allowed for preventative measures to protect the body from potential harm. To prevent an imbalance and restore the body to a natural state, one had to account for a range of elements, such as age, constitution, season, and the appropriate treatment. Though intricate, this was achievable and desirable, as health was valued as 'the most precious of goods.'[49]

1 Graeco-Arabic Medicine

Building upon the foundations of Greek medical heritage, scientific medicine began to flourish centuries later under Islamic civilisation, marking one of the most dynamic phases in the historical development of medicine.[50] The reception and translation of Greek literary and scholarly traditions within the regions that became the Islamic world was crucial for the later integration of Greek arts and sciences into Islamic thought[51] and for the formation of Graeco-Arabic medicine.[52]

During the Umayyad period (661–750 A.D.[53]), translation efforts were largely pragmatic, driven more by administrative and social needs than by scholarly ambition. Following the Arab conquest of Syria, Palestine, and Egypt, the continued use of Greek in government and daily life made translation from Greek into Arabic essential—especially in administrative contexts, as evidenced by bilingual documents and papyri from the seventh and eighth centuries.[54] The lack of scientific, and especially medical, knowledge became evident, and teachings from Greek sources had to be accessed indirectly, first through Syr-

---

49 Nutton, *Ancient Medicine*, pp. 82–83.

50 Isaacs, *Arabic Medical Literature*, p. 342.

51 Goodman, *The Greek Impact on Arabic Literature*, p. 472.

52 While some scholars use the term 'Islamic medicine' to describe the medical tradition that emerged in the Islamic Empire, this term may have limitations and could be perceived as implying an exclusive association with Islam. However, as Pormann & Savage-Smith (p. 2) point out, the term is not limited to practitioners of Islam and does not exclude practitioners of other religions or cultures. I have chosen to use the term 'Graeco-Arabic medicine' instead, which emphasises the continuity of the Graeco-Roman medical tradition in this development. However, I acknowledge that any term could be misunderstood or have limitations. While there currently is no term that explicitly recognises the multiple sources of this tradition, it is important to clarify that the term 'Graeco-Arabic medicine' is not meant to imply that only Greek and Arabic traditions were involved, but rather to highlight the prominent role of these two in the development of the medical tradition.

53 Gutas, *Greek Thought, Arabic Culture*, p. 17.

54 Gutas, *Greek Thought, Arabic Culture*, pp. 23–24.

iac translations and later through Arabic ones.[55] Although some translations took place under the Umayyads—often by Syriac-speaking Christians—they remained limited in scope and lacked the organisation and scale that would come to define the Abbasid period.[56]

Despite the practical approach to translations, there was some interest in Greek learning: for instance, ʿUmar b. ʿAbd al-ʿAzīz, who reigned between 99–102/717–720, is credited with ordering the Arabic translation of a Greek medical work.[57] Some political and advisory texts were rendered into Arabic, and the administrative apparatus was gradually arabicised. However, the translations of scientific texts remained rare, with few confirmed instances.[58] Furthermore, early intellectual activity also encompassed topics like grammar, administration, law, and Islamic thought.[59]

While the Umayyad period laid important groundwork, it was under the Abbasids that the translation of scientific and medical texts truly flourished. The transmission of Greek medical heritage gained significant momentum with the rise of the Abbasid dynasty around 750 A.D. and the subsequent foundation of Baghdad in 762 A.D., which led to an immense translation movement[60]—a deliberate and large-scale scholarly project with far-reaching historical, social, and cultural consequences.[61] In its first century, the translation movement introduced foundational Greek concepts such as the four elements, four humours, and four temperaments into Arabic discourse.[62] Over a period of two centuries, nearly the entire corpus of Greek scientific texts was translated into Arabic.[63] Beyond its own merits, this translation movement was essential because it ensured the survival of numerous Greek works, the original versions of which have since perished.[64]

A central force in this intellectual activity was the work of Syriac-speaking Christians, who served as trilingual intermediaries, often translating from Greek into Syriac and then into Arabic.[65] Among them, Ḥunayn ibn Isḥāq

55 Isaacs, *Arabic Medical Literature*, pp. 342–343.
56 Gutas, *Greek Thought, Arabic Culture*, pp. 20–22.
57 Goodman, *The Greek Impact on Arabic Literature*, p. 473.
58 Gutas, *Greek Thought, Arabic Culture*, pp. 23–24.
59 Goodman, *The Greek Impact on Arabic Literature*, p. 473 ff.
60 Gutas, *Greek Thought, Arabic Culture*, p. xiii.
61 Gutas, *Greek Thought, Arabic Culture*, p. 24.
62 Isaacs, *Arabic Medical Literature*, p. 343.
63 Gutas, *Greek Thought, Arabic Culture*, p. 1.
64 Gutas, *Greek Thought, Arabic Culture*, p. 1.
65 Hoyland, *Seeing Islam as Others Saw It*, pp. 195–196.

(192/808–260/873[66]), a Nestorian Christian active in the 9th-century Baghdad, played a central role. He not only translated much of the *Hippocratic Corpus* and the commentaries of Galen,[67] but also led a circle of disciples, including his family members, who translated numerous other medical works.[68] His method emphasised clarity, precision, and fidelity to the original meaning, prioritising technical accuracy over stylistic ornamentation.[69] The intellectual activity of centres like Alexandria, which had already engaged with Greek medical thought, further facilitated the reception of Hippocratic texts in Baghdad.[70] Prior to Ḥunayn ibn Isḥāq, Arabic lacked a suitable technical vocabulary. His pioneering efforts in translation and terminology became the model for future translators, and profoundly shaped Arabic medical literature.[71]

While deeply rooted in Hellenistic medicine, Graeco-Arabic medicine evolved to incorporate elements from across the vast Islamic Empire, which during the medieval period stretched from Spain and North Africa to India and Central Asia, fostering a society in which different cultures and languages co-existed and collaborated. Thus, Graeco-Arabic medicine was cultivated by scholars from diverse backgrounds, overlooking origin, language, religion, and culture. They would all write in Arabic, a language that connected both medical practitioners and patients.[72] In urban centres like Baghdad, an elite medical culture developed, while rural areas maintained more traditional, pre-Islamic medical practices.[73] The necessity of precise medical communication functioned as an incentive for establishing a comprehensive Arabic technical terminology, ultimately transforming Arabic into the scientific *lingua franca* of the Empire.[74]

In parallel with the translation of medical works, a sophisticated culinary tradition also emerged. Significantly, this Arabic-Islamic culinary culture was built upon the foundations of Greek humoral theory and the existing culinary practices of the ancient Near East. The connection between diet and medicine, rooted in humoral principles, is illustrated for instance in Ibn Sayyār al-Warrāq's culinary manual, *Kitāb al-Ṭabīḫ*, and in the works of the early Abbasid

66 Isaacs, *Arabic Medical Literature*, p. 344.
67 Pormann, *The Cambridge Companion to Hippocrates*, p. 19.
68 Waines, *Dietetics in Medieval Islamic Culture*, p. 101.
69 Isaacs, *Arabic Medical Literature*, p. 344.
70 Pormann, *The Cambridge Companion to Hippocrates*, pp. 19–20.
71 Isaacs, *Arabic Medical Literature*, p. 344.
72 Pormann & Savage-Smith, *Medieval Islamic Medicine*, p. 2.
73 Pormann & Savage-Smith, *Medieval Islamic Medicine*, p. 6.
74 Pormann & Savage-Smith, *Medieval Islamic Medicine*, pp. 31, 33–35.

court physician, Abū Zakariyyā' Yuḥannā b. Māsawayh (d. 857), to whom a culinary manual, alongside medical manuals, is attributed.[75] This reflects the broader integration of medical principles into daily life, which is also reflected in the current work.

Following the translation period, Arab physicians entered a phase of original learning and teaching. Greek methods dominated medical education, which was often rhetorical and debate-oriented. Medical training varied, combining theoretical knowledge with practical skills in diverse ways. The physicians' engagement with the translated texts sharpened their critical skills and powers of observation. Most physicians were usually generalists rather than specialists, and often authored encyclopaedic works, revering ancient Greek authorities and aiming to systematise medical knowledge.[76] A notable example is ʿAlī ibn Rabbān al-Ṭabarī's (3rd/9th century) *Firdaws al-Ḥikma*, a comprehensive manual covering medicine, philosophy, zoology, meteorology, psychology, and astrology. The author explicitly stated that mastering its contents would provide students with the essentials of medical science.[77]

The scholarly character of this period, often referred to as the 'translation movement,' has been the subject of academic debate. For instance, Gutas (1998) uses this term to highlight several key factors that contributed to its success: its sustained nature over two centuries, the broad support it received from all levels of the Abbasid society, the substantial public and private funding it received, and the rigorous scholarly methodology employed by the translators.[78] In contrast, Pormann (2022) argues against a singular movement, pointing out that the role of earlier Syriac translations as intermediaries is often overlooked, and that attributing Arabic versions solely to specific schools or workshops simplifies the reality that scholars built upon prior work. According to him, the diverse styles, motivations, and contexts of translation over time suggest the lack of a unified purpose implied by the term 'movement.'[79]

Regardless of terminology, the intellectual exchange and transmission of Greek medical knowledge into the Arabic-speaking world during the Abbasid era occurred. It undeniably shaped the course of medicine both within the Islamic Empire and later in Europe, where Graeco-Arabic medical texts were introduced in the late medieval period, forming the core of Western medi-

75 Waines, *Dietetics in Medieval Islamic Culture*, pp. 102–103.
76 Isaacs, *Arabic Medical Literature*, p. 345.
77 Isaacs, *Arabic Medical Literature*, pp. 345–346.
78 Gutas, *Greek Thought, Arabic Culture*, p. 2.
79 Pormann, *Translations of Medical and Occult Texts into Arabic and Syriac and Their Contexts After 80/700*, pp. 57–58.

cine.[80] Furthermore, the transmission of medical knowledge continued in medieval Europe through other linguistic channels, for instance among Jewish communities, who faced exclusion from Christian universities, and thus lacked access to Latin medical education and texts. This led to an effort to translate Latin medical works into Hebrew for Jewish physicians. These Hebrew translations, along with translations into various vernacular languages written in Hebrew characters for regional use, not only preserved valuable medical knowledge but also highlight the multifaceted nature of cross-cultural scientific exchange in medieval Europe.[81]

2 Al-Rāzī

Abū Bakr Muḥammad ibn Zakariyyā' al-Rāzī (251/865–313/925[82] or 323/935[83]) was born on the first day of Šaʿbān in Rayy,[84] near present-day Tehran.[85] He studied music, alchemy, and other natural sciences,[86] and played the oud.[87] According to al-Bīrūnī (d. ca. 442/1050[88]), al-Rāzī's interest in medicine was sparked by seeking treatment for eye damage from alchemical experiments involving fire and harmful vapours, a condition possibly worsened by his habit of studying by lamplight and his fondness for beans, which may have contributed to the cataracts he later developed in both eyes.[89] Around the age of thirty, al-Rāzī travelled to Baghdad to study medicine.[90] Although we do not know his medical teacher for certain,[91] Ibn Abī Uṣaybiʿa claims that al-Rāzī studied under ʿAlī ibn Rabbān al-Ṭabarī, which, however, poses a chronological problem.[92] Al-Rāzī was both a prolific author of numerous medical works and a ded-

80 Pormann & Savage-Smith, *Medieval Islamic Medicine*, pp. 3–4.
81 Bos, G., and Fischer, K., *A Glimpse into Medical Practice Among Jews Around 1500*, pp. 1–2.
82 El-Rouayheb & Schmidtke, *The Oxford Handbook of Islamic Philosophy*, p. 63.
83 Stroumsa, *Freethinkers of Medieval Islam*, p. 90. The exact dates of birth and death are not certain.
84 Bīrūnī, *Risāla*, p. 4.
85 Martin, *Encyclopedia of Islam and the Muslim World*, p. 446.
86 Sezgin, *Geschichte des arabischen Schrifttums, Bd. 3*, p. 274.
87 Ibn Ǧulǧul, *Ṭabaqāt*, p. 77.
88 Stroumsa, *Freethinkers of Medieval Islam*, p. 88.
89 Bīrūnī, *Risāla*, pp. 4–5.
90 Ibn Abī Uṣaybiʿa, *Ṭabaqāt*, p. 760.
91 Sezgin, *Geschichte des arabischen Schrifttums, Bd. 3*, p. 275.
92 Ibn Abī Uṣaybiʿa, *Ṭabaqāt*, p. 760. Al-Ṭabarī died when al-Rāzī was just five years old. Perhaps al-Rāzī 'studying under' al-Ṭabarī should be understood as him being trained according to al-Ṭabarī's knowledge, as a disciple.

icated clinical practitioner.[93] Excelling in the study and practice of medicine,[94] he was entrusted with the management of the hospital of Rayy before being selected to direct a hospital in Baghdad.[95] He continued practising medicine in Baghdad before returning to Rayy, and it was also there that he died.[96] His accomplishments in medicine were acknowledged in both Arabic and Latin medical literature, earning him the Latin name Rhazes.[97]

Al-Rāzī was a prolific author who constantly wrote new works.[98] Sezgin attributes 76 works to him,[99] and several other titles in Latin and Hebrew translations are possibly linked to his authorship, though further examination is required to confirm their origin. Additionally, Ibn al-Nadīm, al-Bīrūnī, and Ibn Abī Uṣaybiʿa list more works attributed to al-Rāzī, for which no manuscripts are currently known.[100] According to Ibn al-Nadīm, al-Rāzī was unparalleled during his time, collected information on ancient sciences, and visited various countries.[101] According to Ibn Abī Uṣaybiʿa, al-Rāzī served as a physician to numerous prominent Persian rulers and spent most of his time there, composing several of his books on medicine and other topics,[102] such as *al-Kitāb al-Manṣūrī*[103] composed for al-Manṣūr ibn Isḥāq ibn Aḥmad, the governor of Kirmān and Khorasan, and *al-Ṭibb al-Mulūkī*[104] for ʿAlī ibn Wahzūzān, the son

93 El-Rouayheb & Schmidtke, *The Oxford Handbook of Islamic Philosophy*, p. 63.

94 Ibn Ǧulǧul, *Ṭabaqāt*, p. 77.

95 Ibn Abī Uṣaybiʿa, *Ṭabaqāt*, p. 762. According to Ibn Abī Uṣaybiʿa, al-Rāzī served as the director of the al-ʿAḍudī hospital, attributed to the king ʿAḍud al-Dawla, and played a crucial role in choosing its location by hanging meat around Baghdad and by observing where it did not putrefy quickly (Ibn Abī Uṣaybiʿa, *Ṭabaqāt*, p. 761). However, the story of him working under the king ʿAḍud al-Dawla (936–983) may not be accurate as the king was born after al-Rāzī's death. Most likely, the story refers to a hospital named after the Abbasid caliph al-Muʿtaḍid (d. 902) (*Encyclopaedia of Islam III*, "ʿAḍud al-Dawla"; Iskandar, p. 155).

96 Sezgin, *Geschichte des arabischen Schrifttums, Bd. 3*, p. 275.

97 El-Rouayheb & Schmidtke, *The Oxford Handbook of Islamic Philosophy*, p. 63.

98 Goodman, *Encyclopaedia of Islam*. Consulted online on November 11, 2022.

99 Sezgin, *Geschichte des arabischen Schrifttums, Bd. 3*, p. 274 ff.

100 Sezgin, *Geschichte des arabischen Schrifttums, Bd. 3*, p. 292. For titles attributed to al-Rāzī in early historical sources, see 144 titles in Ibn al-Nadīm, *Fihrist*, p. 701 ff.; 225 titles in Ibn Abī Uṣaybiʿa, *A Literary History of Medicine*, Volume 3–2 [11.5.25] p. 845 ff., and 184 titles in Bīrūnī, *Risāla*, p. 6 ff.

101 Ibn al-Nadīm, *Fihrist*, p. 701.

102 Ibn Abī Uṣaybiʿa, *A Literary History of Medicine*, Volume 3–2 [11.5.14] p. 850.

103 A book on anatomy, physiology, pathology, *materia medica*, general maintenance of health, diet, cosmetics, surgery, toxicology, etc. (Sezgin, *Geschichte des arabischen Schrifttums, Bd. 3*, p. 281).

104 "… on illnesses and the treatment of all diseases through nutrition and the addition of medicine to food where necessary and where the patient is amenable to it" (Ibn Abī

of the governor of Ṭabaristān.[105] Among his other notable works is *al-Kitāb al-Ḥāwī*, a comprehensive medical encyclopaedia that includes quotations from Greek, Syriac, Indian, and Arabic sources.[106] Ibn al-Nadīm notes that al-Rāzī was also known for his compassion towards the ill and poor, offering them financial aid and nursing care, and was generally considered "generous, distinguished, and upright with the people."[107] Al-Rāzī even wrote a book, *Kitāb ilā man lā yaḥḍuruhu ṭabīb*, also known as *Kitāb ṭibb al-fuqarāʾ*, to guide people in treating illnesses when a physician was not available.[108]

Al-Rāzī, being a native speaker of Persian and well-versed in Arabic, certainly had access to texts in various languages and to libraries containing translations of Sanskrit, Pahlavi, and Syriac works. According to Kahl (2015), it is possible that al-Rāzī was even familiar with Syriac and Greek,[109] and he may have been familiar with the Devanāgarī alphabet, if not the Sanskrit language itself, as well as the Chinese writing system.[110] He was unequivocally influenced by Galenic medicine; however, rather than merely implementing the teachings of Galen, he gathered his own observations based on his patients and their response to treatment.[111] He was also committed to scientific progress, conducting his research carefully, identifying areas for further investigation, and expressing his hope that other scholars would collaborate to advance scientific knowledge.[112] Drawing inspiration from Hippocrates' *Epidemics*, al-Rāzī started documenting his own patient histories, including personal details such as names and professions. Notably, his writings reveal an early approach to medical evalu-

---

Uṣaybiʿa, *A Literary History of Medicine*, Volume 3–2, [11.5.25] p. 859). Listed in Sezgin, p. 286, no. 16.

105 The editors of *A Literary History of Medicine* point out that he was rather the governor of Rayy than of Ṭabaristān (Ibn Abī Uṣaybiʿa, *A Literary History of Medicine*, Volume 3–2 [11.5.14] p. 850).

106 Sezgin, *Geschichte des arabischen Schrifttums, Bd. 3*, p. 278.

107 Ibn al-Nadīm, *Fihrist*, p. 702.

108 Ibn Abī Uṣaybiʿa, *Ṭabaqāt*, p. 778. The title is listed in Sezgin as *K. Man lā yaḥḍuruhu ṭ-ṭabīb*, (Sezgin, p. 287, no. 21).

109 However, given that the Syriac and Greek texts had already been translated into Arabic, this is not certain.

110 Kahl, *Rhazes*, p. 6. His book *al-Kitāb al-Ḥāwī* includes a great number of Sanskrit, Syriac, and Persian sources. For more, see Kahl, *The Sanskrit, Syriac and Persian Sources in the Comprehensive Book of Rhazes*.

111 El-Rouayheb & Schmidtke, *The Oxford Handbook of Islamic Philosophy*, p. 63. For more on this topic, see 'Thirty-Three Clinical Observations by Rhazes (circa 900 A.D.)' by M. Meyerhof in *Isis*, Vol. 23, No. 2 (Sept. 1935), pp. 321–372. According to Ibn Abī Uṣaybiʿa, al-Rāzī had a noble friend with whom he used to spend nights reading the works of Hippocrates and Galen (Ibn Abī Uṣaybiʿa, *Ṭabaqāt*, p. 764).

112 Iskandar, *Ar-Rāzī, the Clinical Physician*, p. 215.

ation: in what seems to be an early clinical trial, al-Rāzī applied phlebotomy to one group of meningitis patients and withheld this treatment from a control group to objectively determine its therapeutic value.[113] Other observations of his own, accompanied by the Arabic translations of works of Galen, Hippocrates, and other authors, are gathered in one of his primary contributions to medicine, the aforementioned *al-Kitāb al-Ḥāwī*, 'The Comprehensive Book.'[114] Al-Rāzī acknowledged the views of Galen and other physicians, but only when confirmed by his own practical experience. His writings are filled with evidence of his strong opinions and his reliance on empirical knowledge, showing that he did not blindly follow established authorities.[115] Al-Rāzī's writings demonstrate a critical mindset,[116] as shown for instance in his treatise *Kitāb al-šukūk wa-l-munāqaḍāt allatī fī kutub Ǧālīnūs*, 'Doubts about Galen.'[117] In addition to writing medical handbooks and commentaries, al-Rāzī also composed medical texts on specific topics, such as *Kitāb al-Ǧudarī wa-l-Ḥaṣba*, 'On Smallpox and Measles,'[118] *Kitāb fī l-Qawlanǧ*, 'On Colic,'[119] and *Kitāb al-Taqsīm wa-l-Tašǧīr*[120] on differential diagnosis.

Al-Rāzī recognised the challenges in accurately diagnosing diseases with similar symptoms. In his work 'On how to recognise the Best Physician,' he stressed the crucial need to test a physician's ability to differentiate between conditions such as kidney and colon pains, pleurisy and pneumonia, and various presentations of blood or pus in bodily fluids.[121] Moreover, according to Iskandar, al-Rāzī was not afraid to acknowledge his own mistakes. If persuaded by a different viewpoint, he adopted it. This intellectual honesty clearly reflects his scientific spirit and his ability to overcome pride.[122]

---

113 Young, Latham & Serjeant, *Religion, Learning and Science in the 'Abbasid Period*, p. 377.

114 El-Rouayheb & Schmidtke, *The Oxford Handbook of Islamic Philosophy*, p. 63. See also Sezgin, *Geschichte des arabischen Schrifttums, Bd. 3*, p. 278.

115 Iskandar, *Ar-Rāzī, the Clinical Physician*, p. 221.

116 Iskandar, *Ar-Rāzī, the Clinical Physician*, p. 216.

117 Ibn Abī Uṣaybiʿa, *Ṭabaqāt*, p. 776. In Sezgin listed as *aš-šukūk ʿalā Ǧālīnūs* (p. 292, no. 70). For a recent edition and translation into French, see Pauline Koetschet, *Abū Bakr al-Rāzī, «Doutes sur Galien». Introduction, édition et traduction* (coll. Scientia Graeco-Arabica), Berlin, de Gruyter, 2019. Al-Rāzī justified criticising Galen by stating that "It is more in the spirit of Galen to follow his exhortation to search for truth than to swear by his opinions." (Temkin, p. 118).

118 Sezgin, *Geschichte des arabischen Schrifttums, Bd. 3*, p. 283, no. 3.

119 Ibn Abī Uṣaybiʿa, *Ṭabaqāt*, p. 787; Sezgin, *Geschichte des arabischen Schrifttums, Bd. 3*, p. 286, no. 14. Edited and translated into French by Ḥammāmī, 1983.

120 Ibn Abī Uṣaybiʿa, *Ṭabaqāt*, p. 778; Sezgin, *Geschichte des arabischen Schrifttums, Bd. 3*, p. 284, no. 5.

121 Iskandar, *Ar-Rāzī, the Clinical Physician*, p. 230.

122 Iskandar, *Ar-Rāzī, the Clinical Physician*, p. 222.

While primarily celebrated for his medical authority, al-Rāzī also engaged deeply with philosophy, reportedly studying under al-Balḫī.[123] His largest surviving philosophical work is *al-Ṭibb al-Rūḥānī*, 'The Spiritual Medicine,'[124] written for Manṣūr ibn Isḥāq.[125] Notably, al-Rāzī developed the controversial theory of the 'five eternals'—God, soul, matter, time, and place—suggesting that cosmos derived from these co-eternal principles. This idea, which seemed to place soul, matter, time, and place on a similar eternal footing with God, was widely opposed and ridiculed by other scholars.[126] Unlike his well-preserved medical legacy, most of al-Rāzī's philosophical writings, including the ones explaining the five eternals, are lost, and survive only as fragments in writings by other authors who mostly mention al-Rāzī and his theory with the aim of refuting him:[127] al-Qāḍī Ṣāʿid claimed that al-Rāzī did not understand theology, and thus possessed foolish, malicious beliefs and criticised people he did not understand,[128] and Abū Ḥātim al-Rāzī, a Persian philosopher, also from the city of Rayy, considered him a heretic for his critical views on prophecy.[129]

Despite his potentially unorthodox theological views, the intellectual climate of the time allowed for such radical ideas.[130] Al-Rāzī's philosophical approach was inspired by his scientific interest and background in the natural sciences,[131] drawing influence from Persian, Indian, and Greek thought, though he considered himself an independent philosopher, distinct from established schools of thought.[132] His critical stance on prophecy set him apart and even influenced his scientific work in alchemy: by rejecting the divine qualities often attributed to alchemical substances, al-Rāzī's approach to alchemy leaned towards a more practical investigation of substances, transforming alchemy into chemistry.[133]

Despite producing many works that demonstrate his profound knowledge and exceptional expertise in philosophy,[134] no continuing school of thought

123 Ibn Abī Uṣaybiʿa, *Ṭabaqāt*, p. 763. According to Sezgin, the person in question most likely is Abū Zayd al-Balḫī (236/850–322/934) (Sezgin, *Geschichte des arabischen Schrifttums, Bd. 3*, pp. 274–275).

124 El-Rouayheb & Schmidtke, *The Oxford Handbook of Islamic Philosophy*, p. 64.

125 Sezgin, *Geschichte des arabischen Schrifttums, Bd. 3*, p. 275.

126 El-Rouayheb & Schmidtke, *The Oxford Handbook of Islamic Philosophy*, p. 63.

127 El-Rouayheb & Schmidtke, *The Oxford Handbook of Islamic Philosophy*, p. 63.

128 Ibn Abī Uṣaybiʿa, *Ṭabaqāt*, p. 763.

129 El-Rouayheb & Schmidtke, *The Oxford Handbook of Islamic Philosophy*, p. 63.

130 Stroumsa, *Freethinkers of Medieval Islam*, p. 90.

131 Stroumsa, *Freethinkers of Medieval Islam*, p. 93.

132 Nasr, *Islamic Philosophy from Its Origin to the Present*, p. 144.

133 Nasr, *Islamic Philosophy from Its Origin to the Present*, p. 145.

134 Ibn Abī Uṣaybiʿa, *A Literary History of Medicine*, Volume 3–2 [11.5.14], pp. 849–850.

preserving his philosophical views was established. In contrast, his contributions as a physician and scientist have left their permanent mark in our history.[135] Al-Rāzī was renowned for his knowledge of medicine, alchemy, and philosophy, as well as his studies in physics, mathematics, zoology, and botany. He was a well-respected scholar in the Islamic world, with his reputation resting mainly on his medical achievements.[136] Indeed, he was both a prolific writer of medical works and a dedicated practitioner of clinical medicine.[137] The Latin translations of his *al-Kitāb al-Ḥāwī* and *al-Kitāb al-Manṣūrī* gained wide readership even in Europe where they were used as part of the medical education for centuries,[138] and he was considered the second Galen among his contemporaries and held undisputed authority in Western medicine until the 17th century.[139]

135 Nasr, *Islamic Philosophy from Its Origin to the Present*, p. 145.
136 Sezgin, *Geschichte des arabischen Schrifttums, Bd. 3*, p. 275.
137 El-Rouayheb & Schmidtke, *The Oxford Handbook of Islamic Philosophy*, p. 63.
138 Young, Latham & Serjeant, *Religion, Learning and Science in the 'Abbasid Period*, p. 377.
139 Sezgin, *Geschichte des arabischen Schrifttums, Bd. 3*, p. 275.

CHAPTER 2

The Manuscripts

1 Part 1: Ms. Escorial

The Arabic edition is based on what presumably is the unique copy of al-Rāzī's *Maqāla fī l-Faṣd*, 'On phlebotomy,' Ms. Escorial 857 (fol. 1–22).[1] The treatise is listed by Sezgin (1970) under the name *Kitāb fī l-Faṣd*.[2] Ms. Escorial 857 is preserved in Real Biblioteca del Monasterio de San Lorenzo de El Escorial in Spain. The manuscript consists of 22 folios of Arabic text. The text is divided into 14 chapters, each dealing with a different topic related to phlebotomy: blood in general, how and when phlebotomy is used, prescriptions, cupping, and so on.[3] Ms. Escorial 857 in its totality is a collection of 101 folios, containing several medical works.[4] However, in this book I will refer to the chosen manuscript as Ms. Escorial.

Sezgin lists four additional treatises on phlebotomy attributed to al-Rāzī: *Tehran, Mağlis (1538) 1550 (s. Kat. IV, 252)*, which contains another text; and three other manuscripts: *Tehran, Dānišgāh VIII, 596, No. 1987 (91a–97a, 1075 H.), eb. X, 1667, No. 2830 (ff. 15–22, 12. Jh. H.)*; *Tehran, Malik* (s. *Nağmābādī 145*), *Haidarabad, Āṣaf. II, 914, ṭibb 243 (79a–85a, 12. Jh. H.)*, which may contain fragments of the text of Ms. Escorial or an alternative treatise. The manuscript known as *Tehran, Mağlis (1538)* seems to be the source of a short treatise attributed to al-Rāzī, *Maqāla anšaʾahā Muḥammad ibn Zakariyyāʾ al-Rāzī fī l-Faṣd*, available on the Internet, hereafter referred to as *Alukah*.[5] Consulting both *Tehran, Mağlis 1538* and the online version of *Alukah* led to the conclusion that *Tehran, Mağlis 1538* is a different treatise from Ms. Escorial.

1 Derenbourg & Renaud, *Les manuscrits arabes de l'Escurial 2:2*, p. 65. Sezgin (*Geschichte des arabischen Schrifttums, Bd. 3*, p. 287) dates the manuscript to 1279.

2 Sezgin, *Geschichte des arabischen Schrifttums, Bd. 3*, p. 287. By Ibn Abī Uṣaybiʿa listed as *Kitāb fī šaraf al-faṣd ʿind al-istifrāġāt al-imtilāʾiyya* [...], that al-Rāzī wrote for the emir Abū ʿAlī Aḥmad ibn Ismāʿīl ibn Aḥmad (Ibn Abī Uṣaybiʿa, *Ṭabaqāt*, p. 789)—i.e., Aḥmad II, ruler of the Samanid dynasty between 295/907 to 301/914 (Ibn Abī Uṣaybiʿa, *A Literary History of Medicine*, p. 872, footnote 140).

3 Derenbourg & Renaud, *Les manuscrits arabes de l'Escurial 2:2*, p. 65.

4 Derenbourg & Renaud, *Les manuscrits arabes de l'Escurial 2:2*, p. 67.

5 Alukah.net offers an edited version of a short treatise on phlebotomy attributed to al-Rāzī, *Maqāla anšaʾahā Muḥammad ibn Zakariyyāʾ al-Rāzī fī l-Faṣd*. It is a different treatise that focuses on the method and benefit of cutting each vein, a topic also discussed in chapters 5 and 6 in Ms. Escorial.

As to Ms. Escorial, I have visited the Real Biblioteca del Monasterio de San Lorenzo de El Escorial in November 2022 and consulted the physical copy of the manuscript. Ultraviolet technology was used to check the erased and corrupt parts of the text. Unfortunately, in the parts in which text has been intentionally erased, the paper has been nearly thoroughly destroyed, consequently leaving no traces of whatever had been stated in the manuscript initially.

The folios contain 23 lines of text, and additional notes and corrections are at times added in the margins. The dimensions are 138 × 214 mm. The text is Maghrebi, "Écriture maġribine"[6] and the text size is average. The paper has a lighter shade of brown, and the ink used to write the text is brown. The manuscript employs overlining in reddish-orange ink, a feature observed primarily above headings and key words. The binding of the codex features thread-stitching through ten distinct holes, creating five visible thread segments along the spine.[7] The manuscript contains no illuminations. For a thorough review of the additional signs in the manuscript, see *Principles of edition* below.

As to the date of Ms. Escorial, Sezgin dates it to 1279.[8] As Derenbourg & Renaud (1941) note, the date of *Maqāla fī l-Faṣd* (857/1) is erased, while four other manuscripts in the same volume (857/2–5), according to them, may date from the 12th or 13th century.[9] The last manuscript in the same volume (857/6) is dated to 907/1501–1502.[10] The dating might be further complicated by the codex's mixed composition; catalogues often record only the latest date when a codex contains texts from different periods.[11]

Examination of the manuscript's physical structure reveals further insights that suggest that the current binding is not original. Codicological observations show that the beginning of the codex features unrelated texts: folio 1ʳ contains what appears to be a fragment of a text mentioning botanical substances, and folio 1ᵛ features fragments of another treatise that continues only for two lines on folio 2ʳ before the introduction of al-Rāzī's *Maqāla fī l-Faṣd*. Further indications of additional sewing and rebinding include a text by a different hand,

6 Derenbourg & Renaud, *Les manuscrits arabes de l'Escurial* 2:2, p. 67.

7 A comprehensive codicological analysis of binding and other material aspects was beyond the scope of the research objectives during the visit in Real Biblioteca del Monasterio de San Lorenzo de El Escorial. Detailed observations in these areas were not the focus of data collection.

8 Sezgin, *Geschichte des arabischen Schrifttums, Bd. 3*, p. 287.

9 Derenbourg & Renaud, *Les manuscrits arabes de l'Escurial* 2:2, pp. 65–66.

10 Derenbourg & Renaud, *Les manuscrits arabes de l'Escurial* 2:2, p. 67.

11 Scheper, *The Technique of Islamic Bookbinding*, p. 243, footnote 28.

cut off in the margins at the end of the treatise on folio 21^{r},[12] together with signs of paper repair in the gutter.[13] Scheper (2019) points out that resewing or rebinding, often occurring due to structural damage or the re-assemblage of several manuscripts, can lead to the trimming of textblock edges, potentially causing loss to marginal annotations. Hence, the presence of unrelated texts at the beginning and end, along with the abrupt transition between them, suggest that folios or sections from other manuscripts were incorporated into this codex during a later binding process.[14] These features make it plausible that a re-assemblage occurred. Therefore, the dating of the other treatises within the codex does not necessarily provide a direct indication of the original date of *Maqāla fī l-Faṣd*, and a dedicated codicological analysis, paying attention to signs of rebinding and the physical relationship between the different texts, could provide further insights.

The volume in which Ms. Escorial is extant begins with two folios of irrelevant Arabic text written in a different hand on folios 1^{r} and 1^{v}, reaching folio 2^{r} for one and a half lines. The text then reads: "A book in which a treatise by the wise, skilled Abū Bakr Muḥammad ibn Zakariyyā' al-Rāzī," followed by a smudged word and three Arabic signs, believed to be *hy*, *hā'*, and *'ayn*.[15] The manuscript then contains eight lines of text in Latin: "*Mahamedis Abem Zacharia de chirurgia liber integer cum alijs insertis ad eum Galeni videlicet co[m]mentum super 10 aphorismorum ejusdem tractatus primus de morbis acutis Hypocratis de morbis nationum*". The Latin text is followed by six lines of text in Spanish, containing the same information: Ebubechir Mahamed hijo de Zachaería Errasi de Sangrías y los aphorismos de Hippocrates sin com. de Galeno. Antemedicam. de Hippocrates sin com. Tres tratados de Hipocrates de curar las enfermedades agudas. Otro tratado del mismo sobre las enfermedades de las ciudades por el sitio.

Maqāla fī l-Faṣd begins on folio 2^{v}.

2 Authenticity

It is evident that *Maqāla fī l-Faṣd* is attributed to al-Rāzī, as is clear both in the preface of Ms. Escorial and Ms. Parma, as well as in the catalogues by Sez-

12 Scheper, *The Technique of Islamic Bookbinding*, p. 29.
13 Scheper, *The Technique of Islamic Bookbinding*, p. 39.
14 Scheper, *The Technique of Islamic Bookbinding*, p. 39.
15 For what these may denote, see Gacek, *Taxonomy of Scribal Errors and Corrections in Arabic Manuscripts*, pp. 218, 231.

gin,[16] Derenbourg & Renaud,[17] and Richler (2001),[18] in which the treatise is listed. Likewise, the fact that the *Teheran, Mağlis* manuscript, together with the online version of *Alukah*, contains information that corresponds to chapters 5 and 6 in Ms. Escorial supports its authorship. Additionally, Ibn Abī Uṣaybiʿa mentions that al-Rāzī wrote this treatise on phlebotomy for the emir Abū ʿAlī Aḥmad ibn Ismāʿīl ibn Aḥmad, i.e., Aḥmad II, ruler of the Samanid dynasty between 295/907 and 301/914.[19] Moreover, the content in Ms. Escorial indicates that its author lived one generation after some of the events described in anecdotal stories.[20] These accounts further strengthen the alignment between the narratives and the chronological context of al-Rāzī's lifetime. I have also checked other treatises on phlebotomy, also listed under the name *Maqāla fī l-Faṣd*: an anonymous treatise;[21] *Maqāla fī l-Faṣd* by Ibn al-Tilmīḏ;[22] and *Maqāla fī l-Faṣd*, or *al-Maqāla al-Amīniyya fī Faṣd al-ʿUrūq*, by Ibn al-Tilmīḏ.[23] They all comprise ten chapters. Having conducted a preliminary investigation and review of the content of the three manuscripts in question, it is evident that they are not related to Ms. Escorial.

However, chapter 2, paragraph 7 presents a significant historical and biographical challenge to the established biography of al-Rāzī. The text explicitly describes him treating a Baghdadi man in *Madīnat Miṣr*, most likely referring to al-Fusṭāṭ, a location not usually connected to al-Rāzī. As mentioned earlier, Ibn al-Nadīm notes that al-Rāzī travelled to various countries,[24] and this general indication of wider travels aligns with a claim by al-Khalidi (2013), who in his *Al-Kīmiyāʾ ʿind al-ʿArab* lists Iraq, Syria, Egypt, and al-Andalus as places that al-Rāzī visited in search of knowledge.[25] While al-Khalidi's state-

16 Sezgin, *Geschichte des arabischen Schrifttums, Bd. 3*, p. 287.

17 Derenbourg & Renaud, *Les manuscrits arabes de l'Escurial 2:2*, p. 65.

18 Richler, *Hebrew manuscripts in the Biblioteca Palatina in Parma: catalogue*, p. 451.

19 Ibn Abī Uṣaybiʿa, *A Literary History of Medicine,* Volume 3–2, [11.5.25] no. 197, pp. 871–872.

20 See chapter 2, paragraph 13 for a reference to a relative of an Abbasid vizier who lived a generation prior to al-Rāzī's time, and chapter 9, paragraph 7, where al-Rāzī recounts a story told by his teacher, involving the phlebotomy of the Caliph al-Maʾmūn.

21 An anonymous treatise on phlebotomy, *Maqāla fī l-Faṣd,* Ms. Istanbul, Beyazıt (Umumi) 4161 (2. Teil), fol. 1^r–9^r.

22 *Maqāla fī l-Faṣd,* Amīn al-Dawla Ibn al-Tilmīḏ, edited and translated into French by Subḥī Maḥmūd Ḥammāmī, 1997.

23 According to Qatar Digital Library this manuscript (Arundel Or. 10 ff. 109^r–123^r) is ascribed to Ibn Sīnā, yet the name and information on the first folios reveal its relation to Ibn al-Tilmīḏ.

24 Ibn al-Nadīm, *Fihrist*, p. 701.

25 "*irtaḥala fī ṭalab al-ʿilm ilā l-ʿIrāq, wa-l-Šām, wa-Miṣr wa-l-Andalus*" (Al-Khalidi, *Al-Kīmiyāʾ ʿind al-ʿArab*, p. 21). However, al-Khalidi does not provide sources for this statement.

ment lacks immediate sourcing, supporting arguments could be found in *Al-Kitāb al-Manṣūrī fī l-Ṭibb*, in which al-Rāzī's consistent inclusion of regional synonyms for various substances—in countries such as Egypt, Syria, Morocco, and Iraq—demonstrates a strong familiarity with terminology from diverse geographical areas.[26]

While the passage in Ms. Escorial suggest a direct professional relationship, the absence of supporting evidence leaves several possibilities open: could al-Rāzī indeed have worked in Egypt, thus necessitating a revision of his biography? Or is this a later interpolation or material incorporated by another physician?

Although no certain reports place him in Egypt, there are additional references that suggest some familiarity with the region. For instance, al-Rāzī recounts an anecdote about an Egyptian physician in his *Treatise on the Causes Why Most People Turn Away from Excellent Physicians toward the Worst Ones*.[27] *Maqāla fī l-Faṣd* includes also a passage (chapter 11, paragraph 5) contrasting Iraqi and Egyptian terminology and describing Egyptian customs in a manner similar to his *al-Kitāb al-Manṣūrī fī l-Ṭibb*. These references are not conclusive evidence of travel or work abroad, but they do suggest some degree of familiarity with Egypt.

3 Principles of Edition

The Arabic edition is based on what is presumably the unique text witness of al-Rāzī's *Maqāla fī l-Faṣd*. I have studied a digitised copy of the manuscript and consulted the original manuscript in the Real Biblioteca del Monasterio de San Lorenzo de El Escorial in Spain.[28] To enhance readability, I have made several editorial decisions, such as dividing the text into paragraphs, adding punctuation, and standardising spelling—especially with regard to diacritical points and the *hamza*. Below, I discuss these measures in detail. Additionally, a text-critical apparatus has been included to preserve all relevant information found in Ms. Escorial, including marginal notes and other annotations, and to inform the reader about any editorial interventions, such as emendations.

---

26 See al-Rāzī, *al-Kitāb al-Manṣūrī fī l-Ṭibb*.

27 Pormann & Savage-Smith, *Medieval Islamic Medicine*, p. 92.

28 Quiero expresar mi sincero agradecimiento al personal de la Real Biblioteca del Monasterio de San Lorenzo de El Escorial por su hospitalidad y apoyo durante mi visita de investigación en noviembre de 2022. Su valiosa colaboración para acceder a los recursos de su biblioteca ha enriquecido la profundidad de este estudio y mi experiencia de trabajo con manuscritos.

Chapter division: In Ms. Escorial, the text is divided into fourteen chapters. The chapters are listed at the beginning of the manuscript after the preface. This edition retains the original format of Ms. Escorial but includes captions to clearly indicate the different parts of the manuscript, such as the preface, table of contents, and new chapters. This has been done without altering the essence of the original document.

Paragraphs: I have divided the text into paragraphs for two main reasons. Firstly, to improve readability by providing clear, thematic divisions that make it easier for the reader to follow the text. Some paragraphs are short, while others are longer. Secondly, to facilitate reference to specific parts of the text[29] by using a system where the first number indicates the chapter and the second indicates the paragraph, e.g., § 1:2 means chapter 1, paragraph 2. This system has been applied consistently in both the Arabic edition and the English translation.

Folio numbering: The folios in Ms. Escorial are marked with Arabic numbers in the upper left corner of the recto. This edition retains the same numbering system as used in Ms. Escorial.

Margins: The margins of Ms. Escorial contain marginal notes (*taʿlīqāt*),[30] including corrections, completions of words and sentences, clarifications of smudged text, and notes made by the copyist. In this edition, relevant marginal notes are included and marked with ⟨ ⟩ and a footnote and comment in the critical apparatus, e.g., ⟨[text]⟩ in the margin. To provide an edition as close to the original as possible, irrelevant notes made by the copyist are also marked in the apparatus but not included in the edition.

Diacritical points: Diacritical points, used for differentiating letters that have similar bodies,[31] occur throughout Ms. Escorial. Most diacritical points are in their correct places, though some are occasionally misplaced. In this edition, most of these errors have been omitted from the critical apparatus to avoid an excessive number of unimportant notes. The most common occurrence is *hāʾ* instead of *tāʾ marbūṭa*. As the script is Maghrebi, the letters *fāʾ* and *qāf* are distinguished by the former being written with one point below the body, and the latter with one point above it.

Vowel signs and *muhmal* signs:[32] In Ms. Escorial, the use of vowel signs and *muhmal* signs is inconsistent. While the text is mostly vocalised, the vowel

29 This method is used and supported by, e.g., Samir Khalil Samir, see *Actes du premier Congrès international d'études arabes chrétiennes*, p. 82.

30 Gacek, *The Arabic Manuscript Tradition*, p. 101.

31 Grohmann, *Arabische Paläographie T. 2*, p. 41.

32 For more on *muhmal*-signs, see Grohmann, *Arabische Paläographie T. 2*, pp. 42–46 (Differenten).

signs may sometimes lead to less plausible readings. *Muhmal* signs, intended to ensure correct reading and to differentiate non-dotted from dotted letters of the same form,[33] occur despite the text being written with diacritical points. *Muhmal* signs do not occur coherently, but are found below the letters *ḥā'*, *ṣād*, and *ʿayn*—below *ḥā'* as a small *ḥā'*, below *ṣād* as a small *ṣād*, and below *ʿayn* as a small *ʿayn*. *Tanwīn* can be found in nominative, accusative, and genitive cases, sometimes even when the word is written in the definite form. *Sukūn* occurs occasionally.

Emendations and additions: In the case of emendation in the text, the preferred reading appears first in the critical apparatus, followed by a colon, after which the original word in Ms. Escorial is reproduced. Signs and words omitted from the edition are marked with a + symbol in the critical apparatus. In the event something has been deleted by the scribe from Ms. Escorial, this is indicated either by a slanted line followed by another line with a small circle at one end, or two horizontal lines with a small circle at one end. In some instances, these symbols occur four times above a word that is corrected in the margin.[34] Occasionally, these symbols appear in the text in places where deletion of a word is not deemed necessary. The reader is informed in the critical apparatus when signs of deletion occur.

The spelling of *hamza*: In Ms. Escorial, the spelling of *hamza* varies and is often inconsistent. I have chosen to use the spelling that nowadays is considered standard.

Punctuation: The Arabic text does not contain any punctuation marks. I have added punctuation to clearly separate sentences and to break up longer sentences with discretion to ensure clear and easy reading. As for additional signs in the text, Ms. Escorial also contains reddish-orange lines above certain words, but, as their purpose is unclear, they are included neither in the edition nor in the critical apparatus. At times they seem to serve as markers for catchwords or as if marking the beginning of a sentence, but this theory does not hold throughout the text. Additionally, a circle with a dot inside, ⊙, occurs in the text.[35] The occurrence of this sign is somewhat arbitrary, as it appears, for example, after a proper noun, as if implying that a quote is coming; at the end of a sentence; at the end of a passage; at the end of a quote; in the middle of a

---

33 Grohmann, *Arabische Paläographie T.* 2 p. 42.

34 These correction signs, among several other *signes-de-renvoi*, are described in Gacek (2009), *Arabic Manuscripts: A Vademecum for Readers*, p. 250.

35 For more on punctuation marks, see e.g., Abbott, *Studies in Arabic Literary Papyri II*, pp. 87f., and Gacek, *Taxonomy of Scribal Errors and Corrections in Arabic Manuscripts*, p. 220f.

list of ailments and diseases; at the end of naming a new chapter, or even after a preposition in the middle of a sentence. This circle with a dot inside is marked in the critical apparatus as +o.

Transliteration system: A consistent system of transliteration for Arabic terms, based on the DIN 31635 standard, has been employed throughout this book. However, due to the existence of several recognised systems for the transliteration of Arabic, the original transliteration has been retained in direct quotations from secondary sources to ensure accuracy and fidelity to the cited material.

Weights and measures: This edition does not provide equivalents for the weights and measures that occur in Ms. Escorial, nor does it suggest equivalents in modern units, as they were not standardised and cannot be determined with certainty.[36] A short background and summary of weights and measures can be found in the *indices* section of this work.

Daggers (†) are used to mark erased parts and corrupt or unintelligible words in the text.

4 Remarks on Translation and Commentary

My aim has been to produce a readable English translation that accurately represents the original Arabic text while remaining true to its meaning. Some modifications to the syntax were necessary for improved readability. Any additions I have made as an editor to clarify the text or to improve its flow are indicated in square brackets [].

In the commentary, I have aimed to provide the reader with a comprehensive resource, accessible both to specialists and to those new to the field. This includes providing additional information on the theoretical background, verifying quoted sources, and highlighting the strong influence of the Greek medical tradition. To ensure wide accessibility, the commentary addresses both fundamental medical concepts, providing essential context, and more detailed discussions intended for specialists. It also discusses terminology, alternative interpretations of the text, and recommends further reading on certain subjects to facilitate a deeper understanding. I have primarily utilised English translations of the Greek works and editions of Arabic works by al-Rāzī and Qusṭā ibn Lūqā, as well as Arabic translations of Greek works. Additionally, Ms. Parma has served as a valuable resource for clarifying some challenging pas-

36 Hinz, *Islamische Masse und Gewichte*, p. 1.

sages in Ms. Escorial, and I have noted this in the commentary for the reader's benefit. The overarching goal was to create a resource that can be used for a variety of purposes, serving as both an educational tool and a scholarly reference.

In addition to the Arabic edition with an English translation and commentary, this work includes several indices that cover weights and measures, instruments and utensils, places, personal names, works cited in Ms. Escorial, pharmaceutical forms, terms used in preparations of drugs, prescriptions, *materia medica*, and central medical terminology.

5 Part 2: Ms. Parma

The anonymous Hebrew translation, *Ma'amar baHaqqaza le'al-Rāzī*, is preserved in Ms. Parma, Biblioteca Palatina 2283, cat. Richler 1535, fols. 91^{r}–97^{r}.[37] The text is divided into 14 chapters and covers various aspects of phlebotomy. It was studied using a high-quality digitised copy of Ms. Parma 2283 from the Online Catalogue of Microfilmed Manuscripts of the National Library of Israel.[38] The manuscript is a part of a 15th-century medical miscellany that contains other Hebrew translations of notable works, such as Hebrew translations of Yuḥannā ibn Māsawayh the younger's *Antidotarium*; medical recipes by Armengaud Blaise of Montpellier; *Medicaments*; *Ingenio Sanitatis*, a compendium of Galen's *De prudenti methodo medendi*, written by Ḥunayn ibn Isḥāq; a treatise by al-Rāzī on preference for inferior physicians; and extracts from al-Rāzī's *al-Kitāb al-Manṣūrī*.

The treatise consists of seven folios, each containing 30 lines of text. The text, written in a Sephardic, semi-cursive script, is dark brown, while the paper is light brown.[39] The paper measures 150 × 214 mm.[40] The manuscript contains no illuminations. Additional dots, lines, and round signs are placed in the margins and above certain words in the manuscript. In some cases, an additional line, written with extremely small script, has been added below the bottom line.

It is evident that Ms. Parma is a translation of *Maqāla fī l-Faṣd*, a relationship that is clear from several features. Firstly, its relation to the treatise of al-Rāzī is

37 Richler, *Hebrew Manuscripts in the Biblioteca Palatina in Parma: Catalogue*, p. 451.
38 https://www.nli.org.il, search term מאמר בהקזה לאלראזי. This manuscript belongs to the Biblioteca Palatina of Parma, Ministero per I Beni e le Attività Culturali, Italy, The National Library of Israel. "Ktiv" Project, The National Library of Israel.
39 Richler, *Hebrew Manuscripts in the Biblioteca Palatina in Parma: Catalogue*, p. 451.
40 Richler, *Hebrew Manuscripts in the Biblioteca Palatina in Parma: Catalogue*, p. 451.

explicitly stated in the preface. Secondly, the wording throughout Ms. Parma is almost identical to Ms. Escorial, insofar as the Hebrew language permits. Thirdly, the Hebrew in Ms. Parma is heavily influenced by Arabic: in several instances, the translator has not used Hebrew terms for ailments, body parts, or drugs, but instead frequently resorts to the Arabic expressions used in Ms. Escorial, rendered in Hebrew script.

However, despite largely following Ms. Escorial carefully, many parts differ or are omitted. This is evident simply by comparing the length of the treatises: *Maqāla fī l-Faṣd* consists of 22 folios, while *Ma'amar baHaqqaza le'al-Rāzī* comprises only seven folios. As the reader will notice, the Hebrew text does not include several parts mentioned in Ms. Escorial, including anecdotal stories of other people and their treatment, and prescriptions. Conversely, in a few cases, the content differs. Some deviations appear to be intentional, conscious decisions, while at times they appear to be mistakes. Cases of obvious *lacunae* are noted in the critical apparatus, guiding the reader of Ms. Parma to the corresponding missing passages in the edition of Ms. Escorial.

6 Principles of Edition

In part 2 of this volume, *Ma'amar baHaqqaza le'al-Rāzī*, the Hebrew translation of *Maqāla fī l-Faṣd*, is presented as its own edition, complete with its own translation, commentary, and indices. This approach acknowledges the Hebrew text's divergence from the Arabic original, recognising it as a distinct work deserving its own analysis. I have made several editorial decisions to enhance readability, with many principles corresponding to the edition of Ms. Escorial.

Chapter division: The manuscript consists of fourteen chapters that are listed at the beginning of the manuscript, immediately after the preface. This edition preserves the original format of Ms. Parma but includes captions to indicate the different parts of the manuscript, including the preface, table of contents, and new chapters.

Paragraph division: I have divided the text into corresponding paragraphs to improve readability by providing clear divisions that make the text easier to follow. Consequently, some paragraphs are shorter, and some are longer. Another benefit of this division is enhanced clarity for referencing specific parts of the text by using a system where the first number indicates the chapter, and the second number the paragraph. This system has been applied consistently in both the Hebrew edition and the English translation.

Folio numbering: The folios in Ms. Parma are marked with Arabic numbers on the lower right part of the recto. The same folio numbering is also marked in this edition and translation.

Marginal notes: The marginal notes include notes, additions, or completions of words, and clarifications of smudged text. Marginal notes are given in the critical apparatus. The margins also contain unidentified signs (see *punctuation* below).

Critical apparatus: A critical apparatus has been created to report any operations on the text, as well as deviations, peculiarities, and unclarities. The critical apparatus also presents the multitude of Arabic words borrowed into the Hebrew text, providing the Arabic equivalent for the Hebrew transliteration.

Emendations and additions: In cases of emendation in the text, the preferred reading has been marked in the critical apparatus, followed by a colon, after which the original word stated in Ms. Parma is reproduced. In the few cases where the scribe has deleted something in Ms. Parma, it is marked with a horizontal stroke on the text.

Punctuation: There are elevated dots that occur after some words, seemingly functioning as pausal signs. In most cases, they appear to function as a period, and in some cases as what today would be considered a comma. In many cases, one elevated dot occurs when a new chapter is announced, and one or two dots at the end of a chapter. There are also arbitrary groups of two or three dots or lines in the margins. Two clusters of three dots arranged as a triangle occur at the very end of the treatise. As I am unaware of their significance, they are not included in the edition. I have included modern punctuation to ensure clear and easy reading.

Abbreviations: The Hebrew manuscript contains a great number of abbreviations, *rašei tevot*, common in medieval Hebrew literature.[41] These are divided into two categories: those that serve scholarly interest, and those that do not. The type of abbreviations that are judged to have low scholarly interest are the most frequent type, in which a word is abbreviated by the addition of an elevated dot in the middle or towards the end of the written part of the word.[42] This is especially the case with words such as כאשר abbreviated as כאש׳; אשר abbreviated as אש׳; הנקרא abbreviated as הנק׳; יהיה abbreviated as יה׳׳, or אצטומכא abbreviated as אצטו׳. The same principle applies to several plural endings, with

41 Ashkenazi, Shmuel & Jarden, Dov, *Ozar rashe tevot: Thesaurus of Hebrew Abbreviations*, R. Mass, Jerusalem, 1978, preface.

42 The dots used to mark abbreviations are placed higher than the previously described dots that seem to function as pauses.

an elevated dot instead of the masculine plural ending [ים-] [-im], such as גידים abbreviated as גידי׳, or with feminine plurals, such as הקזות abbreviated as הקזו׳. These abbreviations are not included in the critical apparatus to avoid an unnecessarily large number of footnotes that lack any evident importance. On the contrary, abbreviations of two or several words, understood as authentic *rašei tevot*, are marked, written out fully in the edition, while the abbreviated form is reproduced in the critical apparatus. These abbreviations include cases such as כל שכן, abbreviated as כש׳; the phrase עד שאי אפשר, abbreviated as עד שא״א; and the concluding formula תם ונשלם שבח לאל בורא עולם, abbreviated as תושלבע.

Spelling: I have not had the intention of modernising the spelling of Hebrew in this edition. Consequently, especially the vowels י and ו are mostly absent and at times present, as they occur in Ms. Parma. Moreover, several Hebrew words occur in two different forms throughout the manuscript, which is especially the case for words that end in a ה, in which case an alternative spelling, ending with an א, occurs. For example, the word for 'swelling' occurs both as מורסה and as מורסא. In order to stay true to the essence of the manuscript, I have not interfered with the spelling.

Arabic words: The author of Ms. Parma has in multiple cases used Arabic terms spelled in Hebrew characters instead of translating them into Hebrew. These words also present various spellings. In these cases, the Arabic term in question is given in its Arabic form in the critical apparatus.

Additional signs: Numbers in Ms. Parma are in most cases represented by the numerical values of the Hebrew letters. A dot above the letter indicates that the letter is used as a number, for example א׳ for one, ב׳ for two, ג׳ for three, and so on. In case of a larger number, a long, thin, diagonal line is placed above or after the Hebrew characters, such as יד׳, which may also be expressed by placing a wavy symbol above the characters, as seen on ת״ת. However, marked in my edition by using a *gereš*, they all look the same.

Daggers (†) are used to mark corrupt or unintelligible words in the text.

7 Remarks on Translation and Commentary

My aim has been to produce a readable English translation that accurately conveys the content in Ms. Parma while remaining true to its essence. Some modifications to the syntax were necessary for improved readability. Any additions to clarify the text are indicated in square brackets []. Additional minor notes for enhanced readability are given in the footnotes. The Arabic terms present in Ms. Parma are not challenging to identify, and they are written in *italics* in the translation.

As the Hebrew text is notably shorter than the Arabic original and exhibits deviations, the commentary section focuses on deeper analysis specific to the Hebrew edition. References to the edition of Ms. Escorial are given.

The Hebrew edition also includes its own set of indices. Including Hebrew terms in the Arabic indices would be impractical, as many terms available in the Arabic text do not have direct Hebrew counterparts, in most cases due to them not having been translated in Ms. Parma. Therefore, the indices for the Hebrew edition are designed specifically to facilitate access to relevant information within the Hebrew text, and cover *materia medica*, foods and dishes, weights and measures, personal names, places, works cited, prescriptions, and some central medical terms.

Additionally, the Hebrew indices include their Arabic counterparts where relevant. This inclusion acknowledges the close relationship between the two texts, especially as numerous terms are transliterated rather than translated into Hebrew. This ensures that readers of the Hebrew edition can fully grasp the context and meaning of terms that are derived from or related to the Arabic original.

This dual structure aims to serve both the Arabic and Hebrew readers independently. Each edition is designed to be self-contained, allowing readers to engage with the text without needing to reference the other edition for contextual understanding. The Arabic edition, together with its commentary, remains the comprehensive original, offering extensive information and analysis. The commentary for the Hebrew text is intentionally focused and does not aim to replicate all the details found in the commentary of the Arabic edition. In summary, this method effectively creates two books within one volume, each equipped with its own set of scholarly tools and tailored to the specific needs of its readers.

CHAPTER 3

Survey of the Book and Summaries of the Fourteen Chapters

***Maqāla fī l-Faṣd* consists of the following parts:**

Preface
Table of contents
Chapter 1. Benefits of blood in a human, its generation, and how it flows until it becomes real nutriment.
Chapter 2. Circumstances that must be considered by whoever is determined to perform phlebotomy.
Chapter 3. On the causes that make phlebotomy necessary.
Chapter 4. Quantity of blood that is extracted.
Chapter 5. Phlebotomised veins.
Chapter 6. Method of phlebotomy and the mistake that may occur in order to beware of it.
Chapter 7. Drawing matter.
Chapter 8. Times that are appropriate for extracting blood, and on being careful in its extraction.
Chapter 9. Additional removal of blood.
Chapter 10. The food, drink, and regimen of the phlebotomised person.
Chapter 11. Drugs and foods that extinguish the combustion of blood.
Chapter 12. Benefit of phlebotomy and the indications of the illnesses for which phlebotomy is conducted.
Chapter 13. Treating the mistakes that may happen during phlebotomy.
Chapter 14. Cupping.

Preface: Abū Bakr Muḥammad ibn Zakariyyāʾ al-Rāzī states that he was in the presence of a praiseworthy scholar,[1] wrote down what was said, and promised to compose a treatise on phlebotomy. Al-Rāzī mentions that after the meeting was adjourned, this praiseworthy man came to him, insisting that he would complete the statement about phlebotomy. Thus, al-Rāzī did as he

1 I.e., the emir Abū ʿAlī Aḥmad ibn Ismāʿīl ibn Aḥmad, i.e., Aḥmad II, ruler of the Samanid dynasty between 295/907 and 301/914 (Ibn Abī Uṣaybiʿa, *A Literary History of Medicine*, Volume 3–2, [11.5.25] no. 197, pp. 871–872).

had promised, and composed a treatise by using a method unattained by his predecessors.[2]

Table of contents: The treatise is divided into fourteen chapters. These chapters, numbered 1–14, are summarised in the table of contents, and repeated at the beginning of each chapter, in some cases with slightly different words.

Chapter 1: On the benefits of blood in man, its generation, and how it flows in the parts until it becomes proper nutriment. Al-Rāzī goes through fundamental medical theory and anatomy, explaining the production of blood and how it travels through the parts to become nutriment. Al-Rāzī refers to Hippocrates, introducing the three kinds of nutriment: *nutriment*, i.e., blood, *quasi-nutriment*, i.e., blood affected by an ailment of some sort, thus not nourishing, and *destined nutriment*, i.e., food in the stomach, that is destined to become proper nutriment unless any spoilage or purgation occurs. Medical authorities mentioned in this chapter are Galen, Hippocrates, and Aristotle, although most probably Aristotle is not intended, but Erasistratus.

Chapter 2: On the circumstances that must be considered by whoever is determined to perform phlebotomy. Before conducting phlebotomy, several circumstances must be considered: strength, age, occupation, custom, disposition, season, country, food and drink, and the relation of the humours in the body. Al-Rāzī gives case histories, mentioning the names of ʿAbdallāh al-Rāzī and Muḥammad ibn ʿAbd al-Malik al-Zayyāt. Al-Rāzī also gives a lot of thought to the influence of the geographical location on phlebotomy and mentions which foods and drinks one should eat either before or after being phlebotomised, or instead of it. Medical authorities mentioned in this chapter are Galen, Hippocrates, and Qusṭā ibn Lūqā. In Ms. Parma, a reference to a work by Ḥunayn ibn Isḥāq is mentioned.

Chapter 3: On the causes that make phlebotomy necessary. Al-Rāzī focuses on plethos, i.e., overfilling, and explains that there are two kinds: overfilling relating to the vessels (plethos by filling), and overfilling affecting the strength (dynamic plethos). He explains how the two kinds differ from one another, and how one can distinguish them to offer the patient the right treatment. Al-Rāzī summarises the topic by mentioning that in general one can use phlebotomy or purgation for all the illnesses that are caused by blood or the other humours. Medical authorities mentioned in this chapter are Hippocrates and Rufus of Ephesus, although a lot of the content is identical with Galen's words.

2 For the structure and development of Arabic preface tradition, see Freimark, *Das Vorwort als literarische Form in der arabischen Literatur*.

Chapter 4: On the quantity of blood that is extracted. Al-Rāzī begins with mentioning that knowing the quantity of blood that one should extract is difficult but makes it clear that there is no determined limit on how little or how much blood should be extracted. This depends on the situation, and this topic is briefly discussed in the chapter. If one phlebotomises for over-filling, one should phlebotomise until the patient becomes unconscious. If, on the other hand, one phlebotomises for the combustion of blood, one should phlebotomise until the colour or the consistency of blood changes. No medical authority is mentioned by name in this chapter, although the content is identical with Galen's words.

Chapter 5: On the phlebotomised veins. There are two kinds of phlebotomised veins: pulsatile veins, i.e., the arteries, that originate in the heart, and non-pulsatile veins, i.e., vessels, that originate in the liver. Al-Rāzī mentions 42 veins in the body that can be phlebotomised, notes where they are located, and lists the benefit of phlebotomising each vein or artery. These veins are at times mentioned by their names, at times simply by where they are located. At the end of the chapter, he also mentions Guinea worms—also called *ʿirq*, pl. *ʿurūq*, 'veins'—being aware of them being outside the intention of this work. Medical authorities mentioned in this chapter are Galen and Hippocrates.

Chapter 6: On the method of phlebotomy, and the mistakes that may occur in order to beware of it. Al-Rāzī discusses the differences between veins and arteries, and how the physician should cut them in order to avoid a mistake. He also deals with the matter of phlebotomising a vein that does not become visible, and what reduces the pain of phlebotomy. He also goes through many veins listed in chapter 5 and mentions specifically how each vein is cut properly. Of the medical authorities, Galen is mentioned in this chapter.

Chapter 7: On drawing matters. Al-Rāzī mentions that many physicians have differing opinions on how drawing matters should be conducted, and thus, this chapter should offer some assistance. He states that the phlebotomised sites need to vary depending on the duration of the illness, since in the beginning they are still flowing, while after several days they already will have reached the affected side. Al-Rāzī also mentions that phlebotomising from the contrasting side includes two things: deflection away from the affected site and adapting the matter and preventing its flow. He offers some examples on how this is done in different parts. Medical authorities mentioned in this chapter are Galen and Hippocrates.

Chapter 8: On the times that are suitable for extracting blood, and when to guard against extracting it. Based on Hippocrates, the most suitable time for phlebotomy is the spring. The disposition and regimen of the patient must be considered. Al-Rāzī gives examples on cases when one needs to be cautious with phlebotomy, and when, on the other hand, the patient most certainly will benefit from phlebotomy. He states that one may phlebotomise a patient at any stage of the illness, given that the strength of the patient allows that. Medical authorities mentioned in this chapter are Galen and Hippocrates.

Chapter 9: On epaphairesis. Epaphairesis, i.e., additional removal of blood, is conducted when more blood than would be safe to be extracted in one session has to be extracted. This way the patient may rest, eat, and gain strength between the sessions. Another benefit of epaphairesis is that Nature distinguishes the bad blood from the other parts and dispatches it towards the phlebotomised site due to the weakness caused by the wound. Epaphairesis may take place either on the same day of the first session, or during the following days, depending on why phlebotomy is conducted. The instructions on how this is done are mentioned. No medical authority is mentioned in this chapter, yet the content is very similar to Galen and Hippocrates.

Chapter 10: On the food, drink, and regimen of the phlebotomised. Al-Rāzī begins by briefly describing the optimal surroundings for conducting phlebotomy and mentions what should be eaten and drunk before and after phlebotomy. He also mentions that the intake of food should always be moderate. He proceeds to explain what causes unconsciousness during phlebotomy, and what one can do to treat such a patient. The chapter includes an abundant number of foods and drinks, as well as the prescriptions of melicratum and two types of *mayba*. No medical authority is mentioned in this chapter.

Chapter 11: On the drugs and foods that extinguish the combustion of blood. At times a patient cannot be treated with phlebotomy. This may be due to his disposition, strength, custom, regimen, or a pre-existing illness or condition. Thus, this chapter contains an abundant list of drugs and foods that substitute phlebotomy. Al-Rāzī gives six prescriptions of decoctions and pastilles that either have a purgative effect or extinguish the combustion of blood. Of the medical authorities, Galen, with his case history of a sixty-year-old patient with a swollen tongue, is mentioned in this chapter.

Chapter 12: On the benefit of phlebotomy and the indication of illnesses that are treated with phlebotomy. Al-Rāzī begins by saying that it is time to look at why each vein is frequently used in phlebotomy. Thus, he begins from the frontal vein, continues to the cephalic vein, basilic vein, median cubital vein, *vena salvatella*, the veins in the popliteal fossa, the saphenous vein, and the sciatic vein, offering an extensive list of illnesses and their indications that can be cured by phlebotomy. Of the medical authorities, Galen is mentioned in this chapter.

Chapter 13: On the mistake that occurs during phlebotomy. A mistake may occur when conducting phlebotomy, and thus, in this chapter, al-Rāzī gives seven prescriptions of dressings that cause the flow of blood from the wound to cease. Four of the listed prescriptions are used for stanching the flow of blood from an artery, and the other three prescriptions are for treating a swelling that is generated in the muscle, nerve, and flesh, or if the physician fears that the matters would flow towards the swelling. Of the medical authorities, Galen is mentioned in this chapter.

Chapter 14: On cupping. Cupping is carried out in two manners, with scarification or without scarification. The sites that usually are treated by one of these two are listed, accompanied by the ailments that are cured by using one of the two methods. Al-Rāzī also instructs how cupping is done, the material of the cupping vessels, and what one must consider before conducting cupping. The chapter ends with words that the treatise on phlebotomy is complete. No medical authority is mentioned in this chapter.

***Ma'amar baHaqqaza le'al-Rāzī* consists of the following parts:**

Preface: The author begins by stating that this treatise on phlebotomy is attributed to [Abū Bakr Muḥammad ibn Zakariyyā'] al-Rāzī, as requested by an honoured person who loves science and respects high-ranking individuals.[3] This treatise is a concise summary that discovers the benefits of phlebotomy, appropriate methods, and related topics. This, according to the author, was done by using a method unattained by his predecessors.

Table of contents: The treatise is divided into fourteen chapters. These chapters, numbered 1–14, are summarised in the table of contents, and repeated at the beginning of each chapter, in some cases with slightly different words.

Chapter 1: On the benefits of blood in man, its generation, and how it flows in the parts until it becomes proper nutriment. Al-Rāzī goes through fundamental medical theory and anatomy, explaining the production of blood and how it travels through the parts to become nutriment. He also refers to Hippocrates, introducing the three kinds of nutriment: *nutriment*, i.e., blood, *quasi-nutriment*, i.e., blood affected by an ailment of some sort, thus

---

3 I.e., the emir Abū ʿAlī Aḥmad ibn Ismāʿīl ibn Aḥmad, i.e., Aḥmad II, ruler of the Samanid dynasty between 295/907 and 301/914 (Ibn Abī Uṣaybiʿa, *A Literary History of Medicine*, Volume 3-2, [11.5.25] no. 197, pp. 871–872).

not nourishing, and *destined nutriment*, i.e., food in the stomach, that is destined to become proper nutriment unless any spoilage or purgation occurs. Medical authorities mentioned in this chapter are Galen, Hippocrates, and Erasistratus.

Chapter 2: On the circumstances that whoever is resolute about phlebotomy needs to consider and notice. Before conducting phlebotomy, several circumstances must be considered: strength, age, occupation, custom, disposition, season, country, food and drink, and the relation of the humours in the body—although this chapter in Ms. Parma is incomplete. Medical authorities mentioned in this chapter are Galen, Hippocrates, and Qusṭā ibn Lūqā, and specific to Ms. Parma, Ḥunayn ibn Isḥāq.

Chapter 3: On the causes that make phlebotomy necessary. Al-Rāzī focuses on *plethos*, i.e., overfilling, and explains that there are two kinds: overfilling relating to the vessels (*plethos* by filling), and overfilling affecting the strength (dynamic *plethos*). He explains how the two differ from one another, and how one can distinguish them to offer the patient the right treatment. Medical authorities mentioned in this chapter are Hippocrates and Rufus of Ephesus.

Chapter 4: On the quantity of blood that is extracted. Al-Rāzī begins with mentioning that knowing the quantity of blood that one should extract is difficult, but he makes it clear that there is no determined limit on how little or how much blood should be extracted. This depends on the situation, and this topic is briefly discussed in the chapter. If one conducts phlebotomy for overfilling, one should phlebotomise until the patient becomes unconscious. If, on the other hand, one phlebotomises for the combustion of blood, one should phlebotomise until the colour or the consistency of blood changes. No medical authority is mentioned by name.

Chapter 5: On the phlebotomised veins. There are two kinds of phlebotomised veins: pulsatile veins, i.e., the arteries, that originate in the heart, and non-pulsatile veins, i.e., vessels, that originate in the liver. Al-Rāzī lists 42 veins in the body that can be phlebotomised, notes where they are located, and lists the benefit of phlebotomising each vein or artery. These veins are at times mentioned by their name in Arabic, at times simply by where they are located. Of medical authorities, Hippocrates is mentioned in this chapter in Ms. Parma.

Chapter 6: On the method of venesection, and the mistake deriving from it, and how to avoid it. Al-Rāzī briefly discusses the differences between veins and arteries, and how the physician should cut them to avoid a mistake. He also deals with the matter of hindered flow of blood and phlebotomising a vein that does not become visible. He also goes through some veins listed in chapter 5, mentioning how each vein is cut properly. No medical authority is mentioned in this chapter in Ms. Parma.

Chapter 7: On drawing matters. Al-Rāzī states that the phlebotomised sites need to vary depending on the duration of the illness, since in the beginning they are flowing, while after a few days they are still and stagnant. He offers some examples on how this is done in different parts. No medical authorities are mentioned in this chapter in Ms. Parma. Comparing to Ms. Escorial, this chapter in Ms. Parma ends abruptly.

Chapter 8: On the suitable times for extracting blood, and when to guard against extracting it. The most suitable time for phlebotomy is Nisan, i.e., the spring. The time of the day and the disposition and regimen of the patient must be considered. Al-Rāzī gives examples on cases when one needs to be cautious with phlebotomy, and when, on the other hand, the patient most certainly will benefit from phlebotomy. He states that one may phlebotomise a patient at any stage of the illness, given that the strength of the patient allows that. Medical authorities mentioned in this chapter are Hippocrates—also Galen's words are quoted as if they were words of Hippocrates.

Chapter 9: On epaphairesis. Epaphairesis, i.e., additional removal of blood, is conducted when more blood than would be safe to be extracted in one session has to be extracted. This way the patient may rest, eat, and gain strength between the sessions. Epaphairesis may take place either on the same day of the first session, or during the following days, depending on why phlebotomy is conducted. The instructions on how this is done are mentioned. No medical authority is mentioned in this chapter.

Chapter 10: On the food and drink of the phlebotomised. Al-Rāzī begins by briefly describing the optimal surroundings for conducting phlebotomy and mentions what should be eaten and drunk before and after phlebotomy. He proceeds to explain what causes unconsciousness during phlebotomy, and what one can do to treat such a patient. The chapter includes the prescription of melicratum—for the prescription of *mayba* the reader is referred to *al-Kitāb al-Manṣūrī*. No medical authority is mentioned in this chapter.

Chapter 11: On the drugs and foods that are good to extinguish [the combustion of] blood. As some people have weak composition or are not accustomed to phlebotomy, this chapter contains a list of drugs and foods that can be used in its stead. Prescriptions are given to a purgative decoction and to a pastille with a cooling effect. No medical authority is mentioned in this chapter in Ms. Parma.

Chapter 12: On the benefit of phlebotomy and the indication of illnesses that are treated with phlebotomy. Al-Rāzī begins directly by listing how phlebotomising each vein is beneficial, beginning from the head, then continuing to the cephalic vein, basilic vein, median cubital vein, *vena salvatella*, the veins in the popliteal fossa, the saphenous vein, and the sciatic vein, offering an extensive list of illnesses and their indications that can be cured by phlebotomy. No medical authority is mentioned in this chapter in Ms. Parma.

Chapter 13: On the mistake that occurs during phlebotomy. A mistake may occur when conducting phlebotomy, and thus, in this chapter, al-Rāzī gives two prescriptions of dressings that cause the flow of blood from the wound to cease. Of the medical authorities, Galen is mentioned in this chapter.

Chapter 14: On cupping. Cupping is carried out in two manners, with and without scarification. The sites that usually are treated by one of these two are listed, accompanied by the ailments that are cured by using one of the two methods. The chapter ends with the author mentioning that the treatise on phlebotomy is completed, and that there was an intention to attach another treatise on cauterisation into this treatise. However, that topic was deviating from the purpose of the work and was therefore not attached. No medical authority is mentioned in this chapter.

Edition, Translation, and Commentary

∴

PART 1

Maqāla fī l-Faṣd

كتاب فيه مقالة الحكيم الماهر أبي بكر محمد بن زكرياء الرازي. 2r

٠:١ بسم الله الرحمن الرحيم †.....................†[a] 2v

٠:٢ قال أبو بكر محمد بن زكرياء الرازي قد كان جرى بحضرة رجل فاضل يحب العلم ويكرم أهله ذكر الفصد ومنافعه وقوانين استعماله ووجوه العلاج به.

٠:٣ وأمليت في مجلسه ما حضرني حفظه مما يحتاج إليه ولا غنى له عن الفصد.

٠:٤ ووعدته أن أكون أؤلف مقالة في الفصد يكثر غناؤها للناظرين فيها يغمر نفعها كل من قرأها وعمل بما فيها.

٠:٥ فلما انفصل هذا الرجل الفاضل من سفره ولم يترك ملازما لي يرغب إليّ ويلح عليّ فيما كنت وعدت من إتمام القول في الفصد.

٠:٦ فتقدمت إلى ذلك بقلب مخلص وسلكت في تأليفها مسلكا لم يبلغه من كان قبلنا.

٠:٧ ونسأل الله واهب العقل أن يعصمنا من الزلل فيما تكلفناه وأن يرشدنا إلى سبيل النجاح فيما ألفناه[b] وبالله التوفيق.

أبواب المقالة

٠:٨ وقد قسمنا هذه المقالة على أربعة عشر بابا.

٠:٩ الباب الأول في منفعة الدم في الإنسان وتولده وكيف يصير حتى يكون غذاء بالحقيقة.

٠:١٠ الباب الثاني نذكر فيه الأحوال التي يحتاج أن ينظر فيها من كان عازما على الفصد.

---

a Text erased in Ms. Escorial, see commentary.

b ألفناه: اللفناه

A book in which a treatise by the wise, skilled Abū Bakr Muḥammad ibn Zakariyyāʾ al-Rāzī. 2r

0:1 In the name of God, the Merciful, the Compassionate †.................† 2v

0:2 Abū Bakr Muḥammad ibn Zakariyyāʾ al-Rāzī said: It was in the presence of a praiseworthy man who loves science and honours its scholars that phlebotomy, its benefits, the rules of using it, and the various ways of treatment with it were mentioned.

0:3 I dictated in his salon the things present in my memory that one needs and are not superfluous about phlebotomy.

0:4 And I promised him that I would compose a treatise on phlebotomy, abundant in richness for those who study it, and highly beneficial for everyone who reads it and works with it.

0:5 When this good man came home from his travels, he constantly approached me, asking and insisting that I, as promised, would complete the treatise on phlebotomy.

0:6 Thus I approached it with a sincere heart, and while composing it, I followed a method unattained by our predecessors.

0:7 And we ask God, the giver of intellect, to protect us from making mistakes in what we took upon ourselves, and to guide us to the path of success regarding what we have composed—may God grant us success!

Chapters of the Treatise

0:8 We have divided this treatise into fourteen chapters.

0:9 The first chapter on the benefits of blood in man, its generation, and how it flows until it becomes proper nutriment.

0:10 The second chapter on the circumstances that must be considered by whoever is determined to perform phlebotomy.

٠:١١ الباب الثالث في الأشياء الموجبة للفصد.

٠:١٢ الباب الرابع في كمية ما يخرج من الدم.

٠:١٣ الباب الخامس في[a] العروق المفصودة.

٠:١٤ الباب السادس في كيفية فصد العروق وما يلحق ذلك من الخطأ ليحترس منه.

٠:١٥ الباب السابع في جذب المادة.

٠:١٦ الباب الثامن في الأوقات التي يصلح فيها خروج الدم والاحتراس من خروجه.

٠:١٧ الباب التاسع في التثنية.

٠:١٨ الباب العاشر في غذاء المفصود وشرابه وتدبيره.

٠:١٩ الباب الحادي عشر في الأدوية والأغذية المطفئة للدم.

٠:٢٠ الباب الثاني عشر في منفعة فصد العروق | وعلامة العلل التي يفصد لها. 3r

٠:٢١ الباب الثالث عشر في علاج الخطأ الواقع في الفصد.

٠:٢٢ الباب الرابع عشر في الحجامة.

الباب الأول

١:١ الباب الأول في منفعة الدم في الإنسان وتولده وكيف يصير في الأعضاء حتى يصير غذاء بالحقيقة.

---

a دم + MS

0:11 The third chapter on the causes that make phlebotomy necessary.

0:12 The fourth chapter on the quantity of blood that is extracted.

0:13 The fifth chapter on the phlebotomised veins.

0:14 The sixth chapter on the method of phlebotomy and the mistakes that may occur, in order to beware of it.

0:15 The seventh chapter on drawing matter.

0:16 The eighth chapter on the times that are appropriate for extracting blood, and when to guard against extracting it.

0:17 The ninth chapter on epaphairesis.[1]

0:18 The tenth chapter on the food, the drink, and the regimen of the phlebotomised person.

0:19 The eleventh chapter on the drugs and foods that extinguish [the combustion of] blood.

0:20 The twelfth chapter on the benefit of phlebotomy | and the indications of 3r
the illnesses for which phlebotomy is conducted.

0:21 The thirteenth chapter on treating the mistake that occurs during phlebotomy.

0:22 The fourteenth chapter on cupping.

The First Chapter

1:1 The first chapter on the benefits of blood in man, its generation, and how it flows in the parts until it becomes proper nutriment.

1 I.e., additional removal of blood.

١:٢ قال أبو بكر محمد بن زكرياء الرازي[a] إنه لما كان الدم أعدل الأخلاط وكان ألذها وأولاها بالتقديم على أكثر الأخلاط للحاجة إلى ذلك إذ هو الحار الغريزي الذي هو قوام الحياة بمنزلة الحطب للنار أو بمنزلة الدهن للسراج وبه يخصب البدن ويصح وتذهب الهموم ويمتنع من الأمراض السلية والذبولية وتصح الكبد التي بصحتها نصح كما قال جالينوس: إن نحيا حياة طيبة فبصحة كبودنا. وقد أمرنا بالتدرج في زيادة الغذاء ما لم يقع سرف وإفساد هضم ولا زيادة تمنع البدن من الحركة وتنقله عن فعله الطبيعي إيثارا منه لاجتلاب الدم الذي هو ضد الشيخوخة[b] التي هي الفناء بعينه.

١:٣ وقد حكى جالينوس عن أراسسطراطس[c] أنه كان يمنع من الفصد شحا منه على الدم وكان يرى بالامتناع من الغذاء وتقليله عوضا من الفصد. وهذا كان يمكنه لو لم يفجأه من سورة الدم ما لا يبقى العليل معه إلى أن يقلل غذاءه.

١:٤ والدم أيضا مادة الغذاء الحقيقي الذي ذكره أبقراط حين قال إن الغذاء يكون على ثلاثة أوجه: أحقها وأولاها أن يكون غذاء ما تشبه بالمغتذي واغتذت به الأعضاء من العروق التي يخرج إليها يشبه البخار وهو العوض مما يتحلل دائما.[d]

١:٥ والثاني شبه الغذاء وهو الدم الكائن في العروق ولأن هذا الدم قد يقع به آفة من انتفاخ عروق في[e] أي موضع كان من البدن أو غير ذلك من سقطة أو ضربة | فيقل الدم في البدن 3v
فلا يغذوا.

١:٦ والثالث ما سيغذوا في المستأنف وهو الطعام الكائن في المعدة الذي بالغرض فيه أن يكون مادة الغذاء الحقيقي إلا أن تقع به آفة من قيء أو غيره من إسهال أو يصير في حد ما تشبه بالغذاء ثم تقع به الآفة التي ذكرنا فلا يغذوا أيضا.[f]

---

a +O
b الشيخوخة: الشيخوخية
c أراسسطراطس: أرسطاطيس
d دائما: دايبا
e في: من
f +O

1:2 Abū Bakr Muḥammad ibn Zakariyyā' al-Rāzī said: Indeed, blood is the most balanced of the humours, and it can be preferred to most humours, since it is needed, for it is the innate heat that is the foundation of life, as wood for the fire, or as oil for the lamp. It fattens the body, makes it healthy, makes the worries go away, prevents the illnesses phthisis and marasmus, and cures the liver, in the health of which we are healthy, as Galen said: "if we are healthy, it is due to the health of our liver." He commanded us to gradually increase nutriment as long as there is no immoderateness or spoilage of digestion, nor any excess preventing the body from motion, disturbing its natural activity. This is to be preferred as it attracts the blood that is the contrary of old age, which is cessation of being.

1:3 Galen has reported that Erasistratus[2] used to avoid phlebotomy, sparing blood, and considered abstaining from food and reducing it a substitute for phlebotomy. This would have been possible if he had not been confronted by the surplus of blood that remains in the patient, until he reduces his nutriment.

1:4 Blood is also the substance of real nutriment that Hippocrates mentioned when he said that there are three kinds of nutriment: the most proper and suitable of these three to become nutriment is that which resembles what is being nourished. The parts are nourished by it through the veins to which it flows out similar to vapour. It replaces that which is constantly dissolved from them.

1:5 The second is *quasi-nutriment*, which is the blood that is present in the veins. Since this blood may be affected by an ailment of inflation of veins in any site in the body, or something else, such as a fall or a blow, | then the blood 3v
might be reduced in the body, and they[3] are not nourished.

1:6 The third is *destined nutriment*, and this is the food in the stomach that is destined to be a matter of proper nutriment, unless it is affected by vomiting or some other kind of purgation, or that it reaches the degree of being quasi-nutriment—for then it is affected by the affliction that we have mentioned, and it does not provide nourishment either.

---

2 Ms. Escorial reads Aristotle, see commentary.

3 I.e., the parts.

١:٧ قال: فإن قال قائل كيف يصير الدم إلى الأعضاء على طريق البخار فيغذوها قلنا له إنّ المعدة وضعها كقدر عظيمة حولها مواقد[a] نار كثيرة يمنة منها الكبد ويسرة الطحال ومن فوق الحجاب والثرب مغشى لجميع ذلك ولجميع سائر الأحشاء والأمعاء في الإنسان خاصة وذلك بسبب ضعف هضمه ورقة جلده وعدم شعره بالإضافة إلى سائر الحيوان فعوض بكثرة الثرب كما شاء الباري تعالى.

١:٨ وإذا أحست المعدة بالحاجة إلى الغذاء بالعصب الجاري إليها من الدماغ بامتصاص العروق التي بين أسفل المعدة والكبد ووردها الطعام لزمته واحتوت عليه وانغلق البواب.

١:٩ وفي بعض الحيوان جعل في البواب شبه الغدة ليزيده لزوما فلا يزال كذلك حتى يتم هضمه ويصير الطعام شبيها بعصارة ويدفع حينئذ رديئه ويصلح الباقي. وتجذبه العروق بعد أن يتغير تغيرا قريبا من تغيره في الكبد ودفعها إلى الكبد يكون من طريق واحد يسمى باب الكبد وصورته كصورة عرق إلا أنها لا تجري دما وتتشعب من أصله عروق مفرقة في جرم الكبد وفيها ينطبخ ويتميز من المرتين. ولولا ما يخالط الدم الذي في العروق المتصلة من الأمعاء والمعدة والكبد والعروق المستقيمة من المائية لما وصل الدم في هذه المواضع لضيقها والماء لا يغذوا البتة.[b]

١:١٠ وينبت من حدبة الكبد عرق عظيم منه نبتت إلى جميع العروق الغير ضوارب على ما ذكر | المشرحون وأصل هذا العرق ينقسم في الكبد إلى أقسام شعرية فيلتقي مع الأقسام 4r
المنقسمة من المجرى الذي يسمى الباب فيأخذ منها الدم الذي قد بقي من أكثر المرتين والمائية بالآلات الموضوعة لذلك. ثم إنّ بعضها تأخذ من بعض لأنها متصلة كما قال أبقراط في كتابه في الغذاء.

a مواقد: مواقيد
b +o

1:7 He said: If someone were to say: 'How does blood flow into the parts as a vapour, thus nourishing them?' we would tell him that the position of the stomach is as if it was a large cauldron, around which there are a lot of burning hearths: on the right side of it the liver, on the left side the spleen, and above it the diaphragm. The omentum is covering all that and all the rest of the viscera and the intestines, particularly in the human being. That is because of his weak digestion, delicate skin, and absence of hair in comparison to the rest of the animals. Thus, he was compensated by a large omentum, as the Creator Almighty wanted.

1:8 Whenever the stomach feels the need for nutriment by means of the nerve running to it from the brain, the veins between the lower part of the stomach and the liver attract the food and bring it to it, then it clings to it and holds it [i.e., nutriment], and the pylorus gets closed.

1:9 In some animals, something that resembles a gland has been placed in the pylorus to increase its retention [i.e., of the food]. It remains that way until its digestion is completed, and the food becomes like juice. At that time, it expels what is bad, so that what remains is good. The veins attract it after it undergoes a transformation similar to its transformation in the liver, and its expulsion to the liver takes place via one path that is called the *porta*.[4] Its shape is like the shape of a vein, except that no blood flows in it. Separate veins branch out from its origin in the body of the liver in which it is cocted and separated from the two biles. Had it not been for the watery fluid that mixes with the blood that is in the veins that connect the intestines, the stomach, the liver, and the straight veins, the blood would not reach these sites for the sake of their narrowness, and the water would not nourish at all.

1:10 A large vein grows from the convexity of the liver, from which it grows
into all the non-pulsatile veins, according to what the | anatomists have men- 4r
tioned. The origin of this vein is divided in the liver into capillary parts, so that it meets the parts that separate from the vessel called the *porta*, taking from them the blood that remains from the major portion of the two biles and the watery fluid by the instruments assigned for it. Thereafter, they take from each other, because they are connected, as Hippocrates said in his book, *Nutriment*.

4 Lit. door of the liver.

١:١١ إنّ الإنسان واحد مشترك والعروق إذا تشاعبت وصارت إلى أقاصي البدن اتصل كل عرق منها بعضو يقيم غذاءه أعني أنه يتصل بالطعام عروق دقاق لأنها بطيئة التحليل باردة فهي تحتاج إلى غذاء قليل[a] والقلب وإن كان صلبا فهو يحتاج إلى عروق كبار لكثرة تحليله والدماغ وإن كان لينا فإنه يحتاج إلى غذاء قليل لقلة حرارته وهكذا سائر الأعضاء على هذه النسبة. فسبحن خالق هذا ومدبره.[b]

١:١٢ ثم إن إذا صار هذا الدم في هذه العروق إلى هذه الأعضاء التي ذكرنا لم يكن للدم خروج منها بعد تمام هضمه وبقاء سيره إلا على طريق البخار والرشح. وإن شئت تقول على طريق المجاورة والمماسة كالشيء المسخن أو المجفف أو المرطب أو المبرد لما ماسّه أو جاوره فيجب من هذا أن تكون العروق مبثوثة في البدن إذ هي الموردّة[c] للغذاء إليه.

١:١٣ وكان الإنسان من داخله مطبق بالعروق وذلك أنك لو غرزته بإبرة قد ما يتفق ألا يخرج من موضع الغرزة إلا الدم والدم لا يخرج إلا من عرق. فيدل على هذا أنك حيث تغرز ويخرج الدم تصادف عرقا.

الباب الثاني

٢:١ الباب الثاني في الأحوال التي يجب أن ينظر فيها من كان عازما على الفصد.

٢:٢ أولها القوة والسن والمهنة والعادة والمزاج والزمان الحاضر والبلد وما يؤكل ويشرب وفي نسبة الأخلاط في البدن أهي على التساوي أو مختلفة.[d]

4v ٢:٣ أما القوة فهي ملاك الإنسان وعماد | حياته وهي كالزاد للمسافر[e] الذي لا يقطع مسافة إلا على قدر زاده. فكذلك القوة متى قصرت لم يبلغ المريض منتهى مرضه ولا

---

a +o

b +o

c الموردة: المردية

d corrupt, Ms. Parma: מתחלפות

e خــ للمسافر above the word للراكب

1:11 Indeed the human is one single person [with communicating parts], and when the veins branch out and reach the extremities of the body, each vein connects to a part and provides it with nutriment. I mean, thin veins transport little food to parts that are slow to dissolve and cold, and thus, need little nutriment. But the heart, even if it is solid, needs large veins because it dissolves a lot, and the brain, even if it is soft, needs little nutriment because of its low temperature, and so forth for the rest of the parts in accordance with it. And glory to the Creator who arranged this!

1:12 Then, as this blood flows through these veins into these parts that we have mentioned, the only exit for the blood from them is as vapour and through exudation after it has been completely digested and still flowing. If you desire, you can say [that nutrition occurs] through that which is adjacent and in contact, just as something that heats, dries, dampens, or cools. When it touches or is adjacent, then, due to this, the veins must be dispersed in the body, so that they can supply nutriment to it.

1:13 Veins pervade the inside of a human being. Consequently, if you pierce him with a needle, what occurs is that only blood flows out from the site of the stitch, and blood does not flow out from anything but a vein. What indicates this is that when you pierce and blood comes out, you encounter a vein.

The Second Chapter

2:1 The second chapter on the circumstances that must be considered by whoever is determined to perform phlebotomy.

2:2 The first one of them is strength, [then] age, occupation, custom, disposition, season, country, what is eaten and drunk, and the relation of the humours in the body, whether they are balanced or unbalanced.[5]

2:3 As to the strength, it is the subsistence of the human, and the foundation of | his life. It is as the provisions for the traveller[6] who does not cross 4v
a distance unless by the power of his provisions. Thus, when the strength is reduced, the patient does not reach the end of his illness. One should only

5 Lit. divergent, understood as diverging from balance.
6 See commentary.

يقدم على الفصد والإسهال إلا بثباتها حتى أنّ الطبيب للحاجة إلى القوة ربما رخص للعليل في الغذاء الرديء إذا اشتهاه ويخلط له بجيد عند رجاء حفظ قوته وغذا المحموم في وقت نوبة الحمى لئلا تسقط قوته على أنّ الغذاء في وقت النوبة مما يزيد في الحمى. وقد شهد بذلك أبقراط حين قال: فامنع من الغذاء في وقت النوبة.

٢:٤ وأيضا فقد يغذى العليل إذا تحقق المتطبب أنّ المرض مزمن بالغذاء الغليظ مد يأتي على العليل أربعة عشر يوما وإن كان هذا يزيد في مرضه خيفة أن تسقط القوة قبل منتهى المرض وزواله فيكون ذلك سببا لهلاك العليل وقد يُمنع من الغذاء جملة إذا تحقق أن المرض ينقضي في الأيام الأول وآخرها اليوم الرابع إن تحقق أن القوة تبقى بذلك. وقد شرح ذلك أبقراط حين قال: المرض البالغ في اللطافة جدا ينبغي أن يدبر بالتدبير البالغ في اللطافة جدا[a] ويعني بذلك ترك الغذاء جملة.

٢:٥ فإن علم أنّ القوة لا تبقى بالترك سقي العليل الجلاب فإن علم أيضا أنّ القوة لا يمسكها هذا أعطى ماء الشعير أو اللباب المغسول بالسكر الطبرزدي وما أشبه ذلك.

٢:٦ وأما السن فإن الصبيان ما لم يبلغوا سن الفتيان وهو أربعة عشر سنة لا يجب أن يفصدوا وذلك أنّهم يحتاجون من الوفور وهو الغذاء أكثر وأيضا فيتحلل منهم كثير وأبدانهم رطبة وعصبهم بعد ضعيف. وكذلك المشايخ وهو من حد الستين سنة والفصد ينفع فيما بين هذين السنين. وما فوق ذلك فلا يحتملون الفصد ولا الإسهال على | الأكثر لقلة 5r
دمائهم وضعف هضمهم. وقد ذكر جالينوس أنه فصد شيوخا أبناء سبعين سنة وهذا أقل ما يتفق.

a [*sic*]

undertake phlebotomy or purgation when one is certain [that it will be beneficial]. For the sake of strength, the physician may even permit bad food for the patient in case he has a strong desire for it, and mix it with good [food], hoping to preserve his strength. Someone who suffers from fever should be given food at the time of the paroxysm of fever, so that his strength would not diminish, although nutriment at the time of the paroxysm intensifies the fever. Hippocrates testified that when he said: "Abstain from food at the time of the paroxysm."

2:4 Additionally, if the physician is certain that the illness is chronic, the patient may be fed with coarse food for a period of fourteen days. Should this lead to increased fear that his strength would diminish before the end and cessation of his illness, being the cause of the death of the patient, he may be restrained from food completely. [He may only do so] if he is certain that the illness will be terminated during the first days, maximum on the fourth day, and that the patient will keep his strength anyway. This was explained by Hippocrates when he said: "[in the case of] a very acute illness, one must apply a very restricted regimen," by which he means the complete abandonment of food.[7]

2:5 If he [i.e., the physician] knows that the strength does not remain when [food] is abandoned, he should give the patient julep to drink. If he also knows that this does not retain the strength, he should give [the patient] barley broth or bread pith washed with crystalline sugar and the like.

2:6 As to the age, boys who have not reached the age of adolescence, that is fourteen years, are not to be phlebotomised. They namely need ample [food], a lot of it, and because a lot is dissolved from them, their bodies are moist, and their nerves are still weak. The same holds good for old men, i.e., from the beginning of sixty years. Thus, phlebotomy is beneficial for people between these two ages. Who are above that neither tolerate phlebotomy nor purgation in | most 5r
cases due to their low blood quantity and weak digestion. Galen mentioned that he phlebotomised old men at the age of seventy years, yet this does not happen often.

7 Passage possibly corrupt, see commentary.

٢:٧ وقد كان بمدينة مصر رجل بغدادي يتصرف في خدمة[a] السلطان وكان يلزمني تدبيره وسنه يومئذ نيف وسبعون سنة. كنت أفصده في كل خمسة وعشرين يوما وما قرب منها في جميع الأزمنة. وربما اتفق أن يحتاج إلى الفصد والزمان حديد من الحر والبرد فأمطله بذلك وأشير عليه بأخذ الأشربة المطفئة لسورة الدم كشراب حصرم وشراب رمّانين وشراب عناب ومن الأغذية السكباج والحصرمية والرمانية والسماقية والعدسية. فيفعل ذلك يوما أو يومين فيضطره من الأمر وشدته ما يخيل إليه أنه فاضت منه[b] نفسه ويختنق حتى يسكن ذلك بالفصد. وكان خصيبا ⟨بدنه واللون فيه مشرق جيد البنية⟩[c] وكنت أخرج له من الدم في كرّتين قرب ثلاثة أرطال.

٢:٨ وليس لخروج الدم في الناس حد محدود في القلة والكثرة.[d] فقد ذكر جالينوس أنه استفرغ من قوم من الدم نحو الستة الأرطال فانتفعوا بذلك وآخرين أخرج لهم رطلين أضر ذلك بهم. وحكى قسطاس في المقالة في القوة والضعف عن عبد الله الرازي أنه فصد[e] في خمسة أشهر متوالية ست عشرة فصدة وأخرج له في كثير منها ثماني مائة درهم كيلا وأقل ما أخرج له منها ست مائة درهم كيلا.

٢:٩ وأما المهنة فإنه من كان مباطشا كثير التعب والحركة والجماع والسهر والهم والفكر في العلوم الدقيقة فيجب أن يقلل من إخراج الدم وبالضد.[f]

٢:١٠ وأما العادة فقد قالت فيها القدماء إنها طبيعة مكتسبة فيجب أن لا تقدم على فصد من لم يفتصد قط وقد مد له من عمره | ما يجب له فيه أن يفصد إلا بعد نظر وتوقّف. 5v

---

a MS + في خدمة

b منه added below.

c ⟨⟩ in the margin to complete مشرق جيد البنية

d +O

e إنسانا أظنه هذا وأما الأمر المنتسخ منها هذه فليس فيها شيء in the margin

f +O

2:7 There was a Baghdadi man in al-Fusṭāṭ, working in the service of the sultan, and he charged me with arranging his regimen. At that time, he was around seventy years old. I used to phlebotomise him every twenty-five days or so during all seasons. Sometimes it happened that he needed phlebotomy in a severely hot or cold season, in which case I would postpone it for that sake and advise him to take syrups that quench the surplus of blood, such as verjuice, syrup of both [types of] pomegranates, and jujube syrup, and of the foods *sikbāǧ, ḥiṣrimiyya, rummāniyya, summāqiyya*, and *ʿadasiyya*. He did this for a day or two until he got into a precarious state, so much that one imagined that whilst he was suffocating his soul would depart from him.[8] [This lasted] until this [situation] was alleviated by phlebotomy. His ⟨body⟩ was fat, ⟨its colour healthy, and he was well-built⟩.[9] I used to extract approximately three *raṭls* of his blood in two sessions.

2:8 There is no fixed limit regarding how little and how much blood should be extracted from people. Galen mentioned that he evacuated from people's blood around six *raṭls*, and they benefitted from that, while from others he extracted two *raṭls*, which harmed them. In his treatise, *On Strength and Weakness*, Qusṭās[10] reported that ʿAbdallāh al-Rāzī said that he phlebotomised [a patient] sixteen times during five consecutive months. Many times, he extracted eight hundred *dirhams*,[11] and the least that he would extract was six hundred *dirhams*.[12]

2:9 As to the occupation, someone who is hard-working, with a lot of fatigue, movement, coitus, insomnia, worries, and rational thinking in sciences that require concentration should reduce the evacuation of blood, and the opposite.

2:10 As to the custom, the Ancients have said that it is an acquired nature. Therefore, you ought not to rush into phlebotomising those who have not yet undergone this procedure. [Even] if someone has nearly reached the age | when 5v
one ought to apply phlebotomy, this should only be done after careful consideration and hesitation.

---

8 I.e., die.
9 ⟨⟩ in the margin.
10 Qusṭā ibn Lūqā. See commentary.
11 درهم كيلا
12 درهم كيلا

٢:١١ وأما المزاج فأحمل الأبدان للفصد الحارة الرطبة الخصيبة الكثيرة اللحم المشوبة بحمرة الواسعة العروق الظاهرة المتكاثفة الشعور. وليكن الحذر في الفصد على قدر البعد من هؤلاء والقرب. وقد نرى أبدانا خصيبة سمينة قليلة الدم ومهزولة كثيرة الدم.

٢:١٢ فقد حكى جالينوس في كتاب أفديميا[a] عن امرأة احتبس طمثها ثمانية أشهر وكانت في غاية الهزال ففصدها فعاد بدنها إلى عادته الأولى. وكان الأطباء يمنعون من ذلك سيما أنّ شهوتها كانت مختلفة. وأخرج لها من الدم في ثلاثة أيام نحو ثلاثة أرطال: في اليوم الأول رطل ⟨ونصف⟩[b] وفي اليوم الثاني رطل وفي اليوم الثالث أرجح من نصف رطل. والذي دعاه إلى فصدها سوء احتباس حيضها إنّ عروقها كانت دارّة مملوءة دما يضرب إلى الكمودة. فلما فصدها وأخرج الدم كالزفت السيال استدعاه ذلك إلى الإكثار منه.

٢:١٣ وهل رأيت بمدينة السلام[c] رجلا من ولد محمد بن عبد الملك الزيات[d] وسنه[e] نيف وأربعون سنة وكان من قضافة البدن وصفرة اللون على غاية وكان يعرض له في كل شهر أو ما زاد قليلا أن يحمر جسمه وينخنق ويحس كأن نفسه يمسك حتى يلجأ إلى الفصد وكان يخرج من الدم قرب خمسة عشر درهم كيلا فكان يأنس بالراحة في الوقت. وكان الذي يعرض لهذا احتراق الدم لا كثرته.

٢:١٤ وأيضا كان هذا الرجل قد قرأ كثيرا من كتب جالينوس على معلم ولم تكن له دربة ولا خدمة. وكان يعرض له قديما قبل لقائي إياه اعتقال طبعه فكان يلجأ إلى الأشربة اللينة
6r كشراب البنفسج أو شراب الإجاص أو شراب التين أو شراب القراسيا | أو نحوها. ولم يزل يفعل هذا حتى أمسك طبعه حتى صار لا يجيبه إلا بدواء مسهل. فحين لقيته أخبرني

a أفديميا: أقديميا
b ونصف in the margin
c بمدينة السلام: بمدينة السالم
d محمد بن عبد الملك الزيات: أحمد عبد الملك الزيات
e سنه clarified in the margin

2:11 As to the disposition, the most tolerant bodies for phlebotomy are those that are hot, moist, fat, abundant with reddish flesh, with wide, visible veins, and dense hair. One's caution in phlebotomy should be in accordance with the degree to which the patient's body possesses these properties. We may see bodies that are fat, obese, with a small amount of blood, as well as skinny [bodies] with a lot of blood.

2:12 Galen spoke in [his commentary of] the book *Epidemics*[13] about a woman who suffered from amenorrhea for eight months. She was very emaciated, and thus he phlebotomised her, and her body returned to its former state. The [other] physicians used to abstain from that, especially since her appetite was different [from the usual]. During three days, he extracted around three *raṭls* of blood: on the first day a *raṭl* ⟨and a half⟩,[14] on the second day one *raṭl*, and on the third day most likely half a *raṭl*. What urged him to phlebotomise her was the severity of her amenorrhea, although her veins were filled with copiously flowing dark grey blood. Thus, when he phlebotomised her and extracted the blood [that was] as liquid tar, he was forced to extract a larger quantity [i.e., more than he initially intended].

2:13 Have you seen a man in Baghdad,[15] from the offspring of Muḥammad ibn ʿAbd al-Malik al-Zayyāt, who was forty and some years old, and who had a slender body and was extremely pale?[16] Every month or so it happened that his body turned red and he was unable to breathe, and he felt as if his breath was retained until he resorted to phlebotomy. Nearly fifteen *dirhams*[17] of [his] blood would be extracted, and he would feel relieved immediately. What happened to him was combustion of blood, not its abundance.

2:14 Also, this man surely had studied a lot of Galen's books with a teacher—however, he had no experience nor clinical practice. For a long time before I met him, he would suffer from constipation,[18] and he used to resort to softening syrups, such as that of violet, plum, fig, cherry | or something similar to them. 6r
He became so constipated that only a purgative drug would trigger a reaction.

---

13 Galen's commentary on Hippocrates' *Epidemics*.

14 ⟨⟩ in the margin.

15 *Madīnat al-Salām*.

16 Ms. Escorial reads 'yellow,' understood as 'pale.'

17 درهم كيلا

18 Lit. 'detention of his nature.'

أنه تمتسك طبيعته خمسة أيام حتى يأخذ من حب الإهليلج الأصفر. صفته أن يؤخذ[a] الإهليلج الأصفر المنزوع النوى فيغم في الماء ويجعل في الشمس في وقت القيظ[b] أربعين يوما حتى يذهب الماء وينعقد بعد أن يحرّك في كل يوم مرات. ثم يحبّب ويؤخذ بالسكر والمحمودة.

٢:١٥ وبالجملة الرجال أحمل للفصد من النساء.

٢:١٦ وأما الزمان فإنّ الربيع أفضل الأزمنة للفصد. فقد ذكر جالينوس أنّ كثيرا بمدينة رومية يفتصدون بغير حاجة إلى الفصد في هذا الزمان للعادة وثقتهم فإنّ الخطأ إنْ وقع فيه لم يكن ضره بكثير. والناس في سائر ما رأيناه من البلدان العظام على هذا المنهاج. ثم يليه في الجودة الشتاء ثم الصيف ثم الخريف. وأما الوقت الحاضر فليس يجب أن يستعمل الفصد في يوم شديد الحر والبرد إلا أن تدعو إلى ذلك ضرورة.

٢:١٧ وأما البلدان فإنّ البلدان الواغلة في الشمال ناحية بنات نعش والفرقدين باردة جدا، هي الواغلة في الجنوب نحو سهيل حارة جدا. وكلما قرب أو بعد من هاتين الجهتين فعلى هذه النسبة. وبالجملة البلدان الباردة تصح وأهلها أقوى وأحسن ألوانا وأبدانا والبلدان المائلة إلى الجنوب أحر أبدانا من المائلة إلى الشمال وإن استوت مواضعه من الفلك كما أنّ البلدان قد يحدث لها تغاير من أمور تخصها من قبل الجبال المقابلة والمؤثرة[c] والعلو والانخفاض والبحار والأنهار والأشجار وغير ذلك. وإن استوت عروضها وأحمل الناس للفصد من كان فيما بين هاتين الناحيتين | مائلا إلى الشمال وكان بلده مكشوفا 6v
للشمس مستورا عن المغرب.

٢:١٨ وأما ما يؤكل ويشرب فعلى الأمر الأكثر من أكل اللحم الفتى والحلواء وشرب الأنبذة يكثر دمه.

---

a يؤخذ: يأخذ
b القيظ: القيض
c والمؤثرة: والمواثرة

When I met him, he informed me that he would suffer from constipation for five days until he took one yellow chebulic myrobalan pill. Its prescription is that one takes the yellow myrobalans from which the kernels have been removed, covers them with water and places them in the sun in high summer for forty days until the water is gone, and it thickens after being stirred several times every day. Then it is made into a pill and taken with sugar and scammony.

2:15 In general, men tolerate phlebotomy better than women.

2:16 As to the season, the spring is the most optimal season for phlebotomy. Galen mentioned that many [people] in Rome get phlebotomised without the need for phlebotomy during this season because they are used to doing so and trust [its efficacy]. If a mistake occurred, it did not cause a considerable harm. People in all the other great countries that we have seen follow this manner. The next best season [for phlebotomy] is winter, then summer, and then autumn. As to the current time, one should not use phlebotomy on a very hot or a very cold day, unless necessary.

2:17 As to the countries, indeed the countries high in the north, in the direction of the Big Dipper and the two bright stars of Ursa Minor are very cold. The ones deep in the south, towards Canopus, are very hot. And whatever is near or far from these two sides, correspondingly. In general, cold countries are healthy, and their people are stronger and better in complexion and body, and the bodies [of people in] southern countries are hotter than the [bodies of people] living in the northern countries, even if their positions from the celestial sphere were equal. On the other hand, countries are different because of their specific matters, [e.g.] mountains that face [people] and influence [them], and because of the altitude [of their country], its depth, seas, rivers, trees, and the like. Even if the latitudes were equal, the most tolerant people for phlebotomy are the ones who, regarding these two directions, | live in a northern country 6v
that is exposed to the sun, hidden from the sunset.

2:18 As to what should be eaten and drunk, in most cases blood increases by eating young meat and confections, and by drinking wines.

٢:١٩ وأما من نسبة الأخلاط في البدن أهي على التساوي أو مختلفة فإنّ معرفة هذا صعبة[a] جدا ولا يدرك إلا على التقريب. فقد صرح أبقراط بهذا حين قال معرفة الكمّية صعبة جدا كثيرة[b] المنفعة وذلك أن يعرف مقدار الأخلاط في البدن وزيادة بعضها على بعض ومقدار ما يخرج غير الحاجة إلى ذلك على الحقيقة صعب جدا إلا أنّ الطبيب الكثير القراءة لكتب الأوائل. وما نتجه المربون يدرك على هذا التقريب جدا حتى لا يسمّى ما فاته من معرفة الحقيقة خطأ. فمتى حقق المتطبب أنّ الخلط الغالب في البدن الدم وأنّ الأخلاط في البدن [ليست] على التساوي استعمل الفصد لأنّ الدم تخرج معه جميع الأخلاط. كما قال جالينوس في كتابه في الأدوية المفردة: وإنْ كان الدم الأقل ابتدئ بالإسهال للخلط الغالب في البدن إن شاء الله.

الباب الثالث

٣:١ الباب الثالث نذكر فيه الأسباب الموجبة للفصد.

٣:٢ أؤكد الأسباب الموجبة للفصد.

٣:٣ الامتلاء وهو ينقسم قسمين أحدهما النظر بحسب الأوعية وهي العروق وهو أنْ تكون العروق والشرايين مملوءة دما وروحا وسائر الأخلاط على نسبتها التي كانت عليه قبل زيادة الدم والبدن صحيح ويتبعه التمدد والقربان وكأن العروق تتمزق وتنفتح ويكون الوجه مع ذلك مشرقا كأنه يقطر دما والنوم كثير والتمطي والتثاؤب وثقل الرأس وعظم النبض وغلظ البول وحمرته[c] وكدر الحواس | وبلادة الذهن وحلاوة الفم وتبثيره وخروج 7r
الدم منه والدماميل[d] التي تنفجر بسرعة. فإن انضاف إلى هذا أنْ يكون لمس البدن حارا إلى اللين كأنه قد خرج من الحمام وهو لحم والسن من الفتيان والعروق واسعة والغذاء المتقدم يوجب ذلك كان الدليل أقوى.

---

a صعبة: صعب
b صعبة جدا كثيرة: صعب جدا كثير
c حمرته repeated below the line
d ميل in the margin

2:19 As to the relation of the humours in the body, whether they are balanced or unbalanced,[19] indeed knowing this is very difficult, and can only be grasped approximately. Hippocrates declared this when he said: For to know the quantity of humours in the body, the fact that some exceed others, and the quantity of what flows out unnecessarily, is indeed very difficult. Yet, the physician well-versed in the books of the Ancients and what well educated [scholars] have produced knows [it] approximately, so that when the knowledge of the truth escapes him, this should not be called an error. When the physician verifies that the predominant humour in the body is blood, and that the humours in the body are [not] balanced, he should apply phlebotomy, since all the humours get extracted with blood. As Galen said in his book *On Simple Drugs*: If [the quantity of] blood is less [than the other humours], then begin with the purgation of the dominant humour in the body, God willing.

The Third Chapter

3:1 The third chapter in which we mention the causes that make phlebotomy necessary.

3:2 I confirm the causes that make phlebotomy necessary.

3:3 [It is necessary in the case of] overfilling, which is divided into two parts: one of the two is the one relating to vessels, i.e., the veins, and that is when the veins and the arteries are filled with blood, pneuma, and the rest of the humours in the same proportion that they were before the increase of blood, and the body is healthy. It is followed by tension and contraction, as if the veins are ruptured and opened, and with that the face is shining as if it is dripping blood. There is a lot of sleep, stretching, yawning, heaviness of the head, magnitude of pulse, thick and red urine, troubled sensations, | want of intellect, 7^r^
sweetness of mouth, its vesication, and blood flowing out of it, and boils that burst quickly. If this is combined with the feeling that the body is hot and soft when one touches it, as if he [i.e., the patient] just came out of the bathhouse, and he is corpulent, in the age of adolescence, and the veins are wide, and the preceding food imposes that, then the indication is stronger.

19 Lit. divergent.

٣:٤ وهو يولّد هذه الأحلام كما ذكر أبقراط في كتاب أفديميا[a] وذكر روفس[b] في كتابه فيما يسأل[c] عنه الطبيب العليل وذلك أنه من رأى جراحا ودما سائلا وألوانا حمراء دل على الحاجة إلى إخراج الدم. وهذا يتبين في سائر الأخلاط فإن من رأى ثلجا ومطرا دل على كثرة البلغم.

٣:٥ وأما الامتلاء بحسب القوة فهو الذي تزيد الأخلاط فيه على قدر ما تفي الطبيعة بحفظ الترويح عنه ويتبعه الثقل والكسل والاسترخاء وعسر الحركة وقلة الشهوة للغذاء وضعف القوة عن النهوض بما في البدن من الأخلاط حتى أن الطبيعة لا تقدر أنْ تهضم ما صار إليها في العروق إنْ تصيره غذاء فتنقيه عجزا منها عن إحالته.

٣:٦ وإنْ كانت هذه الأعلام قد تحس للامتلاء بحسب 〈الأوعية فقد يفرق بينهما بالبول〉[d] والنبض وغير ذلك مما قد ذكرناه. فإنَّ النبض في الذي بحسب القوة صغير والبول إلى الفجاجة واللون غير مشرق وفي أكثر الأمر يولّد مرضا قبل أن تتم علاماته.

٣:٧ وكل هذين الامتلاءين يوجبان مرضا ويحوجان إلى الاستفراغ. أما الامتلاء الأول فهو الذي بحسب الأوعية فحاجته إلى الفصد وإلى تقليل الغذاء. وأما الامتلاء الثاني وهو الذي بحسب القوة فقد يحتاج إلى الفصد والاستفراغ ويحتاج إلى توقّف ونظر وأنْ تؤخذ الدلائل التي يجدها العليل من مواضعها المخصوصة بها وذلك أنه قد يكون في البدن من هؤلاء أخلاط | نيئة. فمتى فصد من هذه حاله استرخى وضعف وبرد مزاجه وصار مستعدا 7v للأمراض الباردة حتى لا يمكن أنْ يرد إلى حالته الأولى. والخطر هاهنا عظيم جدا وخاصة إذا كان الوقت صيفا[e] ومعدته وكبده باردتين والمزاج إلى اللين.

a أفديميا: أقديميا
b روفس: روفش
c يسأل: يَسْلُ
d 〈 〉 in the margin; بالبول written once in the text, once in the margin.
e صيفا: ضيقا

3:4 It also brings forth these dreams, as Hippocrates mentioned in his book, *Epidemics*, and as Rufus[20] mentioned in his book, *On What the Physician Asks the Patient*,[21] that if someone sees wounds, flowing blood, and red colours [in his dreams], this indicates the need for extraction of blood. This obviously applies to the other humours [as well], for whoever sees snow and rain, this indicates the large quantity of phlegm.

3:5 As to the overfilling affecting the strength, it is the case in which the humours increase to the extent that [the patient's] nature is not sufficient to ensure a recovery from it. It is followed by heaviness, laziness, feebleness, difficulty of movement, lack of appetite, and weakness of strength to manage the humours in the body, until one's nature cannot digest what has come to it in the veins. If food reaches it, then she cleanses it, since she is unable to transform it.

3:6 Even if these signs [occur], you may feel overfilling relating to ⟨vessels—the two may be differentiated by urine⟩,[22] pulse, and other things that we already have mentioned. For indeed the pulse in the case of overfilling affecting the strength is weak, the urine tends towards yellowish green, and its colour is not bright. Most probably it is generating an illness before its signs are fully developed.

3:7 Both of these two [types of] overfillings cause an illness and require evacuation. As to the first [type of] overfilling, that is the one relating to the vessels, it requires phlebotomy and reduction of food. As to the second [type of] overfilling, the one affecting the strength, it may require phlebotomy and evacuation. It also requires hesitation and consideration: the indications that the patient finds in their specific sites should be taken [into consideration], and that is because the body of such people might contain raw | humours. Whenever one 7v
phlebotomises someone with this condition, he becomes feeble and weak, his disposition becomes cold, and he becomes susceptible to cold illnesses, so that he cannot return to his former condition. The danger here is very great, especially if it is summer, and his stomach and liver are cold, and the bodily disposition tends to softness.

20 Rufus of Ephesus.

21 *Quaestiones medicinales*. See commentary.

22 ⟨⟩ in the margin.

٣:٨ وينفع من كان بهذه الصفة إنْ كان الوقت متمكنا الاستفراغ بالاسطماخيقونات وإيارج الفيقرا على حسب الحاجة والحقن الحادة ودخول الحمام والأدهان المعتدلة وتقليل الغذاء وتلطيفه وأغذية قليلة الغذاء.[a] وقد يخرج لهم من الدم اليسير ويفعل ذلك في مرات.

٣:٩ ومن عرض له نفث دم وبرئ منه فقد يتقدم في فصده في أواني الربيع وإنْ لم يكن في بدنه دليل امتلاء خيفة أن ينهتك في صدره عرق. وكذلك من يتخوّف عليه الصرع أو السكتة الدمويتان أو العروق[b] التي في المقعدة أو الأورام العارضة في الرئة والشوصة والخوانيق وأوجاع المفاصل والنقرس والحميات المطبقة والدموية.

٣:١٠ وبالجملة كل الأمراض التي تتوقع من الدم أو سائر الأخلاط فقد يتقدم فيها بالفصد والإسهال على حسب الحاجة في وقت الربيع وإنْ لم تكن دلائل الكثرة حاضرة توقعا لما يحدث بعد ذلك وذلك أنه قد يستقبل الصيف وتطلب الأخلاط موضعا أوسع. وقد ينتفع أيضا بالفصد وإنْ لم يكن البدن ممتلئا أحد امتلاءين عند ابتداء ورم حار إما بسبب ضربة أو سقطة أو ألم شديد أو ضعف العضو فإنه إذا ألم أو ضعف جذب الدم إليه إذا كانت مادته متهيئة لذلك كما تجذب المحجمة الدم.

الباب الرابع

٤:١ الباب الرابع في كمية ما يخرج من الدم.

٤:٢ أما حقيقة معرفة قدر الدم وسائر الأخلاط في البدن ومقدار | ما يحتاج أن يخرج 8r
منها عند الحاجة بالفصد أو كم مقدار الدواء المسهل المستفرغ بالإضافة إلى الأخلاط فعسر جدا كما ذكرنا إلا أنّ استعمال الفصد أكثر سلامة من استعمال الدواء المسهل لأنك تقطعه متى شئت. وأما الدواء فإذا صار إلى البطن فليس يمكنك أن تنقص منه ولا من فعله.

---

a الغذاء: الأغذاء

b Ms. Parma: פתיחת הגידים

3:8 As for those who are characterised by this, if the season allows, it is beneficial to use evacuation by stomachics and bitter hiera according to the need, as well as sharp enemas, entering the bathhouse, moderate oils, reducing food and making it finer, and [administering] scarcely nourishing food. One may extract a little blood from them, and this may be done in [several] sessions.

3:9 Whoever has suffered from haemoptysis and has healed from it may be phlebotomised in the springtime even if there is no indication of overfilling in his body, because one fears that a vein in his chest might burst open. In the same manner, for anyone suspected to suffer from sanguine epilepsy, sanguine apoplexy, [swollen] veins in the anus, or swellings that appear in the lungs, pleuritis, diphtheria, arthritis, gout, and continuous and sanguine fevers.

3:10 In general, all illnesses expected to arise from blood or the other humours may be tackled by phlebotomy or purgation, as needed during the spring—even if no indications of a surplus are present. This is done in anticipation of what may follow, for as summer approaches, the humours seek a wider space. Phlebotomy may also be beneficial even if the body is not suffering from either of the [two types of] overfillings, at the onset of a hot swelling caused by a blow or a fall, severe pain, or weakness of a part—since when a part aches or weakens, it attracts blood to itself if the matter is predisposed to it, just as the cupping vessel draws blood.

The Fourth Chapter

4:1 The fourth chapter on the quantity of blood that should be extracted.

4:2 Really knowing the quantity of blood and the other humours in the body, as well as the quantity | that needs to be extracted when phlebotomy is required, 8r
or the quantity of a purgative, evacuating drug in relation to the humours, is very difficult, as we have mentioned. However, using phlebotomy is safer than using a purgative drug, because you can end it whenever you want. As to the drug, once it has reached the stomach, you cannot reduce it nor its effect.

٤:٣ ومتى كان في البدن من الدم كثير وغلى وأحدث حمى فاستفرغه دفعة واحدة في وقت انحطاط نوبة الحمى قبل أن ينصب إلى بعض الأعضاء النفيسة لأن هذه الحمى وإن كانت مطبقة فإنما على الأمر الأكثر يكون لها ابتداء وصعود وتزيّد وانتهاء وانحطاط. وليكن الاستفراغ إلى أن يحدث الغشي لأن رديء الدم إذا بقي أفسد غيره وكثيرا ما يبرد بعقب الغشي البدن ويندى وتنطلق الطبيعة وينقضي المرض بسرعة. وليس لخروج الدم في القلة والكثرة حد.

٤:٤ ومن أفضل ما يتعمد في وقت الفصد أن يتفقد نبض العروق من الجانب الغير مفصود ما دام الدم يسيل لئلا يلحق العليل الموت مكان الغشي. فإذا رأيت النبض قد تغير في عظمه واستوائه فضلا عن أن يضعف أو ضعفت حمية الدم فاقطعه على المقام. وكذلك متى تغير لونه وقوامه. وكثيرا ما لا يتغير اللون أو القوام.

٤:٥ ومن كان به ورم قرب الموضع المفصود كالشوصة وغيرها فمن أجود الأشياء أن يخرج له الدم إلى أن يتغير في لونه وقوامه لأن الدم في هؤلاء إنْ كان في حال الصبغ حنيا أو أحمر فإنه يكون في الورم بسبب الغليان وتجنب في الفصد الغشي جهدك ما لم تدفع إليه ضرورة.

٤:٦ ومتى فصدت لكثرة الدم فابلغ إلى الغشي وإن فصدت لاحتراقه فابلغ إلى تغيّر[a] الدم.

الباب الخامس

٥:١ الباب الخامس في العروق المفصودة.

٥:٢ العروق المفصودة صنفان فمنها ضاربة | وهي الشرايين ومنشؤها من القلب ومنها 8v
غير ضاربة وهي الأوراد ومنشؤها من الكبد. وأنا ذاكر مواضعها وأسماءها ومنافعها على التوالي وأبتدئ بذلك من الرأس.

a تغيّر: زخير

4:3 When there is a lot of blood in the body, and it boils, and causes a fever, evacuate it all at once at the time of the decline of the paroxysm of fever before it flows towards some vital parts, because this fever, even if it is continuous, in most cases it will have a beginning, rise, increase, climax, and decline. Evacuation should [last] until the patient loses consciousness, since bad blood, if it remains [in the body], will corrupt the rest [of the blood]. In many cases the body becomes cold immediately after unconsciousness, and moist, and as Nature is not impeded [anymore], the illness terminates quickly. There is no limit regarding how little and how much blood should be extracted from people.

4:4 At the time of phlebotomy it is preferable to proceed by examining the pulse of the veins from the side that is not phlebotomised. As long as the blood is flowing, the patient does not die instead of becoming unconscious. If you see the pulse changing in its magnitude and regularity, in addition to weakening or diminished force, then end it immediately. And likewise, when its colour and consistency change. In many cases the colour and consistency do not change.

4:5 Whoever has a swelling near the phlebotomised site, such as pleuritis and the like, the most suitable thing [to do] is to extract his blood until its colour and consistency change. This is because the blood in these [people], if it is such that it changes colour towards henna or red, it is [generated] in the swelling because of boiling. Avoid phlebotomising until unconsciousness, unless it is necessary.

4:6 When you phlebotomise because there is a surplus of blood, continue until the patient loses consciousness; and if you phlebotomise because of its combustion, continue until the blood changes.

The Fifth Chapter

5:1 The fifth chapter on the phlebotomised veins.

5:2 There are two sorts of phlebotomised veins: the pulsatile | i.e., the arteries, that originate from the heart, and the non-pulsatile, i.e., the veins, that originate from the liver. I mention their locations, names, and benefits consecutively, and I begin from the head. 8v

٥:٣ فمن ذلك أربعة عروق خلف الأذنين في الرأس من كل جانب عرقان واحد يمنة والآخر يسرة. ويحاذيان طرف الأذنين من أعلاهما إذا الصقا بالرأس كان العرق فوق الأذن بقدر يسير وفصد هذين العرقين نافع من البثور والقروح في الرأس والسعفة الرطبة واليابسة والجذام.

٥:٤ وثلاثة عروق وهي[a] شرايين[b] في كل أذن اثنان منهما خفيان وواحد ظاهر وفصدها[c] نافع من السعفة ووجع العين. وذكر جالينوس عن أبقراط في كتاب الأهوية والبلدان أنّ من قطعت له هذه لم ينسل وقال هذا قول مقنع.[d]

٥:٥ عرقان في مؤخر الرأس يليان النقرة وفصدهما نافع من البخار المرتقي وبدء الماء والانتشار.

٥:٦ عرق يأتي الجبهة من وسط الرأس يتشعب هنالك شعبتين وربما أكثر فتصير واحدة يمنة وأخرى يسرة فافصد أبدا أملاءهما وفصدهما نافع[e] من وجع العينين القديم والثقل الكائن في مؤخر الرأس.

٥:٧ عرقان يلتويان في الصدغين وهما شريانان وفصدهما نافع من الصداع الدائم والشقيقة والانتشار ووجع العينين التي يخشى عليها الهلاك وفصدهما يكون بالبتر والسيل.

٥:٨ وبالجملة يجب أن تفصد العروق الضوارب فيما علم من العلل كونه مادة حارة لطيفة ناخسة في الأغشية ووجعها يحس كأنه مركّز ثم ذلك الوجع والنخس ينبسط حول ذلك المركز.

a وهي: في
b شرايين: الشرانين
c وفصدها: وفصده
d +O
e وفصدهما نافع: وهي نافعة

5:3 Four veins behind the ears in the head, two veins on each side, one on the right, and the other on the left. They are aligned with the tip of the ears above them. As the two connect to the head, the vein is directly above the ear. Phlebotomising these two veins is beneficial for pustules and ulcers in the head, wet and dry cradle cap, and leprosy.

5:4 Three veins that are arteries in each ear, two of which are concealed, one visible. Phlebotomising them is beneficial for cradle cap and ophthalmalgia. Galen mentioned Hippocrates' [statement] in the book *Airs and Places*,[23] that 'whoever had these cut, will not procreate,' and commented that this is a convincing statement.

5:5 Two veins in the back of the head near the hollow of the neck: phlebotomising them is beneficial for the rising fumes, watery discharge, and *intišār*.[24]

5:6 A vein comes to the forehead from the middle of the head, dividing there into two branches, sometimes more, and one flows to the right, another to the left. Always phlebotomise them when they are full. Phlebotomising the two is beneficial for chronic ophthalmalgia and the heaviness that is [felt] in the back of the head.

5:7 Two curved veins in the temples, they are two arteries: phlebotomising the two is beneficial for chronic headache, migraine, *intišār*, and ophthalmalgia that make one afraid of dying. Phlebotomising the two is done by making an incision and [letting the blood] flow.[25]

5:8 In general, the pulsatile veins need to be phlebotomised when it is known that the illnesses are caused by a hot, fine, pricking matter in the membranes, and the pain feels as if it is concentrated, then that pain and the pricking sensation spread out around that centre.

23 *Airs, Waters, Places*. See commentary.

24 See commentary.

25 See commentary.

٥:٩ عرقان في المأقين[a] وفصدهما نافع من بقية الرمد والدمعة والعشاوة.[b]

٥:١٠ عرق في طرف الأنف وفصده نافع من الكلف واستحالة اللون والحزاز والبثور والقروح | في الأنف والشفة واحتقان الدم فيهما[c] وهي[d] النواسير[e] والشقاق[f] فيهما. 9r

٥:١١ عرقان في باطن اللسان وفصدهما نافع من تورّم اللسان والخوانيق الدموية.

٥:١٢ عرقان في باطن الذقن وهما الساريان[g] من داخل إذا رفع اللسان رأيت واحدا على اليمن وواحدا على الشمال وفصدهما[h] نافع من اللوزتين وهما ورم العضل الذي عن جنبي المريء.

٥:١٣ عرقان يعرفان بالودجين ومواضعهما العنق وفصدهما نافع من بحّة الصوت ووجع الرئة والربو[i] والجذام في أوّله. ويليهما عرقان متلاصقان للحلقوم ومن قطع أحدهما فقد ذبح المفصود.

٥:١٤ عرقان في العضدين ويعرفان بالإبطين ويوجد كل واحد منهما بين المرفق والإبط من الجانب الإنسي وفصدهما نافع من انصباب الدم إلى القلب ووجع الرئة والصدر والشوصة.

---

a المأقين: المأقيين
b العشاوة: الغشاوة
c فيهما: فيها
d وهي: وفي
e النواسير: البواسير
f +o
g الساريان: الساريين
h وفصدهما: وفصده
i +o

5:9 Two veins in the inner corners of the eye: phlebotomising them is beneficial for remains of ophthalmia, rhyas, and nyctalopia.

5:10 One vein in the tip of the nose: phlebotomising it is beneficial for freckles, discoloration, dandruff, pustules and ulcers | in the nose and the lips, and 9r
congestion of blood, i.e., fistulae and fissures, in them.

5:11 Two veins inside the tongue: phlebotomising the two is beneficial for swelling of the tongue and sanguine diphtheria.

5:12 Two veins inside the chin, and the two begin from [the] inside—if the tongue is lifted, you see one on the right and one on the left: phlebotomising the two is beneficial for the tonsils, that are a swelling of the muscles on the two sides of the oesophagus.

5:13 Two veins that are known as jugular veins, they both are located in the neck: phlebotomising the two is beneficial for hoarseness of voice, lung pain, asthma, and leprosy in its beginning. They are followed by two veins that are connected to the throat, and whoever cuts one of the two, slaughters the phlebotomised.

5:14 Two veins in the upper arms that are known as axillary veins, both of them located between the elbow and the armpit, on the inner side: phlebotomising them is beneficial for the blood flowing to the heart, pain in lungs and chest, and pleuritis.

٥:١٥ ستة عروق في الذراعين في كل ذراع منها ثلاثة عروق أحدها[a] يقال له القيفال وهو اسم يوناني ومعناه الرأس وموضعه الجانب الوحشي وفصده نافع لما فوق اللبة[b] والرأس والوجه لأنه مرتق إليها.

٥:١٦ الباسليق وهو عرق البطن وهو مشتق من الرئاسة وموضعه الجانب الإنسي وفصده نافع لما أسفل اللبة[c] لأنّ مبلغه هنالك ثم ينصب إلى الرجلين.[d]

٥:١٧ الأكحل وهو شعبة من الباسليق وشعبة من القيفال يلتقيان في موضع واحد في الوسط بينهما ويتحدان ويسمى التقاؤهما أكحل[e] وفصده نافع من الأمراض التي تكون في جملة البدن لأنه مؤلف من القيفال والباسليق فمن فصده مكانه فقد فصدهما.

٥:١٨ ومتى كانت العلة في الرأس فافصد القيفال لأنه خصيص بها إلا أن يكون رقيقا فاعدل عنه إلى ما ينوب عنه | كالأكحل بعد أنْ يكون أشد امتلاء منه. وبمثل هذا فقس 9v
في سائر العروق. ولا تفصد ضيقا أبدا إلا إذا أردت جذب المواد. ولتعلم أن فصد العرق الخصيص بينه وبين فصد العرق غير الخصيص فرق كبير.[f]

٥:١٩ عرقان في موضع المعصمين في الذراعين يعرفان بحبل الذراع وهما من الباسليق ويقومان في الفصد مقامه.

٥:٢٠ وشعبة من الباسليق تصير بين البنصر والوسطى وفصده نافع من أوجاع القلب والكبد والطحال والرئة.

---

a أحدها: أحدهما
b اللبة: اللثة
c اللبة: اللية
d رجلين: رحلين
e أكحل: أكحلا
f كبير: كثير

5:15 Six veins in the forearms, three in each forearm, one of them is called cephalic vein, which is a Greek name—it means 'head'—and it is located on the outer side. Phlebotomising it is beneficial for what is above the jugular fossa, the head, and the face, because it ascends to them.

5:16 The basilic vein, i.e., *vena basilica*, derived from *ri'āsa*,[26] and it is located on the inner side. Phlebotomising it is beneficial for what is below the jugular fossa, because its outmost scope is there, and then it flows towards the legs.

5:17 The median cubital vein is a branch of the basilic vein and a branch of the cephalic vein which come together in one place in the middle between the two and unite. Where they come together is called median cubital vein. Phlebotomising it is beneficial for illnesses in the whole body, because it consists of the cephalic vein and the basilic vein. Whoever has phlebotomised it in this place, indeed has phlebotomised the two [veins].

5:18 Whenever the illness is in the head, phlebotomise the cephalic vein, since it is especially intended for it, unless it is thin, for then turn away from it toward something that can replace it, | such as the median cubital vein, because it is 9v
thicker[27] than the other. According to this example, open the rest of the veins. Do not ever phlebotomise a narrow one unless you want to draw matters. You should know that there is a big difference between phlebotomising a specifically intended vein and a vein that is not specifically intended.

5:19 Two veins in the place of the wrists in the arms, known as *vena cephalica pollicis*, that come from the basilic vein and serve in phlebotomy instead of it.

5:20 A branch of the basilic vein runs between the ring finger and the middle finger: phlebotomising it is beneficial for pain in the heart, liver, spleen, and lungs.

---

26 See commentary.

27 Lit. 'fuller.'

٥:٢١ وأخرى تصير بين الخنصر والبنصر وتعرف بالأسيلم اشتقاقا من السلامة لأنها نابت عن الشريان وفصدها نافع من وجع الصدر والكبد والطحال والرئة.

٥:٢٢ عرقان في مأبض الركبتين في باطنيهما[a] ويوجدان أبدا أغلظ وأملأ من سائر العروق التي تقاربها وفصدهما نافع بإذن الله من القروح والبثور التي تطول مدتها في الساقين ومن الدوالي ويدر[b] الطمث.

٥:٢٣ عرقان يعرفان بعرقي النَّسَا وتوجدان في ظاهر الكعبين من الجانب الوحشي وفصدهما نافع من الوجع الشديد الذي يعرض من لدن الورك وظاهر الساق إلى آخر القدم وربما لم يبلغ إلى القدم.

٥:٢٤ عرقان يعرفان بالصافنين ويوجدان على الكعبين من الجانب الإنسي وفصدهما نافع من القروح والبثور وحكة الأنثيين ويدر[c] الطمث.

٥:٢٥ وذلك اثنان وأربعون عرقا سوى شعب الباسليق وقد توجد عروق تعرف بالمدنية وتولدها من الأطعمة والأشربة والمياه الرديئة وخصوصية ذلك البلد وعلاجها خارج عن غرض كتابنا هذا.

الباب السادس

٦:١ الباب السادس نذكر فيه كيفية فصد العروق وما يلحق ذلك من الخطأ ليحترس منه.

10r **٦:٢** إنه لما كانت العروق | المفصودة ضوارب وغير ضوارب نحو ما ذكرنا وكان في فصد الضوارب خطر بسبب غلظ جرمها وعسر انقطاع دمها واندمالها. وهي مركبة من طبقتين إلا العرق الذي يسقي الرئة فإنه وحده مركب من طبقة واحدة وثخن الطبقة الداخلة خمسة

a في باطنيهما corrected in the margin في باطنهما
b ويدر: وتدر
c ويدر: وتدر

5:21 Another [branch] comes towards the little finger and the ring finger, it is known as *vena salvatella*, deriving from *salāma*,[28] since it substitutes the artery: phlebotomising it is beneficial for pain in the chest, liver, spleen, and lungs.

5:22 Two veins in the popliteal fossae,[29] they should always be thicker and fuller than the other veins that are near them. Phlebotomising them is beneficial—with God's permission—for chronic ulcers and pustules in the legs, for varicose veins, and it makes the menstruation flow.

5:23 Two veins that are known as the sciatic veins,[30] that are found on the outer one of the two ankles, on the outside: phlebotomising them is beneficial for the strong pain that occurs from the hip and the external part of the leg, all the way to the tip of the foot. Sometimes the pain does not reach the foot.

5:24 Two veins known as the saphenous veins,[31] and they are on the inner one of the two ankles: phlebotomising them is beneficial for ulcers and pimples, the itching of testicles, and it makes the menstruation flow.

5:25 These are the forty-two veins, excluding the branches of the basilic vein. There are veins that are known as *al-madaniyya*,[32] that are generated from foods, drinks and bad waters, as well as the character of that country—their treatment is outside the intention of this book of ours.

The Sixth Chapter

6:1 The sixth chapter in which we mention the method of phlebotomy, and the mistake this may entail in order to beware of it.

6:2 The phlebotomised veins | are pulsatile and non-pulsatile, as we have men- 10r
tioned, and there is a danger in phlebotomising the pulsatile [veins] due to the coarseness of their substance, the difficulty of stanching the blood flow, and ensuring recovery. They are composed of two tunics, apart from the vein that nourishes[33] the lungs, for it alone is composed of one tunic, and the thickness

28 See commentary.
29 ⟨inside the two⟩ in the margin.
30 See commentary.
31 I.e., the great saphenous veins. See commentary.
32 Lit. 'Medinean veins,' i.e., Guinea worms. See commentary.
33 Lit. 'irrigates.'

أمثال ثخن الطبقة الخارجة. وزعم جالينوس أنه ما أقدم على فصدها إلا لسبب وجع كان يجده قديما في الموضع الذي يتصل فيه الكبد بالحجاب وكان يومئذ غلاما فأُرِيَ في نومه أن يفصد العرق الضارب الذي بين السبابة والإبهام وأن يترك الدم حتى ينقطع ففعل ما أري فسكن عنه الوجع على المكان[a] وخرج من الدم أقل من رطل.

٦:٣ وأفضل فصدها أن تبتر بنصفين على نصف دائرة فينقبض أحد الجانبين إلى منشئه والآخر إلى الجانب الآخر. وقد يعرض هذا بعينه للعرق غير الضارب إلا أنه في العرق الضارب إحدى وأولى.[b]

٦:٤ وأما العرق غير الضارب فأول ما يجب عليك أن تملأه ثم تقيده بعصابة بالقرب منه وادلك الموضع بالدهن فإنْ خفي فحله وعلم على الموضع أعني موضع الفصد بلا تقييد واتركه قليلا ثم شدّه وادلكه. فإنْ خفي فشد جدا وعلّق من اليد شيئا ثقيلا واتركه ساعة. فإنْ خفي ولم يظهر فافصده في موضع العلامة.

٦:٥ وخبّرني بعض من كنت أتعلم عنده الفصد أنه عسر عليه إخراج عرق امرأة فنهرها وضجرها ولكمها فبرزت عروقها ففصدها للوقت واعتذر إليها وأخبرها بحيلته.

٦:٦ ومتى دلكت موضعا ولم تره ممتلئا فاعلم أنّ ليس هناك عرق.

10v **٦:٧** فأما عرق الجبهة | فيفصد بالخنق بعصابة.

٦:٨ وأما الودجان ففصدهما بالنفخ القليل.

٦:٩ القيفال ينبغي أن ينزل عن العضلة نحو اللحم إلى الموضع اللين ولا تفصده ضيقا فإنه يرم.

---

a +O

b +O

of the inner tunic is five times the thickness of the outer tunic. Galen declared that he did not undertake phlebotomising them unless for the reason of pain that he had once felt in the area where the liver connects to the diaphragm. At that time, he was a boy, and it was shown to him in his dream that he should phlebotomise the pulsatile vein that is between the index finger and the thumb and let the blood [flow] until it[s flow] ceases. He did as was shown to him [in his dream], and the pain ceased immediately, with less than a *raṭl* of blood flowing out.

6:3 The best way of phlebotomising them is to cut them into two halves, as a half circle, for then one of the two sides will shrink to its place of origin, and the other to the other side. This very thing may happen to the non-pulsatile vein, but it primarily occurs in the pulsatile vein.

6:4 As to the non-pulsatile vein, the first thing that you need [to do] is to have it filled [with blood], then bind it with a bandage near it and rub the spot with oil. If it [i.e., the vein] disappears, untie it and put a mark on the spot—I mean the spot of the phlebotomy—without binding, and leave it for a moment. Exert pressure on it and rub it. If it disappears [again], put severe pressure to it and fasten something heavy to the hand and leave it for a while. If it remains unseen and does not become visible, then phlebotomise at the site of the mark.

6:5 Someone with whom I was studying phlebotomy informed me that it was difficult for him to extract [blood from] the vein of a woman, thus he scolded her, annoyed her, and punched her, causing her veins to emerge. He then phlebotomised her right away, and apologised to her, informing her about his trick.

6:6 When you have rubbed a spot and do not see it filled, then know that there is no vein.

6:7 As to the frontal vein, | it is phlebotomised by compression with a head- 10v
band.

6:8 As to the two jugular veins, they are phlebotomised with a slight inflation.

6:9 The cephalic vein must go down from the muscle towards the flesh, to the soft spot. Do not phlebotomise it when narrow, for it will swell.

٦:١٠ وليكن الفصد عند احتراق الدم واسعا لغلظ المادة وعند جذب المادة[a] ضيقا ‹ليطول الجذب›[b] وعند الكثرة متوسطا لأنه إنْ كان واسعا خُشِيَ من انصباب الدم بقوة فيحدث في موضع الفصد ورم. ومتى تعذر خروج الدم فإنّ عكر الزيت إذا جعل عليه أكثر من صفائه.

٦:١١ الأكحل يتفقد فإن كان العصب يمنة أو يسرة فصد بشفرة[c] المبضع خلاف جهة العصب. وإن كان بين عصبتين فصد طولا وترك التعميق لأنه ربما بتر معه غير محسوس فيعقب خدرا.

٦:١٢ الباسليق ينبغي أن يتفقد الشريان الذي تحته قبل التقييد ويعلّم عليه وهو أبدا بنفسجي اللون ثم يشد وينظر موضع العلامة فيتنحى عنه. والباسليق أبدا يفارق الشريان أسفل المرفق ويعرض فأنزل الفصد أسفل ما أمكن وجنّب فصده جهدك ما لم يكن ممتلئا. وقد يشرّح الباسليق إذا لم يظهر ويعلّق بسنّارة ويفصد أو يفصد بعض شعبه كالإبطي ونحوه. ومتى شددت الرباط ورأيته ينتفخ ويعلو[d] فتوق فصده فإنه شريان ويكون فصده بمبضع لين قصير الشفرة.[e]

٦:١٣ فإنه عرق عصبي فإن اتفق في حاله أن ترى الدم مشرقا رقيقا يثب وثبا فاعلم أنه من الشريان وعلاجه سأصفه في موضعه.

٦:١٤ حبل الذراع وأما حبل الذراع فإنه كثير الزوال فافصده طولا بمبضع لين له شفرة[f] ويكون غمزك بالمبضع على حسب ما تقدم من صلابة الجلد وصلابة جرم العروق وما عليه من اللحم. واعلم أن الجلد الأسود أبدا أصلب والأبيض أرخى ومتى كان العرق رقيقا فافصده تعليقا بمبضع لا شفر[g] له.

---

a بيان جذب in the margin
b ليطول الجذب أصل in the margin
c بشفرة: بشعرة
d يعلو: يعلوا
e الشفرة: الشعرة
f شفرة: شعرة
g شفر: شعر

6:10 At the time of combustion of blood, phlebotomy should be conducted to a wide [vein] for the coarseness of the matter, to a narrow one when drawing matter ⟨in order to lengthen the drawing⟩,[34] and to an average one when there is a lot, since had it been wide, one would fear that the blood flows out copiously, thus a swelling at the site of phlebotomy would occur. When blood flows with difficulty, it is better[35] to apply the sediment of oil on the spot instead of clear oil.

6:11 [When] the median cubital vein is examined, and if the nerve is on the right or on the left, it is phlebotomised with the blade of the scalpel on the opposite side of the nerve. If it is between two nerves, it is phlebotomised lengthwise, and not deeply, because one might cut with it [a nerve that is] not noticeable, so that numbness follows.

6:12 The basilic vein: one must examine the artery that is below it before binding, and mark it, and it is always purple in colour. Then it is tightened, and one keeps in mind the place of the mark and then takes it away. The basilic vein always separates from the artery below the elbow and becomes visible. Hence, conduct phlebotomy as low as possible, but avoid phlebotomising it unless it is full. If not visible, the basilic vein may be cut open being lifted with a hook and phlebotomised, or one phlebotomises one of its branches, such as the axillary vein, and the like. Whenever you tighten the ligature and see it inflate and elevate, be wary of phlebotomising it, for it is an artery. Phlebotomising it is done by a fine, short-bladed scalpel.

6:13 It is a nerval vein, so should you see that the blood is clear and refined, [and that it is] squirting, then know that it is from an artery. I will describe its treatment in its place.

6:14 *Vena cephalica pollicis*. As to *vena cephalica pollicis*, it withdraws often. Thus, phlebotomise it lengthwise with a fine scalpel that has a blade, and hold the scalpel in accordance with how hard the skin is, and how hard the body of the veins is, and the flesh above it. Know that black skin is always harder, and white softer. If the vein is thin, phlebotomise it by lifting it with a scalpel with no blade.

---

34 ⟨⟩ in the margin.

35 Lit. 'more.' See commentary.

٦:١٥ وينبغي أن ترسل اليد في وقت الفصد | على حالها الطبيعية وتحر في وقت الشد 11r
أن يزول ⟨الجلد⟩[a] عن موضعه عند الفصد فينبغي أن يتسع خروج الدم. وإذا أردت غسل العرق فمد اليد[b] واغسل.

٦:١٦ والفصد يكون في الطول أو العرض أو التأريب. أما الطول[c] فإذا[d] كان بين عصبتين. وأما العرض فإذا أريد أن يلتحم سريعا. والتأريب بين هذين وشكله في خروج الدم أحسن الأشكال وليكن المبضع عند الأمن من العصب قائما ومبطوحا عندما يخاف تحته عصب مفروش ومقلوبا عند الحذر من مقابلة العصب لوجه المبضع.

٦:١٧ ومما يقلل⟨وجع⟩ الفصد[e] لين المبضع ورقته وأن تمتلئ العروق ويكمد الموضع بالماء الحار لا جرم في الشتاء. واحذر أن لا يمس المبضع دهن ولا ما يحويه. وأشد العروق التي في الذراعين وجعا حبل الذراع ثم القيفال لمكان العضلة وصلابة الجلد. فأما الباسليق والأكحل فأقل وجعا لا سيما إن لم يكن فوقهما ⟨لحم⟩.[f]

٦:١٨ وأما الأسيلم فليوضع الكف في ماء حار حتى ينتفخ ويشد المعصم بعصابة ثم يفصد ويعاد في الماء الحار لئلا يجمد الدم.

٦:١٩ عرق النسا توق فصده[g] ما أمكن لأن الخطأ فيه يعقب زمانة[h] لعصب كثير[i] والوجه في فصده أن يشد من لدن الورك على الاتصال إلى فوق الكعب بحبل صوف يكون له عرض قليل فإن لم يتبين فيدخل الحمام أو يدخل الرجل في ماء حار ويعتمد على الرجل العليلة بعد أن يجعلها على طوبة أو آجرة ويرفع الصحيحة. وإنْ لم يظهر فصد بدله

a الجلد above the line
b فمد اليد: فمد ولد/ أظنه فمد اليد in the margin
c فإذا أريد أن يلتحم سريعا + MS
d فإذا: وإذا
e الفصد + MS, وجع الفصد أصل in the margin
f لحم أصل in the margin
g فصده: فصدها corrected in the margin
h لا مجاور possibly deleted in the MS
i ة added below the line

6:15 At the time of phlebotomy it is necessary to let the hand rest | in its natural state, and to be warm at the time of binding. If the ⟨skin⟩[36] withdraws from its place during phlebotomy, the extracted blood volume will necessarily increase. If you want to rinse the vein, extend the hand and rinse. 11r

6:16 Phlebotomy is [performed] lengthwise, widthwise, or obliquely. [It is performed] lengthwise if it [i.e., the vein] is between two nerves.[37] [It is performed] widthwise when I want it to heal quickly. The oblique method is between these two, this is the best manner for the blood to flow out. The scalpel should be secured from the nerve vertically and horizontally when one fears for a nerve spreading under it, and inverted at the risk of encountering a nerve with the front of the scalpel.

6:17 The ⟨pain of⟩[38] phlebotomy is reduced by the scalpel being fine and thin, the veins being full, and a hot compress being applied on the spot, especially in the winter. Be careful that no oil or anything that contains it touches the scalpel. The most sensitive veins in terms of pain in the forearms are *vena cephalica pollicis*, then the cephalic vein due to the site of the muscle and the hardness of the skin. As to the basilic vein and the median cubital vein, [phlebotomising them is] less painful, particularly if there is no ⟨flesh⟩[39] above the two.

6:18 As to *vena salvatella*, the hand should be put in hot water until it swells, and the wrist is tightened with a bandage. It should then be phlebotomised, and put once again in the hot water so that the blood does not coagulate.

6:19 [As to] the sciatic vein, be as wary of phlebotomising it as possible, because a mistake in [phlebotomising] it is followed by chronic damage to many nerves. The method of phlebotomising it is to bind a woollen rope, not very broad, from somewhere below the hip to above the ankle. If it is not clearly visible, he should enter the bathhouse or put his foot in hot water and stand on the ailing foot after putting it on baked bricks or a tile, whereas the healthy one is lifted. If [even then] it does not become visible, phlebotomise one of the

---

36 ⟨⟩ above the line.
37 See commentary.
38 ⟨⟩ in the margin.
39 ⟨⟩ in the margin.

بعض الشعب التي في ظاهر القدم مما يلي الجانب الوحشي وأجودها التي بين الخنصر والبنصر.

٦:٢٠ ولتعلم أن ما في مأبض الركبة عرقان[a] أحدهما عرق النسا والآخر الصافن وإن فصد هذا | العرق على الكعب أو بعض شعبه التي ذكرنا كان أفضل من فصد أصله كثيرا جدا. 11v
وهكذا كلما بعد الفصد من موضع العلة في الأمراض المزمنة كان أفضل من فصد أصله كثيرا جدا.

٦:٢١ وبعد أن يكون المرض لا يبدو للبصر مثل الأورام فإنّ إخراج الدم حينئذ[b] من الموضع نفسه أفضل كما ذكرنا وعلة ذلك طول الجذب فإنَّ الطبيعة حينئذ تتهيأ لدفع رديء الدم في طول المسافة بعد أن يكون الفصد بالعروق المتصلة بموضع العلة. وهذا يجري في سائر الأمراض مثل إن فصد الأسيلم لوجع الطحال أفضل من فصد الباسليق على أن هذين العرقين بينهما وبين الطحال اشتراك إلا أن الأسيلم أبعد ففصده أفضل للعلة التي ذكرنا.

٦:٢٢ وأما الصافن وعروق مأبض الركبة فشد دونهما بعصابة كما تشد اليد وتعتمد[c] بالرجل العليلة على آجرة وتفصدهما.[d]

الباب السابع

٧:١ الباب السابع في جذب المواد.

٧:٢ إنه إذا كانت المواد في أوائل الأمراض الدموية منصبّة وعند منتهاها واقفة وجب أن تختلف المواضع المفصودة بحسب ذلك.

---

a عرقان: عرقين
b حينئذ: حينذ
c +o
d +o

branches in the external part of the foot, close to the outer side of the leg. The best one of those is the one that is between the pinkie toe and the ring toe.

6:20 You should know that there are two veins in the popliteal fossa, one of the
two is the sciatic vein, and the other the saphenous vein. Phlebotomising this
| vein on the ankle, or one of its branches that we have mentioned, is much 11v
better than phlebotomising its origin. Thus, the further away phlebotomy is
[performed] from the site of the illness in the case of chronic illnesses, it is
much better than phlebotomising its origin.

6:21 When the illness is not visible to the eye, as [in the case of] swellings, evacuation of blood at that time from the site itself is better, as we have mentioned. The reason for that is the length of the drawing [of the blood]. For at that time, after phlebotomy, Nature prepares to expel the bad blood all the way, through the veins that are connected to the site of the illness. This applies to all illnesses. For instance, if the *vena salvatella* is phlebotomised for the pain of the spleen, it is better than phlebotomising the basilic vein. This is because there is a connection between these two veins and the spleen, except that the *vena salvatella* is further away, and hence, phlebotomising it is better for the reason that we have mentioned.

6:22 As to the saphenous vein and the veins in the popliteal fossa, tighten below them with a bandage, just as the hand is tightened, while the affected leg is leaning on a tile, and phlebotomise the two.

The Seventh Chapter

7:1 The seventh chapter on drawing matters.

7:2 Since the matters in the first stages of the sanguine illnesses are flowing, and in the end of them stagnant, the phlebotomised sites need to vary according to that.

٧:٣ مثال ذلك أن من عرضت له شوصة دموية في الجانب الأيمن فالوجه في علاجه في أول الأمر أن تنظر: فإنْ كان الدم في البدن كثيرا فصدت العليل من اليد اليسرى وجعلت التثنية من اليد اليمنى. و إنْ كان الدم في البدن قليلا جعلت الفصد من الجانب[a] العليل نفسه. وهذا خارج من الفكر والقياس وصحّحته التجربة. فإذا جاوز العليل أربعة أيام فصاعدا جعلت فصده في[b] جميع الأحوال من الجانب العليل نفسه وذلك أن المواد قد صار أكثرها إلى الجانب العليل.

12r **٧:٤** قد امتحنا هذا في جملة من المرضى في المارستانات | وغيرها فوجدناه نافعا سالما. ورأينا من خالفه كان سببا لهلاك العليل وشيكا وهذا القياس ينسّق في الأمراض الظاهرة والباطنة والأوجاع التي تكون في البدن من سقطة أو ضربة أو غيرها مما يوجب الفصد. والذي قاد إلى هذا ودل عليه حكيم الصناعة أبقراط وتابعه عليه جالينوس حيث يقول: وبالجملة فينبغي في الأورام التي هي بعد في الكون أن تجتذب المادة بالضد وأما الأورام المزمنة فمن الأعضاء أنفسها أو ما قرب منها. وأفضل ما يكون استفراغها بالعروق المتصلة بها.[c] وفصدها[d] من الجانب المخالف فيه أمران أحدهما إمالة عن الموضع العليل وهذا باب جلي والثاني تبليد المادة ومنع انصبابها.

٧:٥ وقد تتفق في جذب المواد اختلافات كثيرة والأصل واحد ونذكر منها ما يليق هذا الموضع ليكن عونا على ما يراد منها.

٧:٦ فمن ذلك أن يكون بإنسان ورم في زنديه أو في معصمه أو ذراعه ويده اليسرى بها وجع أو يعتاده بها ما يتوقع مع ذلك إن فصدت أن تنصب المواد إليها فالوجه في علاجه أن يفصد الصافن من الرجل اليمنى كي تنجذب المادة على استقامة.

a +O
b +O
c +O
d وفصدها: وفصدنا

7:3 For instance, for someone who is affected by sanguine pleuritis on the right side, the manner of treating it is to first observe: if there is a lot of blood in the body, you should phlebotomise the patient from the left hand and conduct the epaphairesis[40] from the right hand. If there is a little blood in the body, you conduct the phlebotomy in the affected side itself. This is beyond rational thinking and analogy, but it has been confirmed by experience. If the [duration of the illness of] the patient exceeds four days or more, you should always phlebotomise him from the affected side itself. This is because most of the matters will already have reached the affected side.

7:4 We have examined this with several patients in hospitals | and the like and 12r
found it to be beneficial and safe. We have seen one who diverged from this and almost caused the death of the patient. This analogy should be drawn in the external and internal illnesses, as well as in pains that occur in the body due to a fall, or a blow, or other things that require phlebotomy. The one who led to this [conclusion] and demonstrated it was the master of the art, Hippocrates, whom Galen followed, as he says: "In general, in the case of incipient swellings, it is necessary that the matter is drawn to the opposite side. As to chronic swellings, from the parts themselves or what is close to them." The best thing is to evacuate them through the veins that are connected with them. Phlebotomising them from the opposite side includes two things: one of the two is the deflection away from the affected site, which is something that is evident, and the second is the adaptation of the matter and preventing its flow.

7:5 Many disagreements concerning drawing matters may happen, but the origin is one. We will mention what seems worthy considering this topic—may this help to achieve its goal.

7:6 For instance, if a person has a swelling in his antebrachiums, his wrist, or his forearm, and there is pain in his left hand, or he is accustomed to this, what might be expected in this case is that if you were to phlebotomise, the matters would flow into them. In that case the manner of treating it is to phlebotomise the saphenous vein in the right leg, so that the matter is drawn correctly.

---

40 I.e., additional removal of blood. See commentary.

٧:٧ وقد يفصد في مثل هذا من اليد اليسرى إذا كان الورم من الجانب الأيمن عظيما أو كان الوجع قليلا ومن الصافن معا أو يقدم فصد اليد اليسرى بالصافن فتدبر هذا واعن بالأخطر والأصعب.

٧:٨ ومتى اتفق أن تفصد العليل ويلزم العلاج ويبقى من الورم بقية وليس معها وجع وكان ظاهرا فاشرطه وعلق عليه العلق. ولا تفعل هذا حتى يجاور المرض ثلاثة أسابيع لأنه حينئذ يدخل في عدد الأمراض المزمنة. ومتى كمد الموضع واخضر فبادر بشرطه لئلا يفسد هو وغيره.

٧:٩ ولقد رأيت في جذب المواد وإمالتها عن المواضع العليلة منافع جمة[a] من ذلك أنه جاءتني بالمارستان جارية شديدة السواد حسنة | اللحم وقد تغرقت ثيابها بالدم من 12v
رعافها ومنخراها[b] ينسكبان دما متصلا فعالجتها بالأدوية التي تجعل في الأنف مما يقطع الرعاف على أنها في أكثر الأمر قليلة الغناء. فلما فعلت ذلك ووثقت بقوتها أمرت بفصدها من الجانبين القيفالين في وقت واحد فما جرى من دمها إلا نحو رطل ونصف حتى انقطع الدم وكان عندي الذي جرى من دمها مع فصدها قدر سبعة أرطال وفوق ذلك.

الباب الثامن

٨:١ الباب الثامن نذكر فيه الأوقات التي يصلح فيها خروج الدم والاحتراس من خروجه.

٨:٢ أفضل[c] الأوقات لخروج الدم وقت الربيع كما ذكرنا ومن الربيع اليوم المعتدل الحر والبرد ومن اليوم الساعة الثانية أو الثالثة من الساعات المستوية وقد يختلف هذا بحسب برد المزاج وحده.

---

a +O

b ها written above the line, repeated in the margin

c أفضل: لفضل

7:7 One may phlebotomise according to this example from the left hand if the swelling on the right side is large, or if there is just a little pain, and from the saphenous vein at the same time, or one may phlebotomise the left hand through the saphenous vein. Thus, you should be concerned with what is more dangerous and severe.

7:8 When it happens that you phlebotomise the patient and treatment is required, and there is a remain of the swelling with no pain, and it is visible, then scarify it and attach leeches to it. Do not do this until the [duration of the] illness is close to three weeks, because at that time it is included in the number of chronic illnesses. When the site becomes discoloured and turns green, then scarify it promptly, so that it or anything else does not putrefy.

7:9 Indeed, I have seen plentiful benefits in drawing matters and their deflection from the affected sites. For instance, a young, deep black[41] and nicely plump slave girl came to me in the hospital | and her clothing was soaked with 12v
blood from her epistaxis, and blood was pouring down from her nostrils continuously. I treated her with the drugs that are put in the nose, causing the epistaxis to cease, even though they are in most cases of little worth. When I did that and I was confident about her strength, I ordered to phlebotomise the cephalic vein on both sides at the same time. When around a *raṭl* and a half of her blood had flowed, the bleeding ceased. The amount of blood that flowed through phlebotomising was seven *raṭls* or more.

The Eighth Chapter

8:1 The eighth chapter in which we mention the times that are suitable for extracting blood, and when to guard against extracting it.

8:2 The best time for extracting blood is the spring, as we have mentioned, and in the spring a day moderate in heat and cold, and of the day the second or the third hour of the average hours. This may vary solely according to the coldness of disposition.

41 I.e., very dark.

٨:٣ فإن كان حار المزاج أو يسرع إليه الجوع فاليبادر بفصده في أول ساعة ومن كان بارد المزاج فليؤخر حتى يحمى النهار قليلا.

٨:٤ وسنذكر ما يجب أن ينال من الغذاء شيئا قليلا قبل الفصد في موضعه وليستعمل قبل استحكام الهضم وخروج الثفل واعتدال الطبع لأن كثيرا ممن تلين طبيعته بعد فصده بسبب أن الحرارة الغريزية تضعف لخروج الدم وبعد أن يستحم من كان قليل التعب غليظ الدم.

٨:٥ ويتركه من تعب وتحرك قبل وقت الفصد أو لم يكن[a] دمه مؤاتيا للخروج ومهتاجا. ومن كان مخلطا في تدبيره فالفصد أولى به من الإسهال والإسهال أولى بمن كان متحفظا.

٨:٦ ومن فصدت فلا تشد له الرباط فإنه يجلب الورم ولا تكثر فوقه الخرق.

٨:٧ ويحترس من الجماع إلا عند الشبق الشديد فإنه أفضل شيء مجتمع وخروجه أفضل من تركه ومن الأغذية الرديئة قبله وبعده بيومين. ويحترس من الفصد من تعتاده منه الأمراض الباردة أو هو ضعيف العصب أو |[b] يغتم أو يسهر ويعنى بالعلوم الدقيقة أو 13r
يجامع كثيرا ومن قرب عهده بالسفر أو الفصد أو التعب العنيف والمعتقل الطبيعة والقريب العهد بانطلاقها أو بالقيء أو سخن بدنه أو برد بأكثر من المعتاد أو المتخوم أو السكران أو الممتلئ من الغذاء أو الجائع أو من فسد هضمه أو †للاض†[c] أو من كانت في بدنه أخلاط فجة.

٨:٨ وبالجملة كل ما يهد القوة ويحلها أو تحيرها إلا أن يفجأ أو يتوقع أمرا عظيما مما هو حاضر كالسكتة أو الخناق أو الخفقان أو السقطة العظيمة. فإن مثل هذه الأمراض وشبهها قد يفصد لها فيها في أي الأوقات أمكن من ليل أو نهار ويجب أن تقيس أبدا بين ما طرأ وسلف وتعنى بالأخطر والأصعب ولا تغفل الآخر ما أمكن.

---

a لم يكن: كان
b Ms. + أو
c Uncertain reading.

8:3 If he [the patient] is of hot disposition, or quickly becomes hungry, one should hurry up to phlebotomise him in the first hour. For whoever is of cold disposition, it may be postponed until the day becomes slightly warmer.

8:4 We will mention the foodstuffs that one should eat a small quantity of before phlebotomy in its proper place, including what one should use prior to strengthening the digestion, outflow of residues, and balancing the disposition. [That is] because in many cases one's stools become soft after phlebotomy, for the innate heat weakens due to the outflow of blood. The same holds good for someone who has been to the bathhouse while being somewhat tired and has coarse blood.

8:5 One should not perform it [i.e., phlebotomy] to someone who is tired and has been exercising before the time of phlebotomy, or whose blood is [not] suitable for being extracted and in a state of commotion. If someone's regimen is irregular, phlebotomy is more appropriate than purgation. Purgation is more appropriate for whoever is cautious.

8:6 If you phlebotomise someone, do not make the ligature too tight, for it brings forth a swelling. Also, do not apply many cloths on it.

8:7 He should be wary of coitus unless in the case of strong sexual desire [when a surplus of semen] has collected—[in this case] getting it out is better than leaving it. The same holds good for bad food two days before and after it. One should [also] be cautious when phlebotomising someone who is accustomed
to cold illnesses, has weak nerves, | is distressed or sleepless, takes an interest 13r
in sciences that require concentration, has a lot of sex, has recently travelled or been phlebotomised, is very tired, suffers from constipation and has recently been purged or vomited, whose body has become hotter or colder than customary, suffers from indigestion, is drunk or full of food, hungry, whose digestion is corrupted, or [?], or in whose body there are raw humours.

8:8 In general, [one should be cautious in the case of] everything that weakens the strength, dissolves it or bewilders it, unless a major incident, such as apoplexy, diphtheria, palpitation, or a severe collapse suddenly befalls or can be expected to happen. For such illnesses and the like, phlebotomy may be performed whenever possible, day or night. You must always weigh the present condition against what has occurred and preceded, and you should be concerned with what is more dangerous and severe, without neglecting the other insofar as possible.

٨:٩ ومتى توهمت بعليل مدنف أو منهوك البدن أو مزمن العلة أنه يحتاج إلى إخراج الدم فافتح العرق فإن رأيت الدم أسود قليل الزبد فأخرج ما هممت بإخراجه فإن كان رقيقا أو أصفر أو رمانيا فشده على المكان فإنَّ في خروجه خطرا.

٨:١٠ ولا تمتنع من فصد عليل قد مر لمرضه أيام كما قد ظن ذلك أقوام إذا كانت معك الدلائل القوية كما أنك تمتنع من فصده إذا لم تكن واثقا بقوته نعم وإن كان في أول يوم. وقد فصد أبقراط مريضا في اليوم الثامن من مرضه وجالينوس يقول: ولا تمتنع من الفصد في اليوم العشرين مثلا مع صحة القوة وتمام الهضم.

الباب التاسع

٩:١ الباب التاسع في التثنية.

٩:٢ من كان الغرض في فصده حفظ صحته فليخرج له من الدم في الساعة التي ذكرناها وليجعل تثنيته بعد الساعة الرابعة من الساعات المستوية من فصده، والأكثر إلى أول الساعة السادسة. وليكن للقوي أسرع وللضعيف أبطأ | لا جرم لمن يغشى عليه. فإنه يخرج 13v
دمه في مرات بعد أن ينال من الغذاء بين الفصد والتثنية.

٩:٣ ومن كان الغرض فيه جذب المواد إلى ضد الجهة التي مالت إليها فيجعل تثنيته في اليوم الثاني. فإن بقيت من مرضه بقية وساعدت قوته إخراج الدم أيضا أخرج في اليوم الثالث بعد أن يقوى فيما بين الأيام وعلى حسب كثرة الدفعات تكون قوة جذب الشيء وتكون القوة أوفر وأجم.

٩:٤ ومتى أردت التثنية فتكتفي أن تشد العصابة وتقبض الكف جدا. فإن لم يخرج الدم لويت الذراع قليلا فإن تعذّر خروجه جذبت الدم بالدلك إلى جانب فم العروق. فإن لم

8:9 If you suspect that a patient who is emaciated, physically exhausted, or chronically ill needs to have blood extracted, open a vein. If you see the blood black and slightly foamy, evacuate what you intended to evacuate. If it is thin or yellow or red,[42] tie it off immediately—extracting it is dangerous.

8:10 Do not abstain from phlebotomising a patient whose illness has gone on for some days, as some people have supposed, when you have strong indications, just as you abstain from phlebotomising when you are not confident about his strength. Truly [this should be so], even if it were on the first day. Hippocrates indeed phlebotomised an ill person on the eighth day of his illness, and Galen says: "Do not refrain from phlebotomy on the twentieth day, for instance, when the strength is sound, and the digestion completed."

The Ninth Chapter

9:1 The ninth chapter on epaphairesis.

9:2 Whoever is phlebotomised with the intention of preserving his health, his blood should be extracted at the time that we have mentioned. Epaphairesis should be conducted after the fourth hour of the even hours after his phlebotomy, no later than at the beginning of the sixth hour. Let it be faster for the strong and slower for the weak, | especially for the ones who lose conscious- 13v
ness. His blood should be extracted in several sessions, and he should consume food between the phlebotomy and the epaphairesis.

9:3 For a person whose matters one intends to redirect contrary to their usual direction, epaphairesis should be conducted on the second day. In case a residue of his illness remains, and his strength also supports the extraction of blood, extract on the third day after he has gained some strength over the days. The power of drawing matter should be in accordance with the number of sessions, it should be more abundant and more plentiful.

9:4 When you want [to conduct] epaphairesis, it is enough that you tighten the band and hold the hand firmly. If no blood flows out, you tilt the forearm a little. If its extraction is difficult, you draw the blood by rubbing the side of the

42 Lit. 'the colour of a pomegranate.'

يخرج الدم أو جمد في فم العرق علق فلا تنقره فإن ذلك ربما أحدث ورما. ومتى حدث ورم في موضع الفصد فلا تعرض للتثنية ولتفصد ما فوقه أو ما قرب منه.

٩:٥ وإن لم تبعث الضرورة إلى التثنية فلتجعلها[a] بعد يومين أو ثلاثة.

٩:٦ وقد رأيت بمدينة السلام من يزيل علق الدم بكاغذة مفتولة وقد يسكب الماء الحار على الموضع فيفتحه.

٩:٧ وأخبرني من كنت أقرأ عليه أن المأمون افتصد فلما أتى وقت التثنية عسر خروج الدم فأحضر المتطببين فكل أشار بما لم يقبله وحضر المجلس من ضمن خروج الدم بأسهل الوجوه بعد أن يزول من حضر فلما زالوا امتص العرق فأنزل في فمه في الوقت.

٩:٨ وليخرج في التثنية نصف ما يخرج في الابتداء. ومن منافع التثنية أن الطبيعة تميز رديء الدم من سائر الأعضاء وتدفعه إلى الموضع المفصود لضعفه لما ناله من الجرح وأيضا لأن الطبيعة لا تحتمل إخراج الدم دفعة وإن فعلنا ذلك خفنا خورها.

٩:٩ ومتى خشيت انسداد العروق عند التثنية إما بسبب غلظ الدم أو لأن الضربة | رقيقة 14r
فاجعل على الرفادة ملحا مسحوقا ملتوتا بدهن ورد وعصبه. وإن كان جلد المفصود رقيقا جعلت دهن ورد وحده لئلا يتقرح الموضع.

٩:١٠ وليس كل عرق يحتمل التثنية لأن منها عروقا لا تجيب إلى ذلك.

a فلتجعلها: فليجعلها

opening of the veins. If [still] no blood flows out, or a blood clot coagulates at the opening of the vein, do not cut it, since this sometimes provokes a swelling. When [such] a swelling occurs at the phlebotomised site, do not conduct epaphairesis. You may phlebotomise what is above or below it.

9:5 If there is no necessity for epaphairesis, you may do so after two or three days.

9:6 In Baghdad,[43] I have seen someone who removed a blood clot with a tightly twisted paper. One might also pour hot water on the site, thus opening it.

9:7 A person under whom I studied informed me that al-Ma'mūn was phlebotomised, and when the time of epaphairesis arrived, the extraction of blood was difficult. Thus, he brought in the physicians, and they all recommended things that he would not accept. Someone who was certain about the easiest way of getting the blood out participated in the council after the others had left, and when they had left, he sucked the vein and made [the blood] come down to his mouth immediately.

9:8 When conducting epaphairesis, one should extract half of the amount of blood that was extracted in the beginning. One of the benefits of epaphairesis is that Nature distinguishes the bad blood from the rest of the parts and pushes it towards the phlebotomised site due to its weakness caused by the wound. Also, because Nature does not tolerate the extraction of [a lot of] blood in one session. If we were to do that, we would be afraid of it getting weak.

9:9 Whenever you fear for an obstruction in the veins when conducting epaphairesis, either because of coarse blood, or because the pulse is | thin, put 14ʳ
ground salt mixed with rose oil on a dressing and bind it. If the skin of the phlebotomised person is thin, you apply only rose oil so that the site does not become ulcerated.

9:10 Not every vein tolerates epaphairesis, since there are veins that do not react positively to that.

43 *Madīnat al-Salām.*

٩:١١ ومن كان سكيرا فليستوثق من شده وتربط لجاما في ذراعه إلى عضده وتتعاهد نومه كي لا ينزف فيدول إلى خطر.

الباب العاشر

١٠:١ الباب العاشر في غذاء المفصود وشربه وتدبيره.

١٠:٢ يكون البيت الذي يفصد فيه معتدل الهواء رفيع النمط[a] مفتوحا إلى الشمال مفروشا بالرياحين والورد وضروب الفواكه.

١٠:٣ وليؤخذ من بعد الفصد السكنجبين السكري أو الجلاب أو شراب الورد وعلى قدر اللذة [b]البيض النيمبرشت [c]وأيضا الخس والهندباء بالخل وقد يكتفي بأحد هذه الأشياء. وليكن الغذاء من لحم جدي أو خروف أو فراريج محمّضات نحو السكباج وحصرمية ورمانية وزيرباجة ويطعم الإسفيذباج لمن كان بارد المزاج.

١٠:٤ فإن كان به سعال أو نخس فليترك السكباج ويحل الباقلاء بالسكر ويأكل[d] منها. وليكن الغذاء في يوم الفصد وغيره متوسطا. ومن أحب تناول من الرمان والسفرجل بعد غذائه.

١٠:٥ ومن كان يضعف عند الفصد أو يتوقع عليه الغشي فإنه يطعم قبل فصده من ماء الفروج وحصرمية أو رمانية أو يبلّ له لباب الخبز بماء رمان حامض ⟨ويسقى من شراب الورد ويخرج منه في مرات كما ذكرنا ويطعم بين كل مرتين ويسقى من شراب العسل⟩[e] والميبة فإنهما ينوبان عن النبيذ وسأذكرهما بعد هذا.

a עליון התקרה Ms. Parma
b MS + و
c النيمبرشت: النيمرشت
d ويأكل: ويوكل
e ⟨⟩ in the margin, ويسقى من شراب العسل both in the margin and the text.

9:11 For whoever is drunk, the binding should be checked, and you should tie a strap on his forearm up toward his upper arm. He should be checked frequently while he is asleep so that he does not bleed profusely, thus being exposed to danger.

The Tenth Chapter

10:1 The tenth chapter on the food, drink, and regimen of the patient who has been phlebotomised.

10:2 The house in which phlebotomy is conducted should have moderate air, high ceiling,[44] be open towards the north, with fragrant herbs, roses, and a variety of fruit spread out in it.

10:3 After being phlebotomised, one should take sugared oxymel, julep, or rose syrup, and according to appetite, soft-cooked eggs, and lettuce and endive in vinegar. One of these things might be sufficient. The food should consist of dishes made from goat, mutton, or soured pullets, such as *sikbāǧ*, *ḥiṣrimiyya*, *rummāniyya*, and *zīrbāǧa*. *Isfīḏbāǧ* should be fed to whoever has a cold disposition.

10:4 If he [the patient] has a cough or a pricking pain, one should leave out *sikbāǧ*, and dissolve fava beans in sugar and eat from it. On the day of phlebotomy, as well as otherwise, food should be moderate. Whoever likes, may eat pomegranate and quince after his meal.

10:5 If someone gets weak when being phlebotomised, or can be expected to faint, he should be fed prior to the procedure pullet broth and *ḥiṣrimiyya* or *rummāniyya*, or one should prepare breadcrumbs in sour pomegranate juice ⟨and give him rose syrup to drink. [His blood] should be extracted in several sessions, as we have mentioned, and he should be fed between every session, and be given melicratum⟩[45] and *mayba* to drink, as they both substitute wine. I will mention the two after this.

44 Uncertain reading, see commentary.

45 ⟨⟩ in the margin.

١٠:٦ ولأن أسباب الغشي كثيرة فعلاجه مختلف وفعله واحد وهو انحلال القوة الحيوانية ومسكنها القلب وإن شئت أن تقول الغشي سقوط يعرض للقوة بحدة وسرعة وقد زعم قوم أن الغشي يعرض لأسباب[a] تعوق الدماغ عن إرساله الحس إلى القلب فيلحق بذلك | القلب الغشي. ولأن غرضنا في هذا الكتاب إنما هو في الغشي الذي يحدث عند 14v
الفصد وبسببه فإن كانت الروح التي في كبده لطيفة فإنه يخرج منها كثير مع خروج يسير من الدم فيحدث للقلب بذلك الغشي بالمشاركة بينهما. وأما من كانت الروح التي في كبده غليظة فليس يخرج منها مع كثير من الدم إلا اليسير فليس يحدث حينئذ الغشي. والوجه في علاجه أنه متى وجد معه غثيان استعمل القيء بالريشة ويسقى الماء الفاتر بالسكنجبين لأنه يدل على خلط انصبّ للمعدة وليرش عليه ماء الورد والماء البارد ويصبّ عليه ويهز ويصاح به وليدلك فم المعدة والبدن ويعرك أنفه.

١٠:٧ فإن أفاق وإلا أشم المسك والغالية وخذ[b] ماء العسل وليعاود الريشة ومتى لم يكن مع الغشي غثيان فهو ينذر بشر فبادر في علاجه بماء اللحم وماء العسل والميبة وتشق في الوجه فراريج مشوية وتقرّب من أنفه الأطعمة الذكية نحو المدققات والطباهجات[c] والمطجنات واللقانق الكثيرة الأفاويه والبزور وينشق المسك وتمسح الغالية من داخل أنفه ويضمخ منها جسده وخاصة صدره ويصندل قميصه ومخدته ويرش عليه ماء الورد ويضرب له بالأصوات العالية والأبواق والنايات.

١٠:٨ ومن عرض له سقوط قوة لكثرة خروج الدم أو لرقة القلب فليدبّر بهذا التدبير خلا الأصوات والأبواق والنايات.

---

a لأسباب: الأسباب
b وخذ: واخذ
c +o

10:6 As there are many causes to losing consciousness, its treatment varies, yet its effect is one, i.e., the dissolution of the animal faculty, the seat of which is the heart—if you want to say, losing consciousness is a collapse that occurs to the faculty violently and rapidly. Some people have claimed that unconsciousness occurs due to causes[46] that hinder the brain from forwarding sensation to the heart, and therefore | unconsciousness affects the heart. [However,] as our 14v
goal in this book is rather the kind of unconsciousness that occurs with phlebotomy and because of it [I state the following]: if the pneuma in the patient's liver is fine, a lot of it gets extracted with a slight extraction of blood, and therefore unconsciousness occurs to the heart by means of the interaction between the two. But, if the pneuma in the liver of a patient is coarse, it does not get extracted [even] with a lot of blood, except slightly, and at that time unconsciousness does not occur. The method of treating it is that when nausea occurs with it, one should induce vomiting by a feather, and give lukewarm water with oxymel to drink, since it indicates that a humour has flowed into the stomach. Rose water and cold water should be sprinkled and poured on him, he should be shaken and shouted at, and one should massage the orifice of his stomach and his body and rub his nose.

10:7 If he regains consciousness [then that is fine], but if not, make him smell musk and *ġāliya*, take melicratum, and apply the feather again. When no nausea occurs with unconsciousness, it is an alarming indication of an injury. Hence, hurry to treat the patient with meat broth, melicratum, and *mayba*. Grilled pullets should be torn in [front of] the face [of the patient], and delicious foods, such as *mudaqqaqāt*, *ṭabāhiǧāt*, *muṭaǧǧanāt* and *laqāniq* with lots of aromatic substances and spices should be brought near his nose. He should smell musk, and the inside of his nose should be anointed with *ġāliya*, and his body, especially his chest, should be anointed with it. Sandalwood should be applied on his shirt and pillow, rose water should be sprinkled on him, and high sounds, horns and flutes should be played for him.

10:8 If someone suffers from a collapse of strength due to the abundance of blood extraction, or due to the delicateness of the heart, he should be administered with this regimen without the sounds, horns, and flutes.

46 See commentary.

١٠:٩ صفة شراب العسل: يؤخذ من العسل الصافي رطل فيصب عليه خمسة أرطال من ماء عذب في قدر حديد[a] ويطبخ بنار لينة[b] وتنزع رغوته فإذا قرب أن يصير في قوام الجلاب يؤخذ من الدارفلفل والزنجبيل والدارصيني وسنبل الطيب ومصطكى وقرنفل | 15r من كل واحد درهم يسحق جدا ويشد في خرقة كتان ويعلّق في القدر ويطبخ حتى يصير في قوام الجلاب وتمرس فيه الخرقة والشراب حار بعد أن تنزله عن النار ويترك[c] ويستعمل.

١٠:١٠ صفة شراب الميبة: يؤخذ من السفرجل الغض الحامض العذب الكثير الماء ويقشر خارجه وينقى داخله ويدق في هاوون حجارة ويعصر من مائه عشرون رطلا ويترك ويؤخذ من عقيد العنب الدقيق عشرة أرطال فينقع به ثفل السفرجل ثانية بشيء من ماء السفرجل ويصفّى وتضاف المياه الثلاثة في قدر نظيفة[d] جديدة ويطبخ برفق على نار جمر وتنزع الرغوة حتى يبقى النصف. ثم ينزل ويروّق أياما ثلاثة في كل يوم[e] مرارا بثوب صفيق مضاعف. ثم يلقى عليه عسل منزوع الرغوة خمسة أرطال ويصيّر في القدر جسد[f] زنجبيل ومصطكى وقاقلة كبيرة وصغيرة ودارصيني وقرنفل وزعفران من كل واحد عشرون درهما مدقوقة جريشا مشدودة جدا في خرقة كتان صلبة رقيقة ولتكن معلّقة ويطبخ الجميع ثانية بنار لينة ويمرس الأفاويه وقتا بعد وقت حتى يبلغ إلى حد الأشربة ويصفى ويفتق فيه ثمن درهم مسكا مسحوقا ويوضع[g] [في] ظرف زجاج وتترك الخرقة معلّقة في الظرف أسبوعين ثم تخرج. وإن شئت تركت الأفاويه ترسب في قعر الزجاجة.

١٠:١١ ميبة أخرى لمثل ذلك: يؤخذ من ماء السفرجل والعسل الصافي منزوع الرغوة من كل واحد جزء وإن شئت جعلت مكان العسل سكر طبرزد لمن كان حار المزاج وخل ثقيف ثلاثة أرباع جزء يطبخ برفق على جمر وتنزع[h] رغوته حتى يصير في قوام الأشربة. ومن أراد قليل الحموضة جعل الخل على حسب إرادته.

---

a حديد: جديد
b لينة: ليينة
c ويترك: وتترك written with diacritical points for both *tāʾ* and *yāʾ*
d نظيفة: نضيفة
e +o
f Uncertain reading.
g يوضع: يود ع
h تنزع: تزع

10:9 The prescription of melicratum: one takes a *raṭl* of clear honey and pours over it five *raṭls* of sweet water in an iron pot. It is cooked on a low fire and skimmed. As it gets close to the consistency of julep, one takes long pepper, ginger, cinnamon, Indian nard, mastic, and cloves, | one *dirham* of each, grinds 15r
them well, compresses it in a linen cloth, suspends it in the pot, and cooks it until it reaches the consistency of julep. The cloth is soaked in the syrup while it is hot after being removed from the fire. [Then] it is left [to cool] and consumed.

10:10 The prescription of *mayba*: One takes fresh, very juicy sweet-sour quince, peels the outer layer, cleanses the inside, pounds in a stone mortar, and squeezes twenty *raṭls* of juice and leaves it. [Then] one takes grape jelly, ten *raṭls*, the sediment of the quince is infused in it for a second time in some of the quince juice, and it is then filtered. The three juices are added in a clean, new pot, and boiled gently on embers, skimming it until half of it remains. Then it is removed [from the fire] to be filtered for three days, a few times every day, in a thick, twofold cloth. Then one adds five *raṭls* of skimmed honey, and adds into the pot ginger root, mastic, big and small [varieties of] cardamom, cinnamon, cloves, and saffron, twenty *dirhams* each, ground, crushed, and tied firmly into a hard, thin linen cloth. It [i.e., the linen cloth] should be suspended, and everything is cooked for a second time on a low fire, and the aromatic substances are soaked time after time until it reaches the state of a syrup and becomes clear. Then one-eighth *dirham* of ground musk is mixed with it, and it is put [in] a receptacle of glass. The cloth is left hanging in the receptacle for two weeks and then removed. If you want, leave the aromatic substances to sink to the bottom of the receptacle.

10:11 Another [prescription of] *mayba* for the similar [condition]: One takes quince juice and clear, skimmed honey, one part of each—and if you want, you can use crystalline sugar instead of honey for whoever is of hot disposition—and three quarters of very sour vinegar. One cooks it gently on embers and skims it until it reaches the consistency of syrup. If one wants it to be less sour, one should add vinegar according to one's will.

الباب الحادي عشر

١١:١ الباب الحادي عشر | في الأدوية والأغذية المطفئة للدم. 15v

١١:٢ ولأنا كثيرا ما ندعى إلى العليل وبه من خور القوة وسورة المرض ما لا يمكن فصده أو لأنه في نفسه خوار أو ليس له عادة بالفصد فلا يجيب إليه.

١١:٣ فقد ذكر جالينوس في كتابه في حيلة البرء أن رجلا من أبناء ستين سنة ورم لسانه في فمه حتى كأنه لا يسعه فأشرت عليه بالفصد فلم يجبني إليه بسبب أنه لم تجر العادة فأسهلته بحب القوقايا بالعشي وأمرته أن يحبس في فمه دواء مبردا إذا تحرك للاستفراغ. وكان بالحضرة طبيب لم يساعدني على ذلك فأخذ العليل الحب ولم يعالج العضو نفسه. فأُرِيَ في نومه أن مشورتي في أخذه الدواء صواب وأنه ينبغي أن يحبس في فمه عصارة الخس فاستعملها فبرئ برءا تاما.

١١:٤ فوجب أن نذكر من الأدوية والأغذية ما ينوب عن الفصد فمن الأشربة المشهورة شراب حماض الأترج وشراب الرمانين وشراب القراسيا وشراب العناب والسكنجبين الساذج الشديد الحموضة أو المتخذ بأصول الهندباء وبزره وشراب الرمانين وماء التمر الهندي وشراب الإجاص وامتصاص فلوس الخيارشنبر العسلي البراق.

١١:٥ ومن الأغذية ماء الشعير المطبوخ مع العناب مضافا إليه بعد طبخه ماء الرمان المر ولباب الخبز المغسول بالسكر الطبرزدي ومن المزورات عدسية وحصرمية وسماقية ورمانية من قرع أو رجلة ومن البقول الخس والهندباء ومن السمك الطري الصغير يصنع منه سكباج ومن الفواكه رمانين وماؤهما وسفرجل وكمثرى وتفاح ⟨وخيار وقثاء ودلاع وأهل العراق يسمونه البطيخ المدني وأهل مصر يسمونه البطيخ الدلسي ويولعون بأكل⟩[a]

a بأكل + ⟨ ⟩ + أصل in the margin, MS

The Eleventh Chapter

11:1 The eleventh chapter | on the drugs and foods that extinguish [the combustion of] blood. 15v

11:2 We are often called to a patient who suffers from fatigue and is very ill, due to which phlebotomy is impossible, or because he himself is weak or not accustomed to phlebotomy, and thus, does not consent to it.

11:3 Galen mentioned in his book, *Method of Medicine*, that the tongue of a sixty-year-old man swelled in his mouth until it could not contain it. So, I advised him to [undertake] phlebotomy, but he did not agree because he was not accustomed [to it]. Thus, I purged him with a *qūqāyā* pill in the evening and commanded him to hold a cooling drug in his mouth, if it would set evacuation in motion. A physician who did not support me in this was present, and the patient took the pill, without treating the part itself. He was shown in his dream that my suggestion about the patient taking the drug was correct, and that he [i.e., the patient] needs to keep lettuce juice in his mouth. Thus, he used it and was completely healed.[47]

11:4 It is necessary for us to mention the drugs and foods that substitute phlebotomy. Thus, of the famous syrups: sour citron syrup, syrup of both [types of] pomegranates, cherry syrup, jujube syrup, plain, very sour oxymel, alternatively with the addition of endive roots and its seeds, and syrup of the two [types of] pomegranates, tamarind juice, plum syrup, as well as sucking the honey-like, glossy pod of cassia fistula.

11:5 Of foods: barley broth cooked with jujube; after boiling it one should add bitter pomegranate juice and crumbs of washed bread with crystalline sugar. Of the *muzawwarāt*: *ʿadasiyya*, *ḥiṣrimiyya* , *summāqiyya* and *rummāniyya*; gourd or purslane; and of other greens lettuce and endive. Of fresh fish the small ones prepared as *sikbāǧ*, and of fruit both [types of] pomegranates and their juice, quince, pear, apple, ⟨and cucumber, squirting cucumber, and melon, that the Iraqis call *al-biṭṭīḫ al-madanī*, which the Egyptians call *al-biṭṭīḫ al-dalasī*, and they are very fond of eating⟩[48] jujube solely and when soaked in julep. They

47 See commentary.
48 ⟨⟩ in the margin.

العناب وحده ومنقعا في جلاب ويشمون الصندل وماء الورد وتضمد أكبادهم بهما ويقلل غذاؤهم وتعدل مجالسهم بالرش والرياحين والجلاب والآس والشاهسبرم ونحوها.

16r **١١:٦** فإن كان يفرغ من تبريد مزاج العليل كثير الدم الأشربة الناقصة الحموضة | والحلوة كالجلاب وشراب البنفسج وشراب الورد وشراب العناب والسكر والترنجبين والسكنجبين البزوري ومن الأغذية سويق الشعير ولباب الخبز المغسول الخشكارمية بالسكر ومن المزورات القطف والخبيزى والإسفاناخ والفاكهة الرطبة وحاول إطلاق الطبيعة قبل الأسبوع لا جرم إن كانت طبيعته معتقلة لأن المادة بعد هذا مهيئة للخروج.

١١:٧ صفة مطبوخ يطلق الطبيعة ويمنع سورة الدم: تمر هندي أوقيتان إجاص وعناب وسبستان كبار من كل واحد عشر حبات ورد يابس أحمر وورق بنفسج أزرق غير مستعمل وعدس مقشور وبرباريس وبزر سريس وبزر البقلة الحمقاء من كل واحد ثلاثة دراهم كزبرة يابسة درهمان ورق هندباء وورق عنب الثعلب من كل واحد جزء. يغلى بنار لينة حتى يحمرّ الماء ويغلظ ويؤخذ من[a] صفو الماء نصف رطل ويمرس فيه أوقية من لب خيارشنبر قصبي منقى من حبه ويصفى ثانية ويشرب. فإن أطلق و إلا اعيد ثلاثة أيام متوالية.

١١:٨ صفة أخرى تطلق البطن وأقل بردا: إهليلج أصفر ستة دراهم[b] زبيب منزوع العجم وتمر هندي من كل واحد أوقية إجاص وعناب وسبستان من كل واحد عشر حبات تغلى بالماء على نار جمر لينة حتى يغلظ الماء قليلا ويصفى ويؤخذ من صفوه نصف رطل ويحل فيه لب خيارشنبر فارسي قصبي أوقية أو أكثر على حسب القوة ويعاد هذا المطبوخ على حسب الحاجة.

١١:٩ ومما يمنع من سورة الدم ماء عنب الثعلب مع خيارشنبر ويمنع من سورة الدم ماء الشعير قد طبخ بعدس مقشور وذلك أنه يطفئ حدة الدم.

a من: في
b دراهم: درهم

smell sandalwood and rose water, dress their livers by the two, reduce their nourishment, and improve their gatherings by sprinkling fragrant herbs, julep, myrtle, *šāhasbaram* mint and the like.

11:6 If one had to evacuate a lot of blood in order to cool the patient's disposition, [then give] sweet syrups with reduced sourness, | such as julep, violet 16^{r}
syrup, rose syrup, syrup of jujube and sugar, manna, and spiced oxymel. Regarding food, barley gruel, crumbs of washed full-grain bread with sugar, and of the *muzawwarāt* orach, mallow, and spinach, and fresh fruit. Try to relieve the bowels [of the patient] a week ahead, especially if he suffers from constipation, because after this [regimen] the matter is ready to be extracted.

11:7 A prescription of a decoction that loosens the bowels and prevents the surplus of blood: [one takes] tamarind, two *ūqiyyas*, large plum, jujube and sebesten, ten grains of each; dry, red rose, unused blue violet leaves, peeled lentils, barberry, endive seed, purslane seed, three *dirhams* of each; dry coriander, two *dirhams*; endive leaves and nightshade leaves, a part of each. It is boiled on low fire until the water becomes red and thickens. Thereafter one takes half a *raṭl* of clear water and soaks in it one *ūqiyya* of the pith of cassia fistula that is cleansed from its seed. It is filtered for a second time, and then one drinks it. If it loosens the bowels, [then that is fine], but if not, it should be repeated for three consecutive days.

11:8 Another prescription that loosens the stomach and is less cold: [One takes] yellow myrobalan, six *dirhams*; seedless raisins, tamarind, one *ūqiyya* of each; plum, jujube and sebesten, ten grains of each, [this is] boiled in water on low fire on embers until the water thickens a little. Then it is filtered, and one takes from its filtered part half a *raṭl*, and dissolves in it the pith of Persian cassia fistula,[49] one *ūqiyya* or more according to the strength. [Consuming] this decoction is repeated according to the need.

11:9 Among what prevents the surplus of blood is nightshade water together with cassia fistula. [Likewise], barley broth cooked with peeled lentils prevents the surplus of blood, for it extinguishes the surplus of blood.

---

49 لب خيارشنبر فارسي قصبي. See commentary.

١١:١٠ وصفة ماء الشعير: جزآن من شعير ومن العدس المقشور جزء أو تجعل بدله إجاص أو | عناب وإذا طبخ قصب الصعتر بالعناب وشرب ماؤه أرقّ الدم الغليظ. وهذه 16v الخاصية منه عجيبة جدا وهو حار يابس في الدرجة الثانية.

١١:١١ صفة أخرى لمن يتخوف عليه أن يبرد مزاجه: إهليلج أصفر منزوع النوى ستة دراهم تمر هندي أوقية زبيب منزوع العجم أوقية ونصف ورد يابس أحمر وورق بنفسج من كل واحد أربعة دراهم[a] إجاص وعناب وسبستان جلالا من كل واحد عشر حبات رازيانج أخضر قبضة يغلى بالماء على نار لينة ويصفى ويؤخذ منه نصف رطل يمرس فيه لب خيارشنبر وترنجبين من كل واحد ثلاثة أرباع أوقية ثم يصفى مرة ثانية.

١١:١٢ فإذا جاوز أربعة عشر يوما استعمل هذه الأقراص ببعض هذه الأشربة الموصوفة. صفة قرص يطفئ سورة الدم ويصفيه ويقوّي المعدة ويفتح سدد الكبد: أخلاطه ورد يابس أحمر عشرة دراهم[b] بزر رجلة بزر هندباء وبرباريس وصمغ عربي وكثيراء بيضاء من كل واحد درهمان صندل أبيض وطباشير من كل واحد درهم ونصف أصل السوس المجرود الأعلى ثلاثة دراهم راوند صيني درهم زعفران نصف درهم فإن كان الحر كثيرا زيد فيه ربع درهم كافورا يدق ويعجن بماء ورق عنب الثعلب مغلى مصفى ويقرّص أقراصا من درهم ويجفف في الظل ويؤخذ منه في كل غداة قرص بأوقية من شراب سكنجبين فإن كان في الصدر خشونة أخذ ببعض الأشربة المائلة إلى الحلاوة كشراب القراسيا أو شراب الرمانين إن شاء الله.

١١:١٣ صفة قرص أقل تبريدا من الأول وفي معناه: ورد أحمر يابس ثمانية دراهم بزر هندباء وبزر برباريس وبزر رجلة وصمغ عربي وكثيراء ونشاء وبزر بطيخ مقشور وسنبل الطيب ومصطكى وترنجبين من كل واحد | درهمين أصل السوس مجرودا أربعة دراهم 17r طباشير درهم راوند صيني درهم ونصف زعفران نصف درهم يحل الترنجبين بالماء ويجمع مع سائر الأدوية منخولة وتقرص أقراصا من درهم ونصف وتجفف في الظل ويؤخذ ببعض الأشربة الموصوفة.

a دراهم: درهم
b دراهم: درهم

11:10 The prescription of barley broth: two parts of barley, one part of peeled lentils, or you use instead of it plum or | jujube. If one cooks a sprig of oregano 16v with jujube and drinks the extract, it refines the coarse blood. This specific property [of this herb] is quite amazing, and it is hot and dry in the second degree.

11:11 Another prescription for whoever one is afraid that his disposition will turn cold: [One takes] yellow myrobalan without kernel, six *dirhams*; tamarind, one *ūqiyya*; seedless raisins, one and a half *ūqiyya*; dry, red rose and violet leaves, four *dirhams* of each; plum, jujube and sebesten of great quality, ten grains of each; green fennel, a handful. One boils it in water on low fire, filters it, and takes half a *raṭl*, and soaks in it kernels of cassia fistula and manna, three quarters of *ūqiyya*. Thereafter it is filtered a second time.

11:12 And if it exceeds fourteen days, use these pastilles together with one of these prescribed syrups. Prescription of a pastille that extinguishes the surplus of blood, cleanses it, strengthens the stomach, and opens the obstructions of the liver: its components: dry, red rose, ten *dirhams*; purslane seeds, endive seeds, barberry, gum Arabic, white gum tragacanth, two *dirhams* of each; white sandalwood, bamboo chalk, one *dirham* and a half of each; the upper part of peeled liquorice root, three *dirhams*; Chinese rhubarb, one *dirham*; saffron, half a *dirham*—and if it is very hot, one adds a quarter *dirham* of camphor. One pounds it and kneads it in boiled, filtered nightshade juice, forms it into pastilles weighing one *dirham* [each], and lets it dry in the shade. One takes a pastille every morning with one *ūqiyya* of oxymel. If one has roughness in the chest, one takes it with one of the syrups that tend towards sweet, such as cherry syrup or syrup of both [types of] pomegranates, God willing.

11:13 Prescription of a pastille that is less cooling than the first one, yet similar: red, dry rose, eight *dirhams*; endive seeds, barberry seeds, purslane seeds, gum Arabic, gum tragacanth, starch, peeled melon seeds, Indian nard, mastic, manna, | two *dirhams* of each; peeled liquorice root, four *dirhams*; bamboo 17r chalk, one *dirham*; Chinese rhubarb, one *dirham* and a half; saffron, half a *dirham*. One dissolves manna in water and puts it with the other drugs [once they have been] sieved, forms them into pastilles of one and a half *dirhams* each. They are dried in the shade and taken with one of the prescribed syrups.

الباب الثاني عشر

١٢:١ الباب الثاني عشر في منفعة فصد العروق وعلامات العلل التي يفصد لها.

١٢:٢ قال أبو بكر محمد بن زكرياء الرازي: والآن قد ذكرنا منفعة فصد العروق على التوالي بقول كلي. رأينا أن من الأفضل أن نذكر فصد العروق التي يكثر استعمالها في الفصد بقول جزئي ليكون بمزايا.[a]

١٢:٣ وتنبيها من ذلك أنّ فصد عرق الجبهة[b] ينفع من وجع العين القديم والثقل الكائن في مؤخر الرأس اللذين معهما حرارة ومن الحمرة التي تعرض في الوجه ويسميها البصريون النخيلة منسوبة إلى لون شجرة تسمى بهذا الاسم. وينفع[c] أيضا من البثر الحمر في الوجه ومن شقاق الشفة ونواسير[d] الأنف ومن السعفة القديمة ومن الكلف. وهذا العرق إنما يفصد بعد القيفال وهكذا كل عرق رقيق لا يفصد إلا بعد عرق كبير.

١٢:٤ فصد القيفال ينفع من الضربة والسقطة الواقعة في الرأس لا سيما إذا لم يجر دم كثير ومن الصداع الذي معه ثقل البدن والرأس واستدارة عند الحركة والسجود وحمرة الوجه والعينين وكثرة النوم ومن الشقيقة التي معها ضربان الأصداغ وامتلاء العروق فيهما مع سخانة واستلذاذ الأشياء الباردة ومن الدم الذي معه حمرة الوجه ودرور العروق والأوداج والعروق التي خلف الأذنين ومن الشرسام الحار وهو ورم يعرض في شبكة الدماغ ويحمرّ معه الوجه والعين ويعظم معه النبض ومن الصداع الذي تمتلئ معه الودجان والوجه وحمرة في وقت الصرع وربما يدر الدم من المنخرين ومن السكتة التي معها حمرة الوجه وكأنه محترق ودرور والأوداج والعروق ومع ذلك غطيط | بلا نوم[e] ومن الخدر الذي تكون[f] معه 17v
حمرة اللون وفوران عند الحركة ومن الزكام والنزلة اللذين معهما حمرة الوجه ودرور العروق

a بمزايا: بمراية
b عرق الجبهة: عرق الجيهة
c وينفع: وتنفع
d نواسير: بواسير
e بلا نوم: بَلْ ندمٌ
f تكون: يكون

The Twelfth Chapter

12:1 The twelfth chapter on the benefit of phlebotomy and the indications of illnesses that are treated with phlebotomy.

12:2 Abū Bakr Muḥammad ibn Zakariyyā' al-Rāzī said: Now we have mentioned the benefit of phlebotomy in general terms. [However], we take the view that it is better to mention phlebotomy of the frequently phlebotomised veins in more specific terms to emphasise their benefits.

12:3 In light of that, phlebotomising the frontal vein is beneficial for long-lasting ophthalmalgia and for the heaviness in the back of the head, the two combined with heat, and redness that occurs in the face—the Basrans call it *al-naḫīla*, attributed to the colour of a tree that is known by this name. It is also beneficial for red pimples in the face; fissures in the lip[s]; polyps in the nose; chronic cradle cap; and freckles. This vein indeed is phlebotomised after the cephalic vein; in this manner, every thin vein should be phlebotomised only after a big vein.

12:4 Phlebotomising the cephalic vein is beneficial for a blow or a fall that occurs to the head, especially if there is no profuse bleeding; for headache combined with heaviness of the body and the head, vertigo while moving and prostrating, redness of face and the eyes, and abundance of sleep; for migraine combined with throbbing pain in the temples and overfilling of veins in them combined with heat, so that one finds cold things delicious; for blood combined with redness of face; [for] the copious flow [of the blood] of the veins, the jugular veins, and the veins that are behind the ears; for hot phrenitis, which is a swelling that occurs in the arachnoid mater of the brain, with which the face and the eye[s] turn red and the pulse intensifies; for headache with which the jugular veins and the face become filled, and redness at the time of epilepsy, with blood sometimes flowing from the nostrils; for apoplexy combined with redness of face as if it is burned; for the flow of the jugular veins and [other]
veins, combined with snoring | without sleeping; for numbness combined with 17v
redness and agitation when moving; for rheum and catarrh combined with red-

ومن البرد الذي معه حمرة العينين وعظمتهما وبحوطهما ومن قروح العين المتشققة ⟨العين التي معها وجع وضربان ومن جرب⟩[a] وغلظ الأجفان ومددهما[b] ومن ريح السبل وسلاق الأجفان المزمن الذي معه حمرة الأجفان وانتفاخها مع حكة ومن انتثار الأشفار التي تكون مع حمرة ومن وجع الأذن الذي معه حمرة الوجه وثقل الرأس والجبهة عند السجود ومن البثرة في الصماخ التي معه ضربان والتهاب الوجه ومن الرعاف إذا كانت القوة ثابتة ومن وجع السن الذي معه ورم اللثة وحمرة الوجه وانتفاخه[c] والاسترواح للأشياء الباردة ومن القلاع الأحمر وهو بثور في الغشاء المستطيل المستبطن ومعها حمرة وحرارة الفم ومن سقوط اللهاة الشديدة الحمرة والحرارة ومن ورم اللسان الذي معه حمرة وحرارة ومن الخوانيق التي تكون[d] معها حمرة الوجه والعين وتمدد البدن ومن تنخع الدم الكثير.

١٢:٥ فصد الباسليق ينفع من ذات الجنب والشوصة وزعم قوم أنهما اسمان لشيء واحد وإن اختلفا فتر بينهما واحد والفرق بينهما قريب والشوصة ورم يحدث في الغشاء الداخل الرابط للأضلاع وقد زعم قوم أنّ هذا ذات الجنب وأنّ الشوصة ما كان من خارج ويتبعها حمى دائمة وسعال وضيق نفس ونخس وإن اتفق في هذا الورم أن ينتهي الوجع إلى الترقوة كان الفصد وكيدا جدا وإن كان الوجع مائلا إلى ناحية الشراسيف كان الإسهال أولى ثم الفصد بعد.

١٢:٦ وينفع من الربو الذي يحمرّ معه الوجه وتنتفخ الأوداج ومن الخفقان | الذي معه 18r
حرارة الصدر وعظم النبض وسرعته ومن ورم المعدة الظاهر الحرارة ومن ورم الكبد الذي معه عطش شديد وحمى لازمة ومن المالنخونيا التي[e] معها تغيّر اللون وفساد الهضم وقيء حامض ورياح دائمة نحو الشراسيف ويجب إذا فصدته أن يكون من اليسار وأن تنظر فإن كان الدم أسود وإلا قطعته ومن وجع الطحال إذا كان ورم وحرارة ومن الاستسقاء اللحمي

a ⟨ ⟩ in the margin.
b MS contains a sign above the word, possibly an emendation.
c حمرة الوجه وانتفاخه: حمرة الوجهو انتفاخه
d تكون: يكون
e التي: الذي

ness of face and flow of veins; for coldness combined with redness of the eyes, their largeness, and protrusion; and for fissured ulcers in the eyes ⟨the eye combined with pain and throbbing pain, and itching⟩;[50] for coarseness of eyelids and their expansion; for wind of pannus and chronic ptilosis of the eyelids with which the eyelids are red, inflated and itching; for *intiṯār* of the palpebral margin combined with redness; for earache combined with redness of face and heaviness of the head and the forehead when prostrating; for pustules in the auditory meatus combined with throbbing pain and inflammation of the face; for epistaxis when the strength is steady; for toothache combined with swelling of gums and redness of face, its inflation, and a desire for cold things; for red aphthae, that is pustules in the lining of the mouth combined with redness and heat of mouth; for prolapse of the uvula that is severely red and hot; for swelling of the tongue combined with redness and heat; for diphtheria combined with redness of the face and the eyes, and tension of the body; for expectorating a lot of blood.

12:5 Phlebotomising the basilic vein is beneficial for pleurisy and pleuritis. Some have claimed that these are two names for one and the same thing, and even if they differ, you should see them as one, for the difference between the two is minor. Pleuritis is an inflammation that occurs in the inner lining that connects to the ribs, yet some have claimed that this is pleurisy, and that pleuritis is what comes from the outside, and is followed by chronic fever, cough, difficulty of breath, and pricking pain. Should it happen that the pain in this swelling ends towards the clavicle, phlebotomy is very certain. But, if the pain is inclining towards the false ribs, purgation is more appropriate, thereafter phlebotomy.

12:6 [Phlebotomising the basilic vein] is also beneficial for asthma in combination with the face turning red and the jugular veins swelling; for palpitation | combined with heat of the chest, magnitude of pulse and its speed; 18r
for evidently hot swelling of the stomach; for swelling of the liver combined with strong thirst and unavoidable fever; for melancholy in combination with change of complexion, bad digestion, sour vomit, and chronic winds towards the false ribs—when you phlebotomise it, it has to be from the left [side], and [you have] to observe whether the blood is black [that is fine], otherwise you should end it—; for pain of the spleen if there was a swelling and heat; for

50 ⟨⟩ in the margin.

الذي يكون سببه احتباس دم البواسير والحيض أو من سبب آخر من الامتلاء ومن المغص الذي يستراح معه إلى الأشياء الباردة ومن اختلاف الدم ومن[a] سحج الأمعاء مع صحة القوة ومن الإسهال الذي يكون سببه خلط سوداوي ينصب إلى المعدة والفصد هاهنا يكون من اليسار ومن القولنج الذي يعرض من ورم في الأمعاء ويسمى إيلاوس ومعناه رب ارحم ويتبعه عطش وقيء مرار وضربان البطن ومن ورم الكلى ويتبعه في ابتدائه حميات على غير نظام وإذا انبطح العليل على بطنه أحس كأنّ ثقيلا مغلقا من بطنه ومن ضعف الكلى الذي معه وجع الصلب وقلة الباه وبول مثل ماء اللحم ومن انفجار الدم من الكلى وهو يجيء عقب البول ومن ورم المثانة الذي معه حمى حارة وشدة[b] وجع المثانة ونحسها ومن حرقة البول الذي يسكن معها العليل إلى الأشياء الباردة ومن كثرة الشهوة الباهية التي ⟨لا⟩[c] تضعف والاحتلام والانتشار الدائم مع حرارة ومن كثرة الطمث الذي يكون مع قوة ومن نواسير[d] الرحم التي يجيء منها الدم بأدوار غير أدوار الحيض ومن ورم الرحم الذي يعرض من احتباس الحيض أو عسر الولادة أو الضربة على الرحم ويتبعه حمى[e] ووجع الرأس وعسر النفس ومن أوجاع | البواسير وشقاق المقعدة وورم الأنثيين مع حرارة ومن وجع 18v
الظهر الذي معه ضربان وحرارة ومن وجع الورك الذي معه أدنى حرارة فإنّ هذا الموضع لخوره قلّ ما تتبين فيه حرارة وبالجملة أوجاع المفاصل التي معها حرارة ومن النقرس الذي يتورم[f] ومعه حرارة ويعرض خاصة في مفاصل الرجل وكثيرا ما يتحلل هذا الورم ولا يجمع وربما يتحجر ويتفقع وتخرج منه رطوبات أو شبه الجص والآجر ومن الدوالي وهي عروق ملتفة بالساقين وتعرض كثيرا للحمالين والشيوخ وقد تفصد أيضا هي أنفسها في مواضع شتى ومن عرق النَّسَا الذي معه حرارة في الساق ومن داء الفيل الذي معه حرارة اللمس وكمودة اللون وهذا مرض يعظم معه الساق والقدم أجمع.

a +O
b وشده بيان in the margin
c لا in the margin
d نواسير: بواسير
e حمى repeated below.
f يتورم: يتروم

fleshy-dropsy caused by the obstruction of the blood of the haemorrhoids and menstruation, or for another cause of overfilling; for gripes which is calmed by cold things; for bloody diarrhoea and for abrasion of the guts combined with soundness of strength; for diarrhoea caused by a melancholic humour flowing into the stomach, in which case phlebotomising should be from the left side; for colic that occurs from a swelling in the guts, and is called *ileus*, which means 'Lord, have mercy', that is followed by thirst, bitter vomit, and throbbing pain in the stomach; for the swelling of kidneys that in its beginning is followed by irregular fevers, and if the patient was made to lay down on his stomach, he feels obscure heaviness in his stomach; for weakness of the kidneys combined with pain of the spinal column, reduced sexual desire, and urine like meat broth; for phleborrhagia from the kidneys that follows the urine; for swelling of the bladder combined with hot fever, severe pain of the bladder, and pricking pain in it; for burning urine with which the patient is calmed by cold things; for the abundance of sexual desire that does ⟨not⟩[51] get weaker; [for] nocturnal emission; chronic *intišār* with heat; for heavy menstrual bleeding that occurs with strength; for polyps in the uterus that bleed in cycles that are not menstrual cycles; for the swelling of uterus that occurs due to amenorrhea, difficult birth, or a blow on the uterus that is followed by fever, headache, and difficult
breathing; for pains | of haemorrhoids and fissures in the anus; swelling of the 18v
testicles combined with heat; for back pain combined with throbbing pain and heat; for pain in the hip combined with minor heat—for indeed this site due to its weakness rarely becomes warm—; in general, arthritis combined with heat; for swelling gout combined with heat, that appears especially in the joints of a man, and often this swelling dissolves and does not increase, and sometimes it petrifies and bursts, and moisture or [something] similar to gypsum and baked bricks go out from it; for varicose veins that are intertwined veins in the legs, which occurs often to carriers and old men—one may also phlebotomise exactly those veins in diverse spots—; for sciatica combined with heat in the leg; and for elephantiasis combined with heat of touch and darkening of complexion—this is a disease with which the whole leg and foot become enormous.

51 ⟨⟩ in the margin.

١٢:٧ فصد الأكحل: فأما الأكحل فإنه كما ذكرنا يعمر الجسم. مثال ذلك أنّا نفصده في الحميات الدموية لأنه شامل لسائر البدن ويجب إذا أردت فصده في مثل هذه العلة أن تنظر فإنْ كان الدم لم يبدأ أن يعفن فليس إقدامك على ثقة لأنه لا يؤمن إذا عفن أن يخرج النقي منه فيفسد الباقي وعلامة العفن نتن البول ونثوره[a] ونتن العرق لأنه يخاف في هذا الوقت أن يكون المرض في صعوده وسورته فيكون خروج الدم عند ذلك ضارا جدا وقد فصد جالينوس في حمى العفن من دم والمالنخونيا التي يحترق معها الدم في البدن كله وذلك متى نحف البدن واسودّ وتقدم في ذلك تعب وكد ومن الحكة التي معها بثور حمر وفتورة[b] البدن كأنه قد خرج من حمام ومتى اتفق أن يكون في الجسم مرضان[c] يوجبان الفصد أحدهما في حد ما يفصد له القيفال والثاني في حد ما يفصد له الباسليق فافصد | الأكحل فإنه ينوب عنهما. 19r

١٢:٨ فصد الأسيلم نافع من وجع الطحال والربو اللذين معهما حرارة بعد فصد الباسليق ومن المالنخونيا.

١٢:٩ فصد المأبض والصافن ينفع[d] من احتباس الحيض قبل وقته بيومين ومن قروح الساقين ومن حك الأنثيين ومن الدوالي ومن الصرع الدموي وقد ذكرنا علامته فيما تقدم ومن القولنج الورمي بعد فصد الباسليق.

١٢:١٠ فصد عرق النسا الذي معه حرارة ينفع من وجعه بعد فصد الباسليق.

---

a Uncertain reading.

b Uncertain reading.

c مرضان ما in the margin

d ينفع: ينفعان

12:7 Phlebotomising the median cubital vein: As to the median cubital vein, it indeed, as we have mentioned, fills the body with life. An example of that is that we phlebotomise it in sanguine fevers because it pervades the whole body. If you want to phlebotomise it, such as in this illness, you need to observe: even if the blood has not begun to putrefy, you cannot proceed with confidence, since if it putrefies, one cannot be certain that the clean part of it is expelled, thus it putrefies the rest. The symptom of the putrefaction is bad smell of urine, and small particles in it, and the bad smell of sweat. As one is afraid of the illness escalating and getting severe at that time, extracting blood at this stage is very harmful, yet Galen phlebotomised the corrupted blood in putrid blood fever. [One may also phlebotomise the median cubital vein for] melancholy combined with the blood combusting in the whole body, and that is when the body is slender and has turned black, and it is preceded by fatigue and hard work; and for itching combined with red pustules and lassitude of the body as if he [i.e., the patient] just got out of the bathhouse. Whenever it happens that there are two illnesses in the body that both require phlebotomy, one of the two at the degree for which the cephalic vein should be phlebotomised, and the other at the degree for which the basilic vein should be phlebotomised, phlebotomise | the median cubital vein, since it substitutes them both. 19r

12:8 Phlebotomising the *vena salvatella* is beneficial for pain in the spleen and asthma, both combined with heat, after phlebotomising the basilic vein; as well as for melancholy.

12:9 Phlebotomising the popliteal fossa and the saphenous vein is beneficial for amenorrhea two days before its time; for ulcers in the legs; for itching of the testicles; for varicose veins; for sanguine epilepsy—we already have mentioned its indication previously—; and for colic with swelling after phlebotomising the basilic vein.

12:10 Phlebotomising the sciatic vein combined with heat is beneficial for pain in it after phlebotomising the basilic vein.

الباب الثالث عشر

١٣:١ الباب الثالث عشر في علاج الخطأ الذي يقع في الفصد.

١٣:٢ متى اتفق في فصد الباسليق أن ترى الدم مشرقا يثب وثبا فاعلم أنه من الشريان فاستعمل فيه دواء جالينوس الذي يقول فيه إنه أفضل الأدوية لقطع الدم.[a]

١٣:٣ وصفته: كندر جزء صبر نصف جزء يضرب ببياض بيض حتى يصير في ثخن العسل ويلتّ بالدواء وبر[b] الأرنب ويلزم الموضع فإنْ عدم جعل مكانه نسج العنكبوت أو قطن لين مدبر وليكن الصبر في الأبدان التي غلب عليها اليبس أكثر ويشد شدا محكما. بعد ثلاثة أيام فإنْ كان محتبسا ترك ونثر من الدواء حواليه ويعاد الشد و إنْ كان متبرئا قلع برفق وجعل الإصبع على موضع فتح العرق ويلزم أيضا الدواء على الرسم الأول ويدبر بهذا حتى يبرأ ويسلم من الفتق الذي يلحق هذا كثيرا.

١٣:٤ آخر لمثل ذلك:[c] صبر وكندر ودم الأخوين أجزاء متساوية تعجن ببياض البيض ويشد ويترك ويجعل على الرسم المذكور. وإنْ حمي أو خيف عليه ذلك رش عليه الوقت بعد الوقت من ماء الورد كي لا يحل.

١٣:٥ آخر لمثل ذلك: رأيت نصرانيا كان من الحذاق بالمارستان أراد فصد | الباسليق 19v
فوقعت الضربة بشريانه فاستعمل هذا الدواء فبرئ وهذه صفته: قلقطار محرق وهو الزاج الأصفر وهو متوسط بين الزاجات الثلاثة في الحدة وصفة إحراقه أن يجعل في كوز فخار ويطيّن رأسه ويدخل في الفرن ويستعمل. وهذا القلقطار اليوم يستعمل في المارستانات في مثل هذا.

a لقطع الدم: في قطع الدم corrected in the margin
b ووبر repeated in the margin, additional و omitted.
c ذلك: دالك

The Thirteenth Chapter

13:1 The thirteenth chapter on treating the mistake that occurs during phlebotomy.

13:2 Whenever it happens while phlebotomising the basilic vein that you see the blood bright and gushing, then know that it is from an artery. In that case, use Galen's remedy of which he says that it is the best remedy for stopping the blood.

13:3 Its prescription: frankincense, one part; aloe, half a part, mixed with egg white until it reaches the consistency of honey, and the drug is compounded with hare's fur, and it is bound on the spot. If it is unavailable, one uses instead of it cobweb or processed cotton—and there should be more aloe for the bodies that are dominated by dryness—and one tightens it firmly. After three days, if the bleeding has stopped, it is left, and some drug is sprinkled around it, and it [i.e., the bandage] is tied on again. If the wound has healed, it [i.e., the bandage] is removed gently, and a finger is placed on the spot of the opening of the vein, and the remedy should be applied as first illustrated. It should be treated this way until it has healed and become safe from the rupture that often follows this.

13:4 Another similar [prescription]: aloe, frankincense and dragon's blood, equal parts, kneaded with egg white. One tightens it, leaves it, and applies it according to the mentioned prescription. If he develops fever, or one fears that this might happen to him, one sprinkles on it rose water time after time, but one should not untie it.

13:5 Another similar [prescription]: I saw a Christian man who was one of the skilled ones in the hospital, and he set out to phlebotomise | the basilic vein. 19v
A blow occurred in his artery, so he used this remedy and recovered. This is its prescription: burned chalcitis, which is the yellow vitriol, that is the medium one among the three vitriols in sharpness, and the prescription of burning it is that one puts it into a ceramic jug, coats its head with clay, inserts it into the oven, and uses it. This chalcitis is today used in hospitals in a similar manner.

١٣:٦ آخر قوي: قشور كندر وزاج أخضر ومر وقلقطار وطين مختوم وعصارة لحية التيس ومصطكى وأقاقيا من كل واحد جزء يسحق الجميع ويطلى على الموضع بشيء من بياض البيض وتنثر عليه الأدوية ويلزق عليه شيء من نسج العنكبوت ببياض البيض ويحكم شده ولا يحل ما أمكن وخاصة في الشتاء.

١٣:٧ وإن اتفق بعد فصد الباسليق وبرئه نتوء عليه لين المغمز ويسمع فيه صفير فاعلم أنه فتق أو نتوء شريان فضمده بأشياء قابضة ليصلب[a] الموضع وبدئ من إحراق الشريان ولا يقرب الموضع شيء حاد لأنه يتوقع أن ينزف دم الشريان.

١٣:٨ فإنْ حدث ورم في العضل والعصب واللحم وخشيت أن تنصب إليه المواد فخذ من الخولان والصبر والمر أجزاء متساوية ومن الطين الرومي وماميثا وصندلين ومرتكا من كل واحد نصف جزء ويدق الجميع وينخل ويعجن بماء الكزبرة ويلطخ حول فم العرق وتجعل عليه خرقة خفيفة ويجعل على فم العرق نفسه قطعة شحم من ألية كبش مفترة على ورقة سلق كي يبقى فم العرق مفتوحا ويجري ما فيه. وهذا الدواء يمنع المواد ويحلل.

١٣:٩ دواء آخر محلل: صفرة بيض مشوية ودهن ورد بقدر الحاجة يعجن معه ويلطخ على الموضع ويلزم بخرقة خفيفة.

20r ١٣:١٠ آخر أكثر منه تحليلا: شحم دجاج ودهن ورد من | كل واحد خمسة مثاقيل شمع أبيض ثلاثة مثاقيل يذاب الجميع على النار وينزل ويلقى عليه كثيراء ومرداسنج وإسفيداج أجزاء متساوية ويستعمل بقدر الحاجة.

١٣:١١ فإن علا الورم وزاد ألزم العليل المزورات والأشربة المطفئة وفصد الأسيلم وإسهال الطبيعة ولا يدخل الحمام كما كان العضو حاميا إن شاء الله.[b]

---

a ليصلب: ليطلب
b +o

13:6 Another strong one: Peels of frankincense, green vitriol, myrrh, chalcitis, *terra sigillata*, goatsbeard sap, mastic, and acacia gum, one part of each, everything is ground and coated on the spot with some egg white, and the drugs are sprinkled on it. One presses some cobweb with egg white on it, and it is firmly tightened. One should not untie it, if possible, especially in the winter.

13:7 Should a protrusion that is soft of touch occur after recovering from phlebotomising the basilic vein, accompanied by a whistling sound, then know that it is a rupture or a protrusion of an artery. Dress it with astringent things in order to induce hardness. Begin with cauterising the artery. Nothing sharp should get near the spot since this can be expected to cause a profuse blood flow from the artery.

13:8 If a swelling occurs in the muscles, nerves, and flesh, and you fear that the matters would flow to it, then take some buckthorn, aloe, and myrrh, equal parts; Roman earth, glaucium, red and white sandalwood,[52] and litharge, half a part of each. All that is pounded, sieved, and kneaded in coriander juice, and rubbed around the opening of the vein. One applies a light cloth on it, and on the opening of the vein itself one puts a piece of fat from a ram's tail on a chard leaf, so that the opening of the vein stays open and what is inside it flows. This remedy prevents the matters and dissolves.

13:9 Another, dissolving drug: the yolk of a roasted egg and rose oil according to the need are kneaded, and it is rubbed on the spot, and made to adhere with a light cloth.

13:10 Another, more dissolving [drug]: chicken fat and rose oil, | five *miṯqāls* 20ʳ
each; white wax, three *miṯqāls*. All that is melted on fire, removed, and one adds to it gum tragacanth, litharge, and ceruse, equal parts, and it is used according to the need.

13:11 If a swelling rises and increases, the patient should be compelled [to take] *muzawwarāt* and syrups that extinguish [the heat], and one should phlebotomise the *vena salvatella* and purge the bowels. He should not enter the bathhouse while the [swollen] part is hot, God willing.

---

52 Lit. 'two sandalwoods,' see commentary.

الباب الرابع عشر

١٤:١ الباب الرابع عشر في الحجامة.[a]

١٤:٢ الحجامة تنقسم قسمين أحدهما مع شرط والثاني بلا شرط والمواضع التي جرت العادة بشرطها هي[b] النقرة والأخدعان وتحت الذقن والكاهل والمعصمان والساقان.

١٤:٣ والحجامة تأخذ الدم من عروق صغار وتخفف عن البدن الامتلاء وقد يتفق في الندرة أن يخرج معها دم كثير سيما في الساقين.[c]

١٤:٤ فأما منافعها فإن حجامة النقرة تنفع من الثقل في الرأس إذا كان معه شيء من الحرارة.

١٤:٥ وأما الأخدعان[d] فتخفف عن الرأس والوجه والعينين وتنفع من وجع أصول الأسنان التي يخرج منها الدم.

١٤:٦ والتي تحت الذقن تنفع من القلاع الأحمر واللثة الدامية.

١٤:٧ وأما الكاهل فمن الخفقان الذي معه حرارة ومعه امتلاء.

١٤:٨ وحجامة المعصمين من البثور التي في الذراعين.

١٤:٩ وحجامة الساقين من السكتة والصرع الدمويين[e] ومن الدوار الذي معه حرارة ومن السلاق المزمن ومن وجع الكلى والمثانة والأرحام ومن الدماميل والبثور التي تكون في الفخذين ومن احتباس الحيض ويدر الطمث. ومن كان من النساء سحنة وجهها حسنة

a +O
b هي repeated in the margin
c في الساقين: الساقان
d بيان صح الأخدعان in the margin
e الدمويين: الدموين

The Fourteenth Chapter

14:1 The fourteenth chapter on cupping.

14:2 Cupping is divided into two categories: one of the two is with scarification and the other without scarification. The sites that usually are scarified are the hollow of the neck, the lateral parts of the neck, below the chin, the interscapular region, the wrists, and the legs.

14:3 Cupping takes the blood from small veins and eases the overfilling in the body. Occasionally, albeit rarely, a substantial amount of blood might be extracted along with it, particularly in the legs.

14:4 As to its benefits, cupping the hollow of the neck is beneficial for heaviness in the head if it is combined with some heat.

14:5 As for [cupping] the lateral parts of the neck, it relieves the head, the face, and the eyes, and it is beneficial for pain in the roots of the teeth with which bleeding occurs.

14:6 [Cupping] what is below the chin is beneficial for red aphthae and bleeding gums.

14:7 As for the interscapular region, [cupping it is beneficial] for palpitation accompanied by heat and overfilling.

14:8 Cupping the wrists [is beneficial] for pustules in the forearms.

14:9 Cupping the legs [is beneficial] for sanguine apoplexy and sanguine epilepsy; vertigo combined with heat; chronic ptilosis; pain in the kidneys, the bladder, and the uterus; for boils and pustules on the thighs; for amenorrhea; and it also makes the menstruation flow. For women whose facial complexion

ولونها أبيض فحجامة هذا الموضع أبلغ لها من الفصد وليكن ذلك قبل حيضتها بثلاثة أيام.

١٤:١٠ ومما يقل وجع الحجامة ألا يبدأ | بمص عنيف بل على تدريج وليكن الشرط 20v
بعد أن يحمرّ الموضع جدا ويليّن الشرط على الجلود اللينة ويمسح الموضع بالدهن.

١٤:١١ ويحترس من الحجامة من كان يصعد البخار الغليظ إلى عينيه أو من يتوقع له نزول الماء فيها.

١٤:١٢ وربما أحدثت الحجامة بياضا في الأخدعين عند موالاتها وذلك إذا تجردت العروق التي في ذلك الموضع بالشرط فلا يجري إليه الدم فيبقى اللحم أبيض لأن احمراره إنما يكون من الدم.

١٤:١٣ وأما الحجامة بلا شرط فمتى تجذب ما يحتاج إلى اجتذابه كرها وتحمل الدم إلى الموضع وهي تستعمل على وجهين إما بالمص وإما بالنار وهي أشد لزوما وأجذب وتستعمل[a] على هذه الصفة[b] وذلك أن تأخذ قطعة عجين وتقرصها وتجعلها على الموضع الذي تريد أن تجعل عليه الحجامة وتشعل كاغذة وتجعلها على ذلك العجين وتكب عليها بسرعة محجمة بعد أن يكون الثقب الذي في المحجمة مسدودا[c] فإن النار تنطفئ وتلزم المحجمة[d] جدا فإن أردت أن تسترخي وتقع فتحت الثقب وقد تسترخي وحدها إذا برد الهوى من داخلها.

١٤:١٤ وإن شئت أشعلت الكاغذ وألقيته في المحجمة وجعلتها على الموضع.

١٤:١٥ وقد تتخذ هذه المحاجم من نحاس أو فضة.

---

a تستعمل: تسعمل
b ⟨ص⟩فة محجمة النار in the margin
c مسدودا: مشدودا
d المحجمة: الحجامة

is fair and whose skin is white, cupping this site is far better than phlebotomising her, and that should be [conducted] three days before her menstruation.

14:10 What reduces the pain of cupping is to not begin | with a rigorous suction, but gradually. Scarification should be done once the site has become very red. The scarification should be gentle on gentle skins, and the site should be anointed with oil. 20v

14:11 One should be cautious about cupping if someone has coarse fumes rising into his eyes or is anticipated to suffer from a defluxion.

14:12 Cupping sometimes causes whiteness in the lateral parts of the neck in continuous practice, and that is since the veins in that site are stripped bare by scarification, so that blood does not flow to it. Thus, the flesh remains white, since it is the blood that makes it red.

14:13 As for cupping without scarification, it is when you draw what needs to be drawn forcedly and transport the blood to the site. It is carried out in two manners, either by suction or by fire, which adheres better and draws better. It is done according to this prescription: you take a piece of dough, make it into a pastille, and put it on the spot that you want to treat with cupping. Then, you set fire to a paper, put it on that dough and quickly place a cupping vessel on it upside down. Once the hole in the cupping vessel has been closed tight, the fire is extinguished, and the cupping vessel adheres very tightly. If you want it to release and fall off, open the hole. It may come off by itself if the air inside it gets cold.

14:14 If you want, you set fire to the paper and throw it in the cupping vessel and apply it to the site.

14:15 These cupping vessels may be made of copper or silver.

١٤:١٦ ومن منافعها أنها متى علقت على الرأس[a] أو دون الشراسيف أو الجنبين[b] بعد الفصد قطعت الرعاف و إن وضعت على القفا فتحت حلق من عرضت له الخوانيق للغذاء والدواء.

١٤:١٧ وهي قوية الفعل في جذب المواد المنصبة إلى العينين إذا وضعت على الرأس[c] و إن علقت على الثديين قطعت سورة الدم أعني دم الحيض والنزف.

١٤:١٨ وتنفع من الوجع إذا كان سببه بخار فإن كان سببه خلط رجع الوجع بعد ثلاثة أيام أو أربعة.

١٤:١٩ وتنفع أصحاب المالنخونيا إذا علقت تحت الشرسوف[d] الأيسر وعلى البطن و إن علقت على | الطحال قطعت الإسهال السوداوي وقد بلغت بها بواسير المقعدة للعلاج 21r
إن شاء الله وهو المستعان لا رب غيره.

١٤:٢٠ تمت المقالة في الفصد بتأييد[e] الله تعالى وحسن عونه والحمد لله رب †...............†[f]

a الرأس: الناس
b أو الجنبين repeated in the margin
c الرأس: الناس
d الشرسوف: الشراسيف corrected in the margin
e بتأييد: تباييد
f One and half lines of erased text follow.

14:16 Among their benefits is that when they are fastened on the head or below the false ribs or the flanks after phlebotomy, they stanch epistaxis. If they are fastened on the back of the head, they open the throat to whomever choking from food and drugs occurs.

14:17 They are very effective in drawing matters that flow towards the eyes if they are applied to the head, and if they are fastened on the breasts, they stop the surplus of blood—I mean menstrual blood and haemorrhage.

14:18 They are beneficial for pain caused by vapour. If its cause is a humour, the pain returns after three or four days.

14:19 They help the melancholic if they are attached under the costal cartilages [of the false ribs] on the left side and on the stomach, and if they are fastened on | the spleen, they stop the melancholic diarrhoea, and even treat the haem- 21r
orrhoids in the anus, God willing, for He is the saviour, no other Lord than Him.

14:20 The treatise on phlebotomy is completed with the support of God Almighty and the goodness of his assistance, praise be to God, Lord †.....................†

Commentary

This commentary has several aims: (1) to discuss terminology; (2) to explain editorial remarks; (3) to suggest an alternative reading or interpretation; (4) to verify the quotations to which Ms. Escorial refers; (5) to offer background into the medical framework; and (6) to suggest further reading when some central medical statements are only briefly mentioned in Ms. Escorial. Drugs, potions and other remedies can be found in the index of *materia medica* and *List of Prescriptions*. The commentary follows the logical order of the paragraphs in the edition of Ms. Escorial.

0:1 †....................†: It is most likely that a phrase praising Allah has been erased from the manuscript. This may have occurred during the manuscript's adaptation to a Christian context when it was brought to Europe[1]—the manuscript is, after all, preserved in a Spanish monastery. Despite using UV technology while consulting the physical copy of Ms. Escorial, no trace of the original wording could be recovered.

0:13 **Phlebotomised veins**: The fifth chapter concerns the phlebotomised veins, not the blood in them, as Ms. Escorial reads: دم العروق المفصودة *dam al-ʿurūq al-mafṣūda*, 'blood of the phlebotomised veins.' Thus, the word *dam* is omitted in this edition.

1:1 **Nutriment**: For Galen's account of how food becomes nutriment, see e.g., Galen, *On the Usefulness of the Parts of the Body*, translated into English by Margaret Tallmadge May (1996); and Galen, *On the Properties of Foodstuffs*, translated into English by Powell (2003).

1:2 **Blood is the most balanced of the humours**: Galen: "Of the humors, the most useful and most familiar is the blood."[2] See also Maimonides, *Aphorisms* 2: "Blood is something composed of all the humors according to a natural ratio. It is called 'blood' because of its dominance over the other humors. And this is 2what comes out through venesection and cupping. When we say that the body

1 Penn, *Monks, Manuscripts, and Muslims: Syriac Textual Changes in Reaction to the Rise of Islam*, Hugoye: Journal of Syriac Studies, Vol. 12.2, 235–257, 2009 by Beth Mardutho: The Syriac Institute and Gorgias Press.

2 Galen, *Temp.*, II, 3, 603K (LCL 546: 158–149).

contains four humors—blood, phlegm, yellow bile, and black bile—by blood we do not mean something composed of all the humors, but something existing, in our conception, unmixed with the other humors."[3]

Humours: Hippocrates explains the principle of the humours as follows: "The body of man has in itself blood, phlegm, yellow bile and black bile; these make up the nature of his body, and through these he feels pain or enjoys health."[4] Different humours dominate in different seasons: "Phlegm increases in a man in winter; for phlegm, being the coldest constituent of the body, is closest akin to winter. […] And in spring too phlegm still remains strong in the body, while the blood increases. For the cold relaxes, and the rains come on, while the blood accordingly increases through the showers and the hot days. For these conditions of the year are most akin to the nature of blood, spring being moist and warm. […] And in summer blood is still strong, and bile rises in the body and extends until autumn. In autumn blood becomes small in quantity, as autumn is opposed to its nature, while bile prevails in the body during the summer season and during autumn."[5]

Innate heat: Innate heat in Galen's system: "There are two kinds of heat; the ordinary variety, which burns things up, and the *innate heat* of living creatures, which makes the body grow instead of consuming it, and also has the power of generation. The innate heat is often equated with nature in Galen's works; it is the life of the body, which dies when it is extinguished. Since it is distributed to every part with the arterial blood, it is often also equated with blood. The innate heat, as its name suggests, is not acquired from outside; it comes to the embryo through the semen, which contains the hot principle, and resides in the arterial blood of the left ventricle when the heart is formed."[6]

As wood for the fire: Corresponds to Galen: "Not only do the parts of the animal derive their nourishment from the blood, but the innate heat also owes its continuance to it, just as the fire on the hearth does to the burning of suitable logs, by which we see whole houses made warm."[7]

---

3 Maimonides, *Aphorisms* 2, 1, p. 26.

4 Hippocrates, *Nat. Hom, IV* (LCL 150: 10–11).

5 Hippocrates, *Nat. Hom. VII* (LCL 150: 18–21).

6 Brain, *Galen on Bloodletting*, p. 8.

7 Galen, *Cur. Rat. Ven. Sect.*, p. 72.

As Galen said: This is clearly a quotation from Galen, although I have not been able to identify the source.

Motion: Galen explains this term as follows: "When, therefore, such and such a body undergoes no change from its existing state, we say that it is *at rest*; but, if it departs from this in any respect we then say in this respect it *undergoes motion*. Accordingly, when it departs in various ways from its pre-existing state, it will be said to undergo various kinds of motion."[8] This can happen with respect to colour, flavour, quality, transference, growth and decay, genesis and destruction.[9]

1:3 **Erasistratus:** Ms. Escorial reads أرسطاطليس *Arisṭāṭalīs*, but it is most certainly not Aristotle who is meant, but Erasistratus, who was notorious for rejecting bloodletting and preferring fasting. See e.g., *Galen's Book on Venesection against Erasistratus*, and *On Venesection against the Erasistrateans at Rome* in Brain, *Galen on Bloodletting*.[10] For this reason, the suggested emendation is أراسسطراطس *Arasisṭrāṭus*, also supported by Qusṭā ibn Lūqā:

إن جالينوس ذكر العلاج بالفصد في كتابه المسمى "حيلة البرء" وفي كتابه "في تدبير الأصحاء" وفي مقالة مفردة ناقض فيها أراسسطراطس وبين فيها بيانا واضحا أنه كان مخطئا في تركه العلاج بالفصد.[11]

1:4 **Hippocrates … three kinds of nutriment**: "Nutriment is what nourishes, what can nourish, and what will nourish."[12] Galen's views on this topic, based on Hippocrates' statement above and introducing the terms 'quasi-nutriment' and 'destined nutriment' used in this edition, are discussed in detail in Galen, *Nat. Fac., I. XI*: "For to that which is already being assimilated he gave the name of *nutriment*; to the similar material which is being presented or becoming adherent, the name of *quasi-nutriment*; and to everything else—that is, contained in the stomach and veins—the name of *destined nutriment*."[13]

---

8 Galen, *Nat. Fac.*, I, II (LCL 71: 4–5).

9 Galen, *Nat. Fac.*, I, II (LCL 71: 4–7).

10 Both works, *Galeni de Venae Sectione adversus Erasistratum Liber* (pp. 15–37), and *Galeni de Venae Sectione Adversus Erasistrateos Romae Degentes* (pp. 38–66) extant in Brain 1986, *Galen on Bloodletting*.

11 Qusṭā ibn Lūqā, *Kitāb fī l-Faṣd*, p. 290.

12 Hippocrates, *Nutriment*, 8 (LCL 147: 328–329). For an Arabic translation of the same work, see Hippocrates, *De alimento*.

13 Galen, *Nat. Fac., I.* XI (LCL 71: 42–43).

That which is constantly dissolved from them: Ms. Escorial reads "وهو العوض مما يتحلل دايبا", corrected to وهو العوض مما يتحلل دائما, supported by Ms. Parma: "והוא יהיה במקום מה שנתך תמיד מהם" "and replaces what is constantly dissolved from them".

1:5 **Inflation**: According to Galen, inflation (*intifāḫ*) is a swelling that arises from thin phlegm. The term is a translation of the Greek ἐμφύσημα, which means inflations of the cellular tissue, or stomach, as well as swellings of the eye and knee. The term *intifāḫ* is also used as a common name for swellings.[14]

1:7 **He said**: Galen is most likely intended, as this passage and those that follow continue with Galenic material: "And if one considers along with this the adjacent viscera, like a lot of burning hearths around a great cauldron—to the right the liver, to the left the spleen, the heart above, and along with it the diaphragm (suspended and in a state of constant movement), and the omentum sheltering them all—you may believe what an extraordinary alteration it is which occurs in the good taken into the stomach. How could it easily become blood if it were not previously prepared by means of a change of this kind?"[15]

Large omentum: Galen on omentum: "Why is this part [the omentum] so very extensive in man, covering all the intestines? Is it that in man the concoctions are very feeble and the skin very soft, devoid of hair, and very easily injured? In other animals, to be sure, the omentum does not cover the stomach alone, but spreads over the intestines to a greater or lesser extent in accordance with the nature of each animal."[16]

1:8 **Whenever the stomach feels the need for nutriment**: understood as it is the attraction (*imtiṣāṣ*) that brings the food to the stomach, and then the stomach clings to the food and thus receives nutriment. Galen says: "And this cannot possibly take place in any other way than by the stomach drawing the food to itself".[17]

---

14 Ibn Ǧanāḥ II, pp. 786–787.
15 Galen, *Nat. Fac.*, III.VII, 163–164 (LCL 71: 254–255).
16 Galen, *UP*, Fourth Book, 210, p. 215.
17 Galen, *Nat. Fac.*, III, VIII (LCL 71: 270–271).

1:9 ***Porta***: Galen discusses this topic in *UP*, IV, 1, pp. 204ff.

Had it not been for the watery fluid that mixes with the blood: Galen: "For the chyle resulting from the food could not be taken up successfully from the stomach into the veins and could not pass easily through the many fine veins in the liver unless some thinner, watery fluid were mixed with it as a vehicle. In fact, this is the reason why water is useful to the animal; for although no part can be nourished by water, nutriment could not be distributed from the stomach if it were not conducted in this way by moisture of some sort."[18]

Straight veins: What is meant with this is unknown. It may be that Ms. Escorial should read *al-ʿurūq al-ʿaẓīma*, 'great veins'—'great vessels' are mentioned in Galen, *UP*;[19] 'great artery' features in Galen, *Meth. Med.* III.[20]

1:10 **A large vein:** i.e., *vena cava*. Galen: "Another vessel, a vein, which is called hollow because of its size [the vena cava], passes from the convexity of the liver upward and downward and resembles a sort of double trunk; for some parts of our body are higher than the liver and some are lower."[21]

Convexity of the liver …: Hippocrates: "Root of veins, liver; root of arteries, heart."[22] Corresponds to al-Rāzī's *al-Kitāb al-Manṣūrī*: "All the veins arise from the convexity of the liver, the liver being concave on the interior side, convex on the exterior side. A large vein grows from its convex side."[23] For a complete chapter on veins, see De Koning, *Trois Traités d'Anatomie Arabes* (pp. 36–43).

By the instruments assigned for it: probably the kidneys. Galen: "When these thin fluids have finished their work, they should no longer be retained in the body because they would become an alien burden to the veins. This is the purpose for which the kidneys have been formed, hollow instruments that attract this thin, watery residue through one set of canals and expel it through another."[24]

18 Galen, *UP*, Fourth Book, 1, p. 207.
19 Galen, *UP*, Sixteenth Book, II, p. 713.
20 Galen, *Meth. Med. III*, XI, 800K (LCL 518: 208–209).
21 Galen, *UP*, II, 378, p. 682.
22 Hippocrates, *Nutriment*, XXXI (LCL 147: 352–353).
23 De Koning, *Trois Traités d'Anatomie Arabes*, p. 36 (my translation).
24 Galen, *UP*, Fourth Book, p. 207.

They take from each other, because they are connected: The closest parallel I have found in Hippocrates' *Nutriment* is: "There is one flowing together, one breathing together: all things are in accord. All things belong to one system, but part by part the parts of each part fulfill their functions."[25] See also Hippocrates, *Places in Man*: "All vessels communicate and flow into one another."[26] See also Galen, *UP*: "All over the body the arteries and veins communicate with one another by common openings and exchange blood and pneuma through certain invisible and extremely narrow passages."[27]

2:1 **The circumstances that must be considered:** This corresponds to what Galen and also Qusṭā ibn Lūqā have written on the topic.[28] In his *Kitāb al-Iklīl*, al-Rāzī states that unlike phlebotomy, cupping may be used during all seasons, for whomever and wherever.[29]

2:2 **Disposition:** *Diathesis*, in Greek διάθεσις, a term that Galen uses for any stable condition of body, whether it be normal or abnormal,[30] to which Montanari gives "disposal, disposition, state, condition, way of being (*of body and spirit*)."[31] It is close to *crasis*, in Greek κρᾶσις, i.e., "the mixture of humours, or of qualities, in the constitution of an individual; temperament",[32] for which Montanari gives "temperament, constitution, nature".[33] In Galen, *Meth. Med. Hankinson*, Galen writes "the conditions of the parts, which some call 'dispositions' ".[34]

Unbalanced: The word in Ms. Escorial is corrupt, but Ms. Parma reads מתחלפות, 'divergent.'

2:3 **Nutriment at the time of the paroxysm intensifies the fever:** Galen: "When movement to the depths prevails without inflammation of a viscus or a surplus of humors, you will do no harm if you nourish a little more quickly during the

25 Hippocrates, *Nutriment*, 23 (LCL 147: 332–333).
26 Hippocrates, *Places in Man*, 3 (LCL 482: 26–27).
27 Galen, *UP*, Sixth Book, p. 303.
28 Galen, *Cur. Rat. Ven. Sect.*, p. 67; Qusṭā ibn Lūqā, *Kitāb fī l-Faṣd*, pp. 330–331.
29 Al-Rāzī, *Kitāb al-Iklīl*, p. 145 (f. 31ª).
30 Brain, *Galen on Bloodletting*, p. 178.
31 Montanari, *The Brill Dictionary of Ancient Greek*, p. 486.
32 Brain, *Galen on Bloodletting*, p. 177.
33 Montanari, *The Brill Dictionary of Ancient Greek*, p. 1171.
34 Galen, *Meth. Med. Hankinson*, p. 30.

paroxysms whereas, if there is either some inflammation or abundance, you must guard against nourishment prior to the paroxysm as this is a very harmful thing [to do]."[35]

Hippocrates …: "Abstain from food at the time of the paroxysm": Hippocrates: "And if through lack of forethought there is an attack of fever, nothing should be given for three days except water. If the fever go down in that time, well and good; if it does not, treat the patient with barley water, and on the fourth or the seventh day he will sweat and be quit of the trouble."[36]

2:4 **Physician**: The Arabic word متطبب *mutaṭabbib* is translated as 'physician,' yet a terminological distinction could be drawn between طبيب *ṭabīb*, 'philosopher-physician,' and متطبب *mutaṭabbib*, 'practitioner.'[37]

Fourteen days: Hippocrates: "Acute diseases come to a crisis in fourteen days."[38] This period also marks a critical limit for prognosis: regarding jaundice, Hippocrates states that the "patient generally dies within fourteen days; if he survives that many, he recovers."[39] For a thorough explanation of how this can be concluded, and how the regimen should be applied, see Galen, *Opt. Med. Ex.*, p. 67 (4, 6–10).

[In the case of] a very acute illness, one has to apply a very restricted regimen: This concept is confirmed both by Hippocrates and Galen. Hippocrates: "Where the disease is very acute, immediately, not only is the pain extreme, but also it is essential to employ a regimen of extreme strictness."[40] Galen referring to Hippocrates: "When the disease is at its height a very restricted regimen must be used."[41]

A very restricted regimen: Ms. Escorial reads: المرض البالغ في اللطافة جدا ينبغي أن يدبر بالتدبير البالغ في اللطافة جدا *al-maraḍ al-bāliġ fī l-laṭāfa ǧiddan yanbaġī an yudabbar bi-l-tadbīr al-bāliġ fī l-laṭāfa ǧiddan*. It is likely that the copyist of Ms. Escorial has copied the words *al-bāliġ fī l-laṭāfa ǧiddan* twice by mistake,

35 Galen, *Meth. Med. III, XI*, 21. 809K (LCL 518: 220–223).
36 Hippocrates, *Regimen III*, LXXII (LCL 150, pp. 390–393).
37 Temkin, *Galenism*, p. 72.
38 Hippocrates, *Aphorisms*, XXIII (LCL 150: 112–113).
39 Hippocrates, *Critical Days*, 9 (LCL 509: 308–309).
40 Hippocrates, *Aphorisms*, I.VII (LCL 150: 102–103).
41 Galen, *Opt. Med. Ex.*, p. 81.

and one wants to refer to an acute, *ḥādd*, illness. The concept should, as seen above, be that a very restricted regimen has to be applied in a very acute illness. 'Very restricted regimen' is attested in Arabic as التدبير ما هو في الغاية من اللطافة *al-tadbīr mā huwa fī l-ġāya min al-laṭāfa*,[42] whereas تدبير لطيف *tadbīr laṭīf* is simply 'a light diet.'[43]

Regimen: Cf. Powell in Galen, *Alim. Fac.*: "The way to this state of excellence, many believed, was through *diaita*, which we usually translate as regimen, and which meant much more than the word diet that is derived from it, embracing as it did virtually everything to do with the lifestyle of the individual. According to Celsus it was one of three forms of therapy available to the physician (although therapy was only a part of its purpose)—the others being surgery and pharmacology. The concerns of regimen were with the whole of an individual's activities, covering such things as how often and when one should bathe; the nature of one's work and leisure; sexual activity; and, of course, the food one ate and its preparation. This was a holistic approach to personal health two millennia before the word was coined and the concept popularized in the twentieth century."[44]

2:5 **Barley broth**: also translated as gruel. It was considered a suitable dish for many ailments. Hippocrates: "Now I think that gruel made from barley has rightly been preferred over other cereal foods in acute diseases, and I commend those who preferred it; for the gluten of it is smooth, consistent, soothing, lubricant, moderately soft, thirst-quenching, easy of evacuation should this property too be valuable, and it neither has astringency nor causes disturbance in the bowels or swells up in them. During the boiling, in fact, it has expanded to the utmost of its capacity."[45]

Bread pith: Ms. Escorial reads لباب *lubāb*, most likely referring to لباب الخبز *lubāb al-ḫubz*, bread pith.[46] Ms. Parma reads לביבות הפת, *levivot ha-pat*.

2:6 **As to the age, boys ...**: Corresponds to Galen: "Those who have large veins, who are moderately slender and neither fair nor soft-fleshed, you will evacuate

42 Translated from Galen by Ḥunayn ibn Isḥāq in Galen, *Opt. Med. Ex.*, pp. 80–81.
43 Translated from Galen by Ḥunayn ibn Isḥāq in Galen, *Opt. Med. Ex.*, pp. 66–67.
44 Galen, *Alim. Fac.*, pp. 4–5.
45 Hippocrates, *Regimen in Acute Diseases*, x (LCL 148: 70–71).
46 Nasrallah, *Annals of the Caliphs' Kitchens*, p. 570.

freely. Those of the opposite type, however, must be sparingly evacuated, since they have little blood and flesh that transpires well. For the same reason you will not phlebotomise children up to the age of fourteen."[47]

Old men, i.e., from the beginning of sixty years: Corresponds to Galen: "Some sixty-year-olds can no longer bear phlebotomy, while some people of seventy still can. But obviously you will remove less from these, even if they appear to be in the same condition as a body in the prime of life."[48]

Galen mentioned that he phlebotomised old men in the age of seventy years: Galen: "You have learned to trust the strong, regular pulse as an infallible sign of strength of the faculties; this applies even more strongly to the large pulse. Thus you will phlebotomise even the seventy-year-olds, if the kind of pulse I have mentioned is present, whenever their condition demands it."[49]

2:7 **Al-Fusṭāṭ:** Ms. Escorial reads *Madīnat Miṣr*, referring to al-Fusṭāṭ, that was the capital of Egypt.[50] However, this location is commonly not connected to al-Rāzī. As discussed in the introduction, Ibn al-Nadīm does mention al-Rāzī visiting various countries,[51] offering a general indication of wider travels that aligns with a claim by al-Khalidi, who in his book *Al-Kīmiyā' ʿind al-ʿArab* specifically mentions Iraq, Syria, Egypt, and al-Andalus as regions that al-Rāzī visited in search of knowledge: "*irtaḥala fī ṭalab l-ʿilm ilā l-ʿIrāq, wa-l-Šām, wa-Miṣr wa-l-Andalus*".[52] However, the lack of additional support and immediate sourcing for al-Khalidi's claim necessitates a cautious approach to this information. Another indication of the author's familiarity with Egypt is evident in § 11:5, where he briefly notes some Egyptian customs and habits, and their distinct terminology in comparison to Iraq.

Verjuice: "An acidic juice obtained by pressing unripe grapes, or a juice of other unripe fruits".[53]

---

47 Galen, *Cur. Rat. Ven. Sect.*, p. 87.
48 Brain, *Galen on Bloodletting*, p. 131.
49 Galen *Cur. Rat. Ven. Sect.*, p. 87.
50 Minorsky, *Ḥudūd al-ʿālam*, p. 151.
51 Ibn al-Nadīm, *Fihrist*, p. 701.
52 Al-Khalidi, *Al-Kīmiyā' ʿind al-ʿArab*, p. 21. However, al-Khalidi does not provide sources for this statement.
53 Liddell & Scott, *A Greek-English Lexicon*, p. 1229a.

Syrup: According to Temkin, syrups were "an Arabic contribution to pharmacology."[54]

Syrup of both [types of] pomegranates: What is meant by this is both sweet (*ḥulw*) and sour (*ḥāmiḍ*) pomegranates.[55]

***Sikbāǧ, ḥiṣrimiyya, rummāniyya, summāqiyya, ʿadasiyya*:** For more on these dishes, see commentary for § 11:5.

2:8 **There is no fixed limit:** Corresponds to Galen: "we cannot lay down in black and white a fixed amount to be removed in each of the conditions mentioned."[56] Furthermore, Qusṭā ibn Lūqā mentions that there is no specific amount of blood one shall extract, but instead, one has to take into account all the distinguishing features of each case, i.e., body type, nature of the illness, mixture of the country, the present time, the age of the patient and their strength.[57] The weights and measures mentioned in Ms. Escorial depend on time and place, introducing a degree of uncertainty regarding their equivalence. For a brief overview of weights and measures, see *index of weights and measures*.

Galen mentioned …: Galen: "I have known myself remove as much as six pounds of blood from some patients, extinguishing the fever forthwith and doing the faculties no harm; yet in others one and a half could not be taken without some slight injury to the faculties, and if two had been taken from these patients, the gravest damage would have resulted."[58]

In his treatise, *On Strength and Weakness*, Qusṭās reported …: Ms. Escorial refers to Qusṭā ibn Lūqā, who indeed wrote the aforementioned treatise which was preserved in the Aleppo Ḥakīm collection and could not be consulted.[59] That ʿAbdullāh al-Rāzī phlebotomised a patient is supported by Ms. Parma: וזכר קוסטאס בשם עבד אללה אלראזי כי הוא הקיז חולה "and Qusṭās reported that ʿAbdallāh al-Rāzī phlebotomised a patient". The marginal note reads: "إنسانا

54 Temkin, *Galenism*, p. 127.
55 Ibn al-Ǧazzār, *Zād al-Musāfir*, 1.10.4 no: 174 (p. 107).
56 Galen, *Cur. Rat. Ven. Sect.*, p. 89.
57 Qusṭā ibn Lūqā, *Kitāb fī l-Faṣd*, p. 364.
58 Galen, *Cur. Rat. Ven. Sect.*, p. 89.
59 Sezgin, *Geschichte des arabischen Schrifttums, Bd. 3*, p. 273.

أظنه هذا وأما الأمر المنتسخ منها هذه فليس فيها شيء", "A human, I suppose, and as for the thing that is copied from this [مقالة, treatise], there is nothing in it."

2:9 **Hard-working**: Ms. Escorial reads من كان مباطشا, *man kāna mubāṭišan*. The root conveys senses of 'seizing violently,' 'assaulting,' 'labouring,' 'struggling,'[60] understood as an overworked, hard-working person. Ms. Parma reads: מי שיהיה רופא *mi še-yihye rofe*, 'who is a physician.'

Rational thinking in sciences that require concentration: Ms. Escorial reads *al-ʿulūm al-daqīqa*, 'exact sciences,' understood as 'exact*ing* sciences,' i.e., sciences that require concentration.[61] On the other hand, in their book *Islamicate Occult Sciences in Theory and Practice*, Liana Saif and Francesca Leoni mention that the term *al-ʿulūm al-daqīqa*, i.e., 'the intricate sciences,' is synonymous with the occult sciences.[62] This sort of an interest comes with a risk: "No-one who devotes too much effort to thinking about a certain science (*fikr fī ʿilm mā*) can avoid ending up with melancholy."[63]

2:10 **Those who have not yet undergone this procedure:** Galen: "someone who is not used to bleeding [should not proceed to perform venesection]."[64]

2:11 **The most tolerant bodies for phlebotomy are …**: Galen: "Those who have large veins, who are moderately slender and neither fair nor soft-fleshed, you will evacuate freely. Those of the opposite type, however, must be sparingly evacuated, since they have little blood and flesh that transpires well."[65]

We may also see bodies that are fat …: Galen in Maimonides, *Aphorisms 24*: "There are bodies that are extremely emaciated and [yet] have much blood, and there are other bodies that are obese and fat and [yet] have little blood."[66]

60 Lane, *An Arabic-English Lexicon*, book 1 part 1, p. 218.
61 For clarifying what is meant by this term, I want to thank Professor Tzvi Langermann.
62 Saif, *Islamicate Occult Sciences in Theory and Practice*, p. 2.
63 Swain, *Social Stress and Political Pressure: On Melancholy in Context*, pp. 121–122.
64 Quote from Galen's *Method of Medicine to Glaucon* in Maimonides, *Aphorisms 12*, 5, p. 29. In *Method of Medicine to Glaucon*, Galen seems to be talking about purging in this statement. See Galen, *Meth. Med. G*, 15, 45K (LCL 523: 404–407).
65 Galen, *Cur. Rat. Ven. Sect.*, p. 87.
66 Maimonides, *Aphorisms 24*, 17, p. 79.

2:12 **A woman who suffered from amenorrhea for eight months**: I have not been able to consult this specific book in Galen's commentary on Hippocrates' *Epidemics*, but the case is documented in other sources. "Galen reports [the case] of a woman whose menstruation was retained for eight months and who was extremely emaciated. When he saw that the blood was flowing copiously in her vessels but that it had a livid color, he bled her and extracted on the first day a quantity of one and a half *raṭl* of dark blood resembling liquid tar. On the second day he extracted one *raṭl* and on the third day eight ounces. And he said that she was cured and her body returned to its [normal] condition in a short time."[67]

2:13 **Muḥammad ibn ʿAbd al-Malik al-Zayyāt**: Ms. Escorial reads Aḥmad ʿAbd al-Malik al-Zayyāt, probably referring to Muḥammad ibn ʿAbd al-Malik al-Zayyāt (d. 243/847), who was a vizier in the Abbasid period under the caliphs al-Muʿtaṣim and al-Wāṯiq, and an important sponsor of the translation of the works of Galen.[68]

2:14: **Experience**: It was highly important that the physician was educated and has experience, as already Hippocrates mentioned: "Life is short, the Art long, opportunity fleeting, experiment treacherous, judgment difficult. The physician must be ready, not only to do his duty himself, but also to secure the co-operation of the patient, of the attendants and of externals."[69] In *Epidemics* I, he says: "The art has three factors, the disease, the patient, the physician. The physician is the servant of the art. The patient must cooperate with the physician in combating the disease."[70]

Scammony: The Arabic word in Ms. Escorial, المحمودة, *al-maḥmūda*, is a synonym for السقمونيا, *al-saqmūniyā*, i.e., *convolvulus scammonia*. The resin of the dried, milky sap extracted from its living roots has a strong laxative effect.[71]

2:16 **Spring is the most optimal season for phlebotomy**: Galen: "The first point is that the health of the primary body parts consists on the balance of the mixture of hot, cold, dry and wet. The second is that spring is the most balanced

67 This story features in book 6 of Galen's commentary of Hippocrates' *Epidemics*, see Maimonides, *Aphorisms 24*, 17, p. 79.
68 Ibn Abī Uṣaybiʿa, *Literary History of Medicine*, 9.49, p. 554, footnote 62.
69 Hippocrates, *Aphorisms* I, 1 (LCL 150: 98–99).
70 Hippocrates, *Epidemics* I, 11 (LCL 147: 170–171).
71 Dietrich, *Dioscurides Triumphans*, IV 160, pp. 674–675.

season in (terms of) mixture when it maintains its characteristic mixture, and blood therefore increases during it."[72]

Galen mentioned … Rome: I have not managed to locate this quotation.

2:17 **Countries:** Content identical to information given in several long passages in Hippocrates' *Airs, Waters, Places* (LCL 147), chapters III, IV, and V. See also Galen, *Meth. Med. G.*, Book I, chapter 15 (LCL 523: 402 ff.).

The Big Dipper: The asterism of Big Dipper consists of seven bright stars that belong to the larger constellation of Ursa Major, i.e., Dubhe (α), Merak (β), Pherkad (γ), Megrez (δ), Alioth (ε), Mizar (ζ), and Benetnash (η).[73]

Ursa Minor: The constellation of Ursa Minor consists of three bright stars, α, β and γ, of which the Arabic term *farqadān*, acc. and gen. *farqadayn*, refers to the stars named Kochab (β) and Pherkad (γ).[74]

Canopus: Canopus (α) is the brightest star in the constellation of Carina, and the second brightest of all stars in the night sky.[75]

2:18 **Blood increases by eating young meat and confections, and by drinking wines:** Foodstuffs discussed in detail in Galen: *On the Properties of Foodstuffs*, edited and translated by Powell (2003). According to Galen, the flesh of animals from the pig family is the best meat,[76] but it is understandable that al-Rāzī due to Islamic influences does not hold this view. Young meat in general, according to Galen, is superior to the meat of older animals.[77] Of wines, thick, red wines are the most beneficial for producing blood.[78]

Wine: Wine, in Arabic نبيذ *nabīḏ*, is defined as either grape or date wine in al-Kindī, *Aqrābāḏīn*.[79]

72 Galen, *Com. Hip. Ep.*, I, p. 77.
73 Bakich, *The Cambridge Guide to the Constellations*, p. 300.
74 Bakich, *The Cambridge Guide to the Constellations*, p. 302.
75 Bakich, *The Cambridge Guide to the Constellations*, p. 168.
76 Galen, *De Alim. Fac.*, III:1.
77 Galen, *De Alim. Fac.*, III:18.
78 Galen, *De Alim. Fac.*, III:39.
79 Al-Kindī, *Aqrābāḏīn*, p. 339. For more on wines, see Galen, *Alim. Fac.*, III:39 (pp. 149–150); Galen, *Meth. Med. II, XII*, chapter 4; Dioscorides, *GHD*, Book V; and Hippocrates, *Regimen III* (LCL 150: 324–327).

2:19 **Hippocrates declared this ...**: I have not managed to locate this quotation.

The humours in the body are [not] balanced: Since the principle of phlebotomy is to restore the balance in the body when the humours are out of balance, most likely a negation was missing.

As Galen said in his book *On Simple Drugs*: I have not been able to locate this quotation.

3:2 **The causes that make phlebotomy necessary**: Galen in *Cur. Rat. Ven. Sec.*: "Those who intend to use phlebotomy must consider first of all how many states of the body there are that call for evacuation. The next question is, which of these states require evacuation by phlebotomy; for there are many conditions, some of which need some other sort of evacuation, and certainly not bloodletting."[80]

3:3 **Overfilling**: In *Galen on Bloodletting*, Brain translates this as *plethos*, or *plethora*, from the Greek πλῆθος, that stands for excessive quantity or surplus.[81] Galen: "Whenever the humors are increased to an equal degree to each other, [doctors] call this 'abundance' or 'plethora'. On the other hand, whenever the body is already full of yellow or black bile, or phlegm, or the serous humors, they call such a condition *kakochymia* and not plethora. Plethora is treated by the letting of blood, and by numerous baths, exercises and rubbings, as well as by discutient medications, and in addition by all fastings, which I covered comprehensively in the treatises on health. *Kakochymia*, however, is treated by the specific evacuation appropriate for each of the humors in excess."[82] Every excess is harmful, as stated by Hippocrates: "all excess is hostile to nature."[83]

Overfilling, which is divided into two parts: i.e., overfilling relating to vessels, and overfilling affecting the strength. In *Galen on Bloodletting*, Brain translates these as *plethos by filling* and *dynamic plethos*: "It has been shown in my book on plethos that plethos is of two kinds, both in origin and in terminology. One set of signs indicates dynamic plethos, another the variety due to dilatation of the vessels containing the humours, which some call plethos by filling."[84]

80 Galen, *Cur. Rat. Ven. Sect.*, p. 67.
81 Montanari, *The Brill Dictionary of Ancient Greek*, p. 1681.
82 Galen, *Meth. Med. III, XIII*, 891K (LCL 518: 344–345).
83 Hippocrates, *Aphorisms* II, LI (LCL 150: 120–121).
84 Galen, *Cur. Rat. Ven. Sect.*, p. 71.

Overfilling relating to vessels: Galen: "The other sort, which is known as plethos by filling, also frequently rushes down into parts, leading to swellings, but it is a cause of apoplexies and rupture of veins as well; it is therefore essential to try to evacuate plethos quickly, before it has a chance to do the patient some grave harm."[85]

Pneuma: Galen identifies three types of pneuma: vital pneuma that is generated in the heart and the arteries, that is produced from the inhalation and vaporisation of the humours; psychic pneuma, that is generated from a further refinement of the vital pneuma in the retiform web through the carotid arteries, reaching the ventricles of the brain;[86] and natural pneuma, generated in the liver and distributed through the veins.[87]

The body is healthy: Galen: "when the faculties are oppressed by plethos, it may be that the person has not yet become ill."[88]

Magnitude of pulse: In general, pulse is a strong prognostic sign. For more about pulse in prognostics, see, e.g., Maimonides, *Aphorisms 4*, "Containing aphorisms concerning the pulse and the prognostic signs to be derived from it".[89]

Urine: Urine in general is a bodily fluid from which prognostic signs can be derived. See, e.g., Hippocrates, *Prognostics*, Iyōḇ Urhāyā's *Kitāb fī l-Bawl* in al-Rāzī's *The Comprehensive Book*,[90] and Maimonides, *Aphorisms 5* "Containing aphorisms concerning the [prognostic] signs to be derived from the urine".[91]

Indication: Galen attests that the term 'indication' is "the discovery of the truth about the thing in question arising out of the nature of the thing and made through following out the clues given by what is clearly observable".[92] Kieffer

---

85 Galen, *Cur. Rat. Ven. Sect.*, p. 74.
86 Galen, *PHP* VII 3, pp. 444–445. For an explanation how this works, see Galen, *PHP* VII 3–4, pp. 442–453.
87 Galen, *UP*, p. 48.
88 Galen, *Cur. Rat. Ven. Sect.*, p. 71.
89 Maimonides, *Aphorisms 4*.
90 Kahl, *The Sanskrit, Syriac and Persian Sources in the Comprehensive Book of Rhazes*, p. 276 ff.
91 Maimonides, *Aphorisms 5*, p. 71 ff.
92 Galen, *Inst. Log.*, p. 42.

writes that the term 'indication,' in Greek *endeixis*, is "a medical term and is preserved in the modern medical use of the word".[93]

3:4 **These dreams, as Hippocrates mentioned**: In *Epidemics I*, Hippocrates gives a story of Erasinus, who manifested a fever after supper, and suffered from delirium, distress, exacerbation, convulsions with sweating, discomfort, fear, and dreams. His urine was dark with round particles in it, and towards the end of the fifth day he died.[94] The symptoms resemble the indications of overfilling described in this paragraph. Dreams indicating multitude of blood are not mentioned in *Dreams* or *Regimen IV* by Hippocrates. In *Epidemics VI*, Hippocrates mentions the following: "Overfullness is apparent, the blood vessels are visible."[95] Perhaps the word 'dreams,' أحلام, should be read as 'signs,' أعلام, in this case. It is also very possible that what al-Rāzī is referring to is Galen's commentary on Hippocrates' *Humours*, see below.

Whoever sees snow and rain, this indicates the large quantity of phlegm: The quoted part in Ms. Escorial does not correspond to the content of Rufus' *Medical Questions*. On the contrary, the passage does look very similar to Galen in his commentary on Hippocrates' *Humours*: "Dreams belong to the things that regularly indicate the disposition of the body. If someone see fire in a dream, then this man suffers from yellow bile. If rain appears, then know that cold liquid is in overabundance. Likewise also if [someone see] snow, ice, or hail, this indicates cold phlegm; if he thinks that he is in a malodorous place, this indicates the putrefaction of the humours. If he sees the crests of cocks, or something flaming red, this indicates that blood is in overabundance. If he sees something dark-coloured or thinks that he is in a dark place, then this indicates breaths [i.e., flatulence.]."[96]

Dreams: Dreams too are a strong prognostic sign. "For Rufus the way melancholy affects the mind is not simply that it leads to odd, morbid, anxious thoughts or dreams."[97] In the quoted work, *Medical Questions*, Rufus of Ephesus provides many examples in which dream interpretation has been used in

93 Galen, *Inst. Log.*, p. 100.
94 Hippocrates, *Epidemics I* (LCL 147: 207–209).
95 Hippocrates, *Epidemics VI*, Section III, 17. (LCL 477: 230–231).
96 Galen's Commentary on Hippocrates' *Humours*, 2.2 [16.219.9–220.3 Kühn]. I am very grateful to Professor Peter Pormann for his help with identifying the quote in this passage.
97 Swain, *Social Stress and Political Pressure: On Melancholy in Context*, p. 121.

diagnostics of overfilling.[98] Cf. Mattern: "Following Hippocrates and other predecessors, Galen recognized several sources of dreams, including some that might make sense to modern readers. A dream could reflect an imbalance of the humours, and a wrestler suffering from an excess of blood, for example, dreamed of standing in a cistern of blood; snow or ice would represent the cold, wet humour of phlegm, and so on."[99]

3:5 **Overfilling affecting the strength**: Galen: "If, then, some people who are still engaging in their usual occupations complain of feeling heavy, slow, lazy and sluggish, this is dynamic plethos."[100]

3:6 **Even if these signs [occur] …**: Understood as even if the signs that are characteristic for overfilling affecting the strength occur, it may be the case of overfilling relating to the vessels, and whether it is the first or the second, the two can be differentiated in the urine, pulse, and other things already mentioned.

Yellowish green: Ms. Escorial reads فجاجة, *fağāğa*, meaning acerbic, understood as yellowish green, as for an unripe fruit.[101] Iyōḇ Urhāyā: "Urine that resembles olive oil, combined with acute fever, is an indication of (looming) mental confusion and death, for it suggests that the intensity of the fever has consumed (most of) the moisture (in the body), to the point of melting the fat, in which case the brain dries out very much."[102]

3:7 **Both of these … evacuation**: Galen: "Both kinds call for evacuation, whether they occur in a sick man or in one in health."[103]

Raw humours: "Crude or raw humour is material, derived from nutriment, that has not been properly cooked or concocted by the innate heat."[104]

Especially if it is summer: Ms. Escorial clearly reads "وخاصة إذا كان الوقت ضيقا" *wa-ḫāṣṣatan iḏā kāna al-waqt ḍayyiqan* 'if the time is limited,' but it is likely

98 Rufus, *Quaestiones medicinales*, §§28–33 (pp. 74–77).
99 Mattern, *Prince of Medicine*, p. 174.
100 Galen, *Cur. Rat. Ven. Sect.*, p. 71.
101 Dozy, *Supplément aux dictionnaires arabes*, p. 242.
102 Kahl, *The Sanskrit, Syriac and Persian Sources in the Comprehensive Book of Rhazes*, p. 298.
103 Galen, *Cur. Rat. Ven. Sect.*, p. 71.
104 Galen, *Cur. Rat. Ven. Sect.*, p. 76, footnote 29.

that 'صيفا' *ṣayfan* 'summer' is meant, referring to warm weather, as in Galen's writings: "But where there is heavy oppression by plethos it is not always desirable to remove blood. It is possible for crude humour to collect in the body, in which event it is necessary to consider precisely, not only to what extent the faculties are in good condition, but also to what extent the humour has increased. For when the faculties have already been broken up by such conditions, they are liable, if phlebotomy is used, to sink to their last extremity, so that it is no longer possible to restore them. When this happens the danger is great, and particularly when, in warm weather, there is an attack of fever while the stomach is disordered, or when the whole body is by nature soft and damp in its temperament."[105] Reading is also supported by Qusṭā ibn Lūqā, *Faṣd*.[106]

3:8 **Stomachics:** الاسطماخيقونات *al-usṭumāḫīqūnāt*, compound purgative pills. See prescription in the index of prescriptions.

Bitter hiera: *iyārağ fiqrā*, from the Greek ἱερὰ πικρά = bitteres Heiligmittel,[107] i.e., 'divine bitter';[108] ἱερά, a name for several medicines in the Greek pharmacological tradition, e.g., ἱερὰ πικρά.[109] Prescription in the index of prescriptions. According to Sābūr ibn Sahl, it is "useful against headaches, moistness of the stomach, rheumatic pain, colic, vomiting that results from colic and moisture, hemiplegia, paralysis of the facial nerve, laxity of the organs, and dumbness".[110]

Entering the bathhouse: For more on bathing, see Galen, *Meth. Med. III, X* (LCL 518).

Moderate oils: Ms. Escorial reads only 'moderate oils.' Ms. Parma adds 'משיחים עם השמנים הישרים,' 'massages with moderate oils.' For more on rubbing and anointing with oils, see, e.g., Galen, *Meth. Med. III, XII*, chapter 3 (LCL 518). The rubbing can be moderate too, see Galen: "the rubbing is moderate in these cases so as to warm the body".[111]

---

105 Galen, *Cur. Rat. Ven. Sect.*, p. 76.
106 Qusṭā ibn Lūqā, *Kitāb fī l-Faṣd*, p. 314.
107 Fellmann, *Das Aqrābādīn al-Qalānisī*, p. 216.
108 Kahl, *Sābūr ibn Sahl; The Small Dispensatory*, p. 72.
109 Liddell & Scott, *A Greek-English Lexicon*, Vol I, p. 820.
110 Kahl, *Sābūr ibn Sahl; The Small Dispensatory*, p. 72.
111 Galen, *Meth. Med. II, VII* 491K (LCL 517: 288–289).

scarcely nourishing foods: Cf. Nasrallah, *Annals of the Caliphs' Kitchens*: Foods with poor nutrition include those low in density, excessively dry foods like salted meat, and those producing too much excretion such as trotters, tripe, intestines, tallow, ears, lungs, poultry, barley bread, bread with bran, and all vegetables. Astringent foods such as olives, pistachios, walnuts, and almonds also offer poor nourishment. Fish, gourd, pomegranate, mulberry, plums, and apricot are poor sources of nutrition due to their high moisture content and rapid nutrient dissolution.[112] This is in contrast with highly nourishing foods that are dense and nourishing when fully digested, even in small amounts. Travellers and convalescents who cannot eat a lot need such foods. Highly nourishing foods include beef, brain, heart, gizzards of all birds, fish with thick flesh, fine white flour, fava beans, chickpeas, beans, lentils, dates, acorn, chestnut, turnip, milk, and red sweet wine.[113]

3:9 **Whoever has suffered from haemoptysis ...**: Galen: "Those who have been temporarily cured by spitting blood, but nevertheless have a condition in the parts round the chest and lungs by a virtue of which, if a slightly increased amount of blood should accumulate in them, some vessel will again have its mouth forced open or be ruptured—these patients must be phlebotomised at the beginning of the spring, even if there are as yet no symptoms anywhere in the body."[114]

In the same manner, for anyone ...: Galen: "it is better to phlebotomise in advance rather than wait for some clear sign of plethos to show itself."[115] In general, according to Qusṭā ibn Lūqā, one has to phlebotomise the patient before a severe illness is being generated, given that the symptoms of plethos suggest that one of the mentioned illnesses would befall.[116]

[Swollen] veins in the anus: Ms. Escorial reads "veins in the anus", while Ms. Parma reads פתיחת הגידים 'burst veins' [in the anus].

Continuous and sanguine fevers: Maimonides in *Aphorisms 23*: " "Continuous" fevers and "perpetual" [fevers] are synonyms. Similarly, the [fever] called

112 Nasrallah, *Annals of the Caliphs' Kitchens*, p. 735.
113 Nasrallah, *Annals of the Caliphs' Kitchens*, p. 732.
114 Galen, *Cur. Rat. Ven. Sect.*, p. 77.
115 Galen, *Cur. Rat. Ven. Sect.*, p. 77.
116 Qusṭā ibn Lūqā, *Kitāb fī l-Faṣd*, pp. 332–333.

"synonchous" is continuous, as is the continuous burning [fever]. The term "burning" has been given to it only because of severe heat."[117] According to Bos, blood fever is synochous fever.[118] See also Hippocrates in *Critical Days*: "About critical days, I have already spoken before. Fevers have their crises on the fourth day, the seventh, the eleventh, the fourteenth, the seventeenth, and the twenty-first; and subsequent to these acute diseases, on the thirtieth, the fortieth, and then the sixtieth. When it goes beyond these numbers, the state of the fevers is already chronic."[119]

3:10 **Spring:** Galen: "And as for those who go down every year in summer with plethoric diseases, they too should be evacuated at the onset of spring."[120] For more on the impact of seasons, see commentary for §1:2.

Purgation: This can be done in two manners, either *per os*, or *per rectum*. Galen: "This is also what we were taught from the position of the parts: to insert something *per rectum* for the intestines situated below and to give something from above (*per os*) for those structures above—the stomach itself, the spleen, and the esophagus."[121] "Ulcers in the large intestines have a greater need for medications inserted *per rectum* because this is nearer. Ulcers in the small intestines need both because this is further on and is in the middle in terms of position for medication taken from above (*per os*) and inserted from below (*per rectum*)."[122]

Phlebotomy may also be beneficial …: Galen in *Cur. Rat. Ven. Sect.*: "Not only is phlebotomy of great benefit in the presence of plethos, either of the dynamic variety or of the kind known as plethos by filling, but it is useful also when inflammation is beginning in the absence of plethos, as a result either of a blow, or pain, or atony of the parts; for the pain attracts blood to it".[123] Galen in *Meth. Med. III*: "Phlebotomy, since it does not dissipate the capacity, is not among those [treatments] directed against a symptom, but is one of those which eradicates the whole condition."[124]

117 Maimonides, *Aphorisms 23*, 30, p. 35.
118 Maimonides, *Rules*, p. 15.
119 Hippocrates, *Critical Days*, 11 (LCL 509: 310–311).
120 Galen, *Cur. Rat. Ven. Sect.*, p. 88.
121 Galen, *Meth. Med. II, XIII*, 922K (LCL 518: 390–391).
122 Galen, *Meth. Med. I, IV*, 297K (LCL 516: 450–451).
123 Galen, *Cur. Rat. Ven. Sect.*, p. 78.
124 Galen, *Meth. Med. III*, XII, 819K (LCL 518: 238–239).

Weakness of a part: Galen in *Meth. Med. III*: "I call a weak part either one that is very *dyskratic* in nature (for such parts are different in different ways), or one that has become *dyskratic* during some preceding disease, or one brought to a *dyskrasia* at the present time."[125]

4:2 **Really knowing the quantity**: Galen: "Nothing shows so clearly that the medical art is in practice a matter of guesswork as the question of the amount of each remedy. We often know exactly that the time for administering food or drink, whether cold or hot, is at hand; we cannot be sure, however, of how much we ought to give. It is the same with purgatives; we sometimes know for certain that a drug purging yellow bile, black bile, phlegm or serous superfluities should be given to the patient; yet we do not know with any certainty the amount that should be administered. A dose of such preparations cannot be corrected. Once the drug has been swallowed and has entered the belly it must of necessity all be digested; nor can one, if the patient has already been purged more than is desirable, remove any part of what has been administered. The greatest advantage of phlebotomy is that you can stop the evacuation when you wish, and afterwards at any time you choose allow it to flow again up to whatever quantity may seem good to you."[126]

4:3 **When there is a lot of blood in the body … vital parts**: Corresponds to overfilling relating to vessels; see commentary for § 3:3. Galen: "For in those patients who appear to you to have a plethos of seething blood, you must try to evacuate it as quickly as possible, before it descends on some vital part".[127] According to Temkin, the principal parts are "brain, heart, liver, and testes".[128] For the dangers of too much blood in the body, see Qusṭā ibn Lūqā, *Kitāb fī l-Faṣd*, pp. 304–305.

This fever, even if it is continuous …: Maimonides identifies four periods of illness:[129] "أوقات المرض الكلية أربعة: ابتداء وتزيد وانتهاء وانحطاط." Perhaps in Ms. Escorial the words 'rise' and 'increase' are denoting the same period, in which case this number, four, would match. Otherwise, the words in Ms. Escorial are

125 Galen, *Meth. Med. III*, XI, 805K (LCL 518: 214–217).
126 Galen, *Cur. Rat. Ven. Sect.*, pp. 84–85.
127 Galen, *Cur. Rat. Ven. Sect.*, p. 85.
128 Temkin, *Galenism*, p. 102.
129 Maimonides, *Aphorisms II*, 1, p. 20.

identical: beginning, rise, increase, climax and decline ابتداء صعود تزيّد انتهاء انحطاط *ibtidāʾ, ṣuʿūd, tazayyud, intihāʾ, inḥiṭāṭ.*

Evacuation should [last] until the patient loses consciousness: Galen: "When, however, there is a plethos of seething blood, enkindling a very acute fever, there is need for copious evacuation. One must try to evacuate this blood to the point of fainting".[130]

The body becomes cold immediately after unconsciousness: "Venesection can extinguish the flame of continuous fevers, in which it is particularly useful if the veins are distended. It cools the body and abolishes or reduces the fever, particularly if pressed to the point of loss of consciousness."[131]

4:4 **Examining the pulse**: Galen: "It is good, however, to pay attention to the diminution of the pulse, feeling it while the blood is still flowing, as is usually done in all patients who are being phlebotomised, so that you will never negligently cause your patient death instead of loss of consciousness, a thing I know has happened to three doctors."[132]

Colour and consistency: "It is often possible to judge it from a change in colour, which may be of two kinds: sometimes from the actual colour of the blood as it flows, sometimes from the colour of the patient's complexion."[133]

4:5 **Whoever has a swelling… change**: Galen: "In patients who have a large inflammatory focus near the vein that has been opened, it is best to await a change both in the colour and in the consistency of the blood, as Hippocrates has also explained in his book *Regimen in Acute Diseases*, speaking of pleurisy."[134] Hippocrates in *Regimen in Acute Diseases*: "Venesection, however, does not relieve the pain so well unless it extends to the collarbone. If the pain does not give way before the hot applications, do not continue them for long; continued heat dries the lungs and is apt to cause empyema. Should, however, the pain show signs of extending to the collarbone, or should there be a weight in the fore-arm, or in the region of the breast, or above the diaphragm, you must open the inner vein at the elbow, and do

130 Galen, *Cur. Rat. Ven. Sect.*, p. 85.
131 Brain, *Galen on Bloodletting*, p. 128.
132 Galen, *Cur. Rat. Ven. Sect.*, p. 86.
133 Brain, *Galen on Bloodletting*, p. 30.
134 Galen, *Cur. Rat. Ven. Sect.*, p. 88.

not hesitate to take away much blood until it flows much redder, or until it becomes livid instead of clear and red. Either of these may occur."[135] The same is stated in Qusṭā ibn Lūqā, *Kitāb fī l-Faṣd*, where Qusṭā refers to Hippocrates.[136]

Henna: حناء, *ḥinnāʾ*, a reddish-orange colour;[137] could thus be read in Ms. Escorial as حنائيا, *ḥinnāʾiyyan*.

5:2 **That originate …**: Hippocrates confirms that the pulsatile veins originate from the heart, and the non-pulsatile veins from the liver. See Hippocrates: "Root of veins, liver; root of arteries, heart."[138] Corresponds to al-Rāzī's *al-Kitāb al-Manṣūrī*: "The arteries arise from the left cavity of the heart."[139] For a complete chapter on arteries, see De Koning, *Trois Traités d'Anatomie Arabes*, chapter 6 (pp. 42–47).

Benefits: Understood as "and the benefits of phlebotomising them."

I begin from the head: Arranging the diseases from head to foot, as seen in Ms. Escorial, was common for Graeco-Arabic medical literature.[140]

5:3 **Four veins behind the ears**: Possibly posterior auricular vein, that is behind the ear, and superficial temporal vein, that is on the other side. The two connect above the ear.[141] Qusṭā ibn Lūqā mentions that phlebotomising the veins behind the ears is beneficial for treating vertigo, as well as other chronic illnesses in the head.[142]

Leprosy: Ullmann[143] defines the Arabic term جذام *ǧuḏām* as both leprosy and elephantiasis, yet in Ms. Escorial the latter is distinguished from leprosy by a different term, داء الفيل *dāʾ al-fīl*. For a broader discussion on this, see commentary for § 12:6.

---

135 Hippocrates, *Regimen in Acute Diseases*, XXII (LCL 148: 80–81).
136 Qusṭā ibn Lūqā, *Kitāb fī l-Faṣd*, p. 358 ff.
137 Wehr, *A Dictionary of Modern Written Arabic*, p. 244.
138 Hippocrates, *Nutriment*, XXXI (LCL 147: 352–353).
139 De Koning, *Trois Traités d'Anatomie Arabes*, p. 42.
140 Perho, *The Prophet's Medicine*, p. 63.
141 Netter, *Atlas of Human Anatomy*, plate 10.
142 Qusṭā ibn Lūqā, *Kitāb fī l-Faṣd*, pp. 401–402.
143 Ullmann, *Islamic Medicine*, p. 88.

5:4 **Three veins that are arteries**: Ms. Escorial reads وثلاثة عروق في الشرانين *wa-ṯalāṯat ʿurūq fī l-šarānīn*, suggested correction وثلاثة عروق وهي شرايين *wa-ṯalāṯat ʿurūq wa-hiya šarāyīn*, 'three veins that are arteries,' as stated in Ms. Parma: וג׳ גידים והם שרינים, 'and three veins that are arteries.' These are possibly anterior auricular arteries and posterior auricular artery, alternatively one of the anterior auricular arteries, posterior auricular artery, and superficial temporal artery.[144]

Phlebotomising them is beneficial: Ms. Escorial seems to refer to the latest mentioned artery, i.e., the visible one. Ms. Parma reads ותועיל הקזתם *ve-toʿil haqqazatam*, "phlebotomising them is beneficial", supporting the view that it is the question of all these three arteries. The reference to Hippocrates below supports the view that it is three arteries in question.

Whoever had these [veins] cut, will not procreate: Hippocrates talking about the Scythians: "They cure themselves in the following way. At the beginning of the disease they cut the vessel behind each ear. After the blood flows out, sleep comes over them from their weakness, and they go to bed. Later they wake up, some being cured and others not. Now, in my opinion, by this treatment their seed is destroyed; for by the side of the ear are vessels which, when someone cuts them, make the person cut sterile, and so I believe it is these vessels they are cutting."[145] I have not been able to consult Galen's commentary on the work in question. According to Nutton (2004), the account of the infertility of the Scythians can be traced back to an eyewitness report, likely written by the author himself, and could potentially be explained by modern medical knowledge regarding the high iron content in certain local rivers.[146]

5:5 **Two veins in the back of the head near the hollow of the neck**: Possibly occipital artery and occipital vein, or alternatively occipital vein, and mastoid emissary vein or meningeal branch of occipital artery.[147]

The hollow of the neck: the Arabic word النقرة *al-nuqra* is translated both as 'occiput' and 'nape of the neck' by Spink and Lewis;[148] نقرة القفاء *nuqrat al-qafāʾ*

144 Netter, *Atlas of Human Anatomy*, plate 10.
145 Hippocrates, *Airs, Waters, Places*, Chapter 22. (LCL 147: 132–133).
146 Nutton, *Ancient medicine*, p. 76.
147 Netter, *Atlas of Human Anatomy*, plate 10.
148 Albucasis, *Albucasis on Surgery and Instruments*, p. 656 ff.

as 'hollow of the neck' by Fonahn.[149] When talking about cupping this region, Galen seems to use the term 'occiput.'[150]

Watery discharge: Johnston explains the term 'discharge' as "A disease of the eye causing continual watery discharge."[151]

Intišār: This term requires a thorough discussion. Both *intišār* and *intiṯār* appear in Ms. Escorial. Ullmann translates the Arabic term *intišār* as Liderweiterung.[152] The term is spelled as *intišār* in al-Rāzī's *al-Kitāb al-Ḥāwī*, book II, 'On the illnesses of the eye.'[153] However, in one instance, we find the term انتثار *intiṯār* with the following explanation (with my translation):

وأما انتثار الأشفار فضربان إما من رطوبة حادة يصير إليها كالحال في داء الثعلب وإما لعدم غذائها كالحال في الصلع وهذان لا حمرة ولا صلابة معهما في الأجفان ومنه نوع آخر يعرض معه غلظ الأجفان وحمرة وصلابة فيها.[154]

"As for *intiṯār* [i.e., dispersal] of the palpebral margin, it is of two kinds: either due to acute moisture that reaches it as in the case of alopecia, or either due to the lack of its nutriment as in the case of baldness, and no redness nor hardness in the eyelids occurs with these two, and there is another type with which coarseness of the eyelids with redness and hardness occurs."

This is similar to that described by Ḥunayn ibn Isḥāq in his book *On the Symptoms of Eye-Diseases*, where *intiṯār* is translated as 'falling out of the lashes,' and two kinds are given: one with acrid moisture resulting in alopecia, in Greek *madarosis*; or the other accompanied by thickening, hardness and ulceration of the lids, in Greek *ptilosis*.[155] The ailment in question has other explanations too: "(synchysis, lit. 'widening/extension') of the eye is a dilation (*ittisāʿ*) of the pupil (*ḥadaqa*). [...] In modern ophthalmology the term synchysis stands for an ailment of the vitreous body. This is in accordance with a definition in another writing by Galen. The Arabic term *intishār*, which was regularly defined as a dilation of the pupil, may also stand for other diseases of the

149 Fonahn, *Arabic and Latin Anatomical Terminology: Chiefly from the Middle Ages*, 103.
150 Galen, *Meth. Med. II, V*, 6., 332K, LCL 517: 40–41 (pp. 40–41).
151 Galen, *Dis.*, p. 60.
152 Ullmann, *Die Medizin im Islam*, p. 142.
153 Rhazes, *Ḥāwī II*, p. 168 ff.
154 Rhazes, *Ḥāwī II*, p. 36.
155 Ḥunayn ibn Isḥāq, *ʿAšr maqālāt fī l-ʿayn*, Book 6, p. 61—Arabic equivalent p. 133.

eye with similar symptoms, such as amaurosis and mydriasis."[156] In *Aphorisms 23*, Maimonides defines *intišār* as follows: "The cataract that occurs in the eye and that the physicians call "extension" lies between the crystalline humor and the hornlike tunic."[157] In his book, *Amrāḍ al-ʿayn wa-ʿilāğātuhā min kitābay al-Muʿālağāt al-Buqrāṭiyya wa-Firdaws al-Ḥikma*, al-Ṭabarī explains *intišār* as *tawassuʿ al-ḥadaqa*, i.e., mydriasis, as the editors of the work in question have added.[158]

5:6 **A vein comes to the forehead**: The frontal vein, *vena frontalis*.[159]

Phlebotomising the two: Galen: "Similarly when a vein in the forehead is cut, heaviness of the head and pains that have become chronic as a result of plethos are usually noticeably relieved. [...] In the same way pains in the back of the head, whether incipient or already established, are relieved by cutting the vein in the forehead."[160]

Phlebotomising the two is beneficial: Ms. Escorial reads وهي نافعة *wa-hiya nāfiʿa*, 'they are beneficial.' It is mentioned that the branches are two, or sometimes more, and directly referred to in the dual form. Therefore, the suggested correction is وفصدهما نافع *wa-faṣduhumā nāfiʿ*. Correction supported by Ms. Parma: ותועיל הקזתם *ve-toʿil haqqazatam*, 'phlebotomising them is beneficial'—Hebrew, with a more restricted usage of the dual form, uses the plural form.

5:7 **Two curved veins in the temples**: Probably the frontal branches of superficial temporal artery, or one branch of the superficial temporal artery and zygomaticoorbital artery.[161] Qusṭā ibn Lūqā mentions that the arteries in the temples should be phlebotomised in case warm, fine matter is flowing into the eyes,[162] which corresponds to what al-Rāzī states in his *The Book of the Crown* (*Kitāb al-Iklīl*): "bleeding them is useful against a thin, hot residue inside the eye, and chronic headache".[163]

---

156 Ibn Ğanāḥ II, pp. 785–786.
157 Maimonides, *Aphorisms 23*, p. 53.
158 Al-Ṭabarī, *Amrāḍ al-ʿayn*, p. 201. I would like to express my gratitude to Scarlett Wood for identifying this source.
159 Fonahn, *Arabic and Latin Anatomical Terminology: Chiefly from the Middle Ages*, p. 76.
160 Galen, *Cur. Rat. Ven. Sect.*, p. 94.
161 Netter, *Atlas of Human Anatomy*, plate 10.
162 Qusṭā ibn Lūqā, *Kitāb fī l-Faṣd*, p. 401.
163 Al-Rāzī, *Kitāb al-Iklīl*, p. 143 (f. 30^b).

Phlebotomising the two is done by ...: Cf. al-Rāzī, *Kitāb al-Iklīl*, "in order to prevent unstoppable bleeding caused by a retraction of their two ends, these veins must only be punctured, and opened up with an arrowhead".[164]

5:8 **Hot, fine, pricking matter in the membranes:** What in Ms. Escorial is called 'fine,' Galen calls 'spirituous.' These, among many other medical statements found in Ms. Escorial, sound very much like Galen's words: "These experiences persuaded me often to open arteries in the extremities of the limbs, and indeed in the head too, in the case of all pains that seemed to have their origin from a hot and spirituous quality, and particularly in the membranes. In these, the pain has a pricking quality and spreads out gently, since the pricking sensation is located in one part as if this were the centre of the affected region, and the whole part round this centre has a sensation of tension."[165]

5:9 **Two veins in the inner corners of the eye**: By Spink and Lewis translated as 'lachrymal veins'.[166] Galen: "So too cutting the vein alongside the greater canthus is good for the crusts on the eyes that remain after inflammations."[167]

Ophthalmia: The Arabic word رمد *ramad* is either ophthalmia, i.e., eye inflammation, or more specifically conjunctivitis, Bindehautentzündung.[168]

Rhyas: Maimonides: "If the flesh in the inner angle of the eye disappears, it is an illness that is called *dam'a* [rhyas]."[169] The term 'rhyades' features in Galen, *Meth. Med.* III: "Also from this same class are the rhyades involving the greater canthus [of the eye] when the canthus is either reduced still more or destroyed altogether. When it is destroyed altogether, the disease becomes completely incurable; when it is reduced, it is treated by moderate astringents along with prior purging, first of the whole body and second of the head."[170]

164 Al-Rāzī, *Kitāb al-Iklīl*, p. 143 (f. 30^{b}).
165 Galen, *Cur. Rat. Ven. Sect.*, pp. 98–99.
166 Albucasis, *Albucasis on Surgery and Instruments*, p. 630.
167 Galen, *Cur. Rat. Ven. Sect.*, p. 94.
168 Ullmann, *Die Medizin im Islam*, p. 235.
169 Maimonides, *Aphorisms* 23, 71, p. 55. The word 'rhyas' appears in brackets in the cited edition.
170 Galen, *Meth. Med.* III, XIV 1002K (LCL 518: 508–511).

5:10 **One vein in the tip of the nose**: Possibly external nasal artery or lateral nasal artery.[171]

Polyps: Ms. Escorial reads 'haemorrhoids,' in Arabic *bāsūr*, in plural *bawāsīr*, in the nose, but probably what is meant is polyps, in Arabic *nāsūr*, in plural *nawāsīr*. Cf. Maimonides, *Aphorisms 23:* "The tumor that forms inside the nose as if it were a fleshy excrescence is called *nāṣūr* and also 'polypus'." For the sake of clarity, I have chosen to limit the usage of *bāsūr* to haemorrhoids, and use the term *nāsūr* for polyps in this edition.

5:11 **Two veins inside the tongue**: possibly deep lingual artery and vein.[172] As to phlebotomising them, see Galen: "Parts in the region of the throat and trachea which are much inflamed are greatly benefited at the beginning by venesection at the elbow, but after the beginning by letting blood from the tongue; both the veins in it are cut."[173]

5:12 **Two veins inside the chin**: Possibly lingual vein, one on each side.[174]

5:13 **Jugular veins**: *vena jugularis interna*, and *vena jugularis externa*, discussed in Galen, *UP*, II, 436, p. 723.

Two veins that are connected to the throat: possibly common carotid arteries, *arteria carotis communis*, discussed in Galen, *UP*, II, 436, p. 723.

5:14 **Axillary veins**: الإبطي *al-ibṭī*, axillary vein, that according to ʿAlī ibn al-ʿAbbās is synonymous to basilic vein.[175] Possibly brachial artery, one in each arm, unless basilic vein running along the brachial artery is meant.[176] Galen suggests different veins to be cut, cf. Galen, *Meth. Med. III:* "So too is it better to open a vein if these parts are affected; the (humero-)cephalic vein in the arm or, if this is not visible, the median cubital [vein], and if the liver, thorax, lungs or heart [are involved], the inner (basilic) vein."[177]

171 Netter, *Atlas of Human Anatomy*, plate 42.
172 Netter, *Atlas of Human Anatomy*, plate 65.
173 Galen, *Cur. Rat. Ven. Sect.*, p. 94.
174 Netter, *Atlas of Human Anatomy*, plate 70.
175 Fonahn, *Arabic and Latin Anatomical Terminology: Chiefly from the Middle Ages*, p. 72.
176 Netter, *Atlas of Human Anatomy*, plate 419.
177 Galen, *Meth. Med. III, XIII*, 904K (LCL 518: 362–363).

5:15 **A Greek name:** It surely means 'head' in Greek: κεφαλή: head.[178]

Jugular fossa: In 5:17 Ms. Escorial reads اللثة *al-liṯa*, and in 5:18 اللية *al-liyya*. Both are deemed corrupt, supported by Ms. Parma that reads אללבה *al-labba*, i.e., the jugular fossa.[179] For *labba*, Ullmann gives σφαγή,[180] throat.[181] In Qusṭā ibn Lūqā, *Kitāb fī l-Faṣd*, the terms are دون الرقبة *dūn al-raqaba* (below the neck) and فوق الرقبة *fawq al-raqaba* (above the neck).[182] See also Galen: "There are three ways on performing phlebotomy at the elbow: inner, outer, and middle. The inner is helpful for those who suffer from conditions of the lower part of the neck; the outer where parts above this, or the face or head, are involved."[183]

5:16 **Basilic vein:** in Ms. Escorial described as عرق البطن *ʿirq al-baṭn*, another name for *vena basilica*.[184]

Riʾāsa: The Greek term for basilic vein is derived from the Greek word *basilikos*, that translates to kingly, regal, royal.[185]

5:17 **Median cubital vein:** also known as median antebrachial vein.[186] Galen: "The middle site sometimes has both the branching veins extending to the end of the arm, and uniting there, and sometimes running to unite quickly with each other at the bend of the elbow. Sometimes one of them is prominent, the other indistinct. When, therefore, the vein that ought to be used for the parts affected is indistinct, you may have recourse to one of the middle ones; try, for preference, to cut the one that branches from the proper vein."[187]

5:19 ***Vena cephalica pollicis***: *ḥabl al-ḏirāʿ*, lit. 'cord of the arm,'[188] in Latin *vena cephalica pollicis*, or *funis brachii*.[189]

---

178 Montanari, *The Brill Dictionary of Ancient Greek*, p. 1120.
179 Fonahn, *Arabic and Latin Anatomical Terminology: Chiefly from the Middle Ages*, p. 81.
180 Ullmann, *Wörterbuch zu den griechisch-arabischen Übersetzungen des 9. Jahrhunderts*, p. 926.
181 Liddell & Scott, *An Intermediate Greek-English Lexicon*, p. 784.
182 Qusṭā ibn Lūqā, *Kitāb fī l-Faṣd*, p. 371.
183 Galen, *Cur. Rat. Ven. Sect.*, p. 91.
184 Fonahn, *Arabic and Latin Anatomical Terminology: Chiefly from the Middle Ages*, p. 75.
185 Montanari, *The Brill Dictionary of Ancient Greek*, p. 379.
186 Netter, *Atlas of Human Anatomy*, plate 406.
187 Galen, *Cur. Rat. Ven. Sect.*, p. 91.
188 Albucasis, *Albucasis on Surgery and Instruments*, p. 651.
189 Fonahn, *Arabic and Latin Anatomical Terminology: Chiefly from the Middle Ages*, p. 67.

5:20 **A branch of the basilic vein**: Possibly one of the intercapitular veins.[190]

Phlebotomising it is beneficial: Galen is more specific on which side to phlebotomise in order to treat the spleen and liver. Galen: "When the liver is starting to become inflamed, [cut] the veins in the right arm and, when the spleen is involved, the opposite (i.e. in the left arm)."[191]

5:21 ***Vena salvatella***: i.e., الأسيلم *al-usaylim*, the *vena salvatella*, which is a specific vein between the little finger and the ring finger. The word only occurs in the diminutive form.[192] Possibly one of the three intercapitular veins.[193] The Arabic word surely is derived from the word *salāma*, which means soundness, safety, security,[194] as stated in Ms. Escorial. As to phlebotomising it, see Galen: "So also when the spleen is affected, incision of the vein in the ring finger of the left hand is of benefit, just as it would be if you were to cut the inner vein at the elbow; for evacuation of blood from the left hand helps a disordered spleen considerably."[195] Qusṭā ibn Lūqā adds that while phlebotomising the *vena salvatella* in the left hand is beneficial for pain in the spleen, phlebotomising the same vein in the right hand is beneficial for pain in the liver.[196]

5:22 **Two veins in the popliteal fossae**: Possibly popliteal vein, one in each leg.[197]

Phlebotomising them: Galen: "In respect to the kidneys, bladder, genitalia and uterus, [cut] those in the legs, especially those in relation to the popliteal fossa; if not, cut those beside the ankle."[198] Qusṭā ibn Lūqā mentions that phlebotomising the veins in the arm for problems of the uterus, on the contrary, causes severe damage, as drawing the blood to the opposite direction causes the menstrual blood to be withheld.[199]

---

190 Netter, *Atlas of Human Anatomy*, plate 406.
191 Galen, *Meth. Med. III*, XIII, 904K (LCL 518: 362–363).
192 Lane, *An Arabic-English Lexicon*, p. 1416.
193 Netter, *Atlas of Human Anatomy*, plate 406.
194 Wehr, *A Dictionary of Modern Written Arabic*, p. 496.
195 Galen, *Cur. Rat. Ven. Sect.*, p. 90.
196 Qusṭā ibn Lūqā, *Kitāb fī l-Faṣd*, p. 369.
197 Netter, *Atlas of Human Anatomy*, plate 475.
198 Galen, *Meth. Med. III*, XIII, 904K (LCL 518: 362–363).
199 Qusṭā ibn Lūqā, *Kitāb fī l-Faṣd*, pp. 377–378.

… makes the menstruation flow: Galen: "When the menses are suppressed, however, those [veins] in the legs are invariably used."[200] See also commentary for § 14:9.

Chronic ulcers: Galen says doctors call these *kakoethical* ulcers. Galen: "It is not actually this chronicity itself, or being called and being chronic, which indicates the appropriate treatment, but from this [chronicity] it is possible to infer the bad state of the ulcerated part. [---] Chronicity in ulcers is, then, a sign of *kakochymia*. The discovery of what is useful is not, however, from the chronicity but from the *kakochymia*. Therefore, there are these three signs that follow each other: the sign, the condition, and the treatment. Chronicity is the sign, *kakochymia* is the condition, and the evacuation of the *kakochymia* is the treatment."[201]

5:23 **Sciatic vein**: in Arabic عرق النَّسَا *ʿirq al-nasā*,[202] which Fonahn translates as "*vena saphena externa*, the external saphenous vein."[203]

Phlebotomising the sciatic vein at the ankles: In this case al-Rāzī seems to differ from Galen, as al-Rāzī seems to suggest phlebotomising the ankles, while Galen has stated rather the contrary. Galen: "I have known diseases of the hip cured in one day by an evacuation through the legs; such of them, that is, as have not arisen as a result of cold, but through blood having collected in the veins in the ischial region. Hence phlebotomy from the ham is more effective than from the ankles in patients thus affected, and scarification brings them no obvious benefit."[204]

5:24 **Saphenous vein**: *al-ṣāfin*, i.e., *vena saphena*,[205] by which most likely the great saphenous vein, running along the inner side of the leg, is meant.[206]

… makes the menstruation flow: see commentary for § 5:22 and § 14:9. Specifically for the ankles, see Galen: "By evacuations from the legs, however, it is possible not only to revulse, but also to urge on the menses. When you

200 Galen, *Cur. Rat. Ven. Sect.*, p. 95.
201 Galen, *Meth. Med. I*, IV, 276K (LCL 516: 418–419).
202 Albucasis, *Albucasis on Surgery and Instruments*, p. 652.
203 Fonahn, *Arabic and Latin Anatomical Terminology: Chiefly from the Middle Ages*, p. 76.
204 Galen, *Cur. Rat. Ven. Sect.*, pp. 93–94.
205 Fonahn, *Arabic and Latin Anatomical Terminology: Chiefly from the Middle Ages*, p. 130.
206 Netter, *Atlas of Human Anatomy*, plate 475.

wish to achieve this at the time when the woman's period is due, start about three or four days in advance by cutting a vein or scarifying the malleoli of one leg, and draw off a little blood; then on the next day evacuate in the same way from the other leg, at the same time prescribing a reducing diet for the days on which you evacuate thus, and in the four or five days preceding them."[207]

5:25 ***Al-madaniyya***: i.e., Guinea worm. Cf. Ullmann, *Islamic medicine*: "Among the parasites, bilharziasis, intestinal roundworms, pineworms and Guinea worms (*al-ʿirq al-madanī*) were the most common."[208] Ullmann's study reveals that Arab physicians consistently called this *al-ʿirq al-madanī*, 'the Medinan vein' due to its prevalence in the area. Moreover, he cites ʿAbdallāh ibn Yaḥyā, a ninth-century physician, who in his *Kitāb al-Iḫtiṣārāt* connected the Medinan vein to hot climates and the consumption of bad water.[209] For a full chapter on the treatment of Guinea worms, see Qusṭā ibn Lūqā's *Medical Regime for the Pilgrims to Mecca, The Risāla fī Tadbīr Safar al-Ḥaǧǧ*, edited with translation and commentary by Gerrit Bos (1992), and al-Rāzī, *Ḥāwī* XI, pp. 291–296.

6:2 **Danger in phlebotomising the pulsatile:** Galen: "Since, however, the arteries are hard to stanch, doctors do not dare to cut them, and where some, while performing phlebotomy, have inadvertently wounded an artery, they have had difficulty in stopping the haemorrhage. When they do the best they can, an aneurysm develops in the incision scar."[210]

They are composed of two tunics, apart from the vein that nourishes the lungs: Galen: "It is perfectly evident to everyone that an arterial vessel cannot possible [*sic*] be derived from a venous one; for a vein has one tunic, and that a thin one, whereas the tunic of an artery is neither single nor so thin. It has, in fact, two tunics. The inner one is exceedingly thick, dense, and hard, and is divisible into transverse fibers; the outer one is soft, fine, and loose-textured, like that of a vein."[211] Ms. Escorial reads "irrigates the lung", understood as a vein that nourishes the lung, bringing nutriment to it, and what is meant with it is *arteria pulmonalis*, cf. Galen: "the vein that nourishes the lung itself [a. pul-

207 Galen, *Cur. Rat. Ven. Sect.*, p. 93.
208 Ullmann, *Islamic Medicine*, p. 1.
209 Ullmann, *Islamic Medicine*, p. 82.
210 Galen, *Cur. Rat. Ven. Sect.*, p. 97.
211 Galen, UP, Sixth Book, p. 304.

monalis]."[212] Galen: "Now when Nature, who is wise in all things, interchanged the tunics of the pulmonary vessels, making the vein [*a. pulmonalis*] like an artery and the artery [*v. pulmonalis*] like a vein, she was not acting in any idle or haphazard manner, any more than she ever does in making any other structure in any animal. Though an artery may be similar to a vein in all its other parts, in the thickness of its tunics it is not the same. On the contrary, it is so different that Herophilus seems to have calculated correctly when he declared that an artery is six times as thick as a vein. Of all the instruments and parts the lung is the only one in which the artery has the tunics of a vein and the vein those of an artery."[213] There is a reason why the ancients thought the aforementioned; cf. Hankinson: "the ancients, lacking the concept of circulation of blood, confused the pulmonary veins with the pulmonary arteries, hence the problem of accounting for why they resembled veins rather than arteries in the first place."[214]

It was shown to him in his dream: Galen: "Urged by certain dreams I had, two of which were particularly vivid, I went for the artery in the space between the index finger and thumb of the right hand, and allowed the blood to flow until it stopped of its own accord, as the dream commanded. Not quite a pound escaped. Forthwith a long-standing pain was relieved which had oppressed chiefly the part where the liver meets the diaphragm. This happened to me in my youth."[215] As seen earlier, dreams were considered highly beneficial in diagnostics, and Galen followed this too: "Like most people, Galen believed that the gods spoke in dreams and he followed their commands."[216]

The pulsatile vein that is between the index finger and the thumb: Possibly radial artery or one of the two dorsal metacarpal arteries that flow between the index finger and the thumb.[217]

6:3 **The best way of phlebotomising them …**: Perhaps a continuation of an indirect Galenic quote that started in § 6:2. Galen: "Even if the artery is larger, however, it will also cicatrise without an aneurysm if it is cut completely

---

212 Galen, *UP*, Sixth Book, p. 303.
213 Galen, *UP*, Sixth Book, pp. 296–297.
214 Hankinson, *Galen's Theory of Causation* in ANRW II 37:2 (1994), pp. 1757–1774, footnote 46.
215 Galen, *Cur. Rat. Ven. Sect.*, p. 98.
216 Mattern, *Prince of Medicine*, p. 38.
217 Netter, *Atlas of Human Anatomy*, plate 459.

through, and this procedure also often prevents the danger of haemorrhage. It can be clearly seen that the whole artery is cut obliquely right through its whole substance, and the two parts are drawn up away from each other, the one above the site, the other below it. This also happens with veins, but only to a moderate degree, and always far more with arteries than with veins."[218]

6:4 **Rub**: About rubbing, see Galen, *Hygiene*, Part II, 91K (LCL 535: 132–133 ff.).

6:9 **narrow**: Al-Rāzī, *Faṣd Alukah*, has similar content, yet instead of *ḍayyiqan*, it reads *ṣayfan*, 'in the summer.' However, like Ms. Escorial, Ms. Parma reads 'narrow.' See also commentary for § 3:7.

6:10 **Better**: Ms. Escorial: أكثر *akṯar*, 'more'; Ms. Parma: יותר טוב *yoter ṭov*, 'better.'

6:12 … **and the like**: Galen: "You must draw off and evacuate by phlebotomy the blood carried to the liver, incising the inner vein in the right antecubital fossa, since this is on a level and connects by a wide channel with the so-called [inferior] vena cava. If this [vein] is not visible, cut the medial vein, and if this is not visible, the remaining third vein."[219]

6:13 **It is a nerval vein**: Ms. Escorial reads فإنه عرق عصبي *fa-innahu ʿirq ʿaṣabī*, "it is a nerval vein", perhaps meaning that it is a vein adjacent to a nerve. There indeed are nerves both under and on the basilic vein: medial brachial cutaneous nerve with all its branches, and intercostobrachial nerve.[220] Describing the basilic vein as *ʿirq ʿaṣabī* appears also in al-Rāzī's *Faṣd Alukah*, in which it is also mentioned that nerval veins can be identified by the touch under the finger.

6:14 **A fine scalpel that has a blade**: understood as a scalpel with a sharp blade.

A scalpel with no blade: understood as a scalpel that has a blunt blade, that does not cut. Perhaps a similar tool that is featured in § 6:12 as 'hook.' A variety of scalpels presented in Bliquez, *The Tools of Asclepius*, p. 72 ff.

---

218 Galen, *Cur. Rat. Ven. Sect.*, p. 98.
219 Galen, *Meth. Med. III*, XIII, 901K (LCL 518: 358–359).
220 Netter, *Atlas of Human Anatomy*, plate 405.

6:16 **When I want it to heal quickly:** It is possible that the phrase "if I want it to heal quickly" is copied twice by mistake. The three manners of phlebotomy are present in al-Rāzī, *Kitāb al-Iklīl* as well: lengthwise as the most recommendable procedure; widthwise, possible for broad veins not overlying a nerve, very risky and requires caution; and crosswise, much less risky than cutting widthwise.[221]

Nerve spreading: Ms. Escorial reads عصب مفروش *ʿaṣab mafrūš*, translated as 'expanded,' cf. Dozy: "*se dilater*, occuper un plus grand espace."[222]

6:17 **Hot compress**: Cf. Maimonides, *Aphorisms 23*: "[The term] "hot compress" applies to everything that warms the body externally. There are five kinds of it: moist, dry, biting, intermediate, and moderate."[223]

Be careful: In contrast, Albucasis recommends the surgeon to wipe the scalpel with some olive oil.[224]

6:19 **لا مجاور**: this seems to be deleted from Ms. Escorial by the copyist. If it was included in the text, perhaps it could be read as 'a mistake in [phlebotomising] it causes a chronic damage to several faraway nerves.'

6:21 **When the illness is not visible to the eye**: An invisible swelling could refer to inflammations (see entry below). It is also possible that the negation here is a mistake, thus the passage should be read 'when the illness is visible to the eye,' if a visible swelling is meant. Thus, it is worth looking at the term.

The reason for that: The Arabic word علّة, *ʿilla*, can mean 'cause,' 'reason,' and 'illness.' Since Ms. Escorial uses another word for 'cause,' namely سبب, *sabab*, I have—in most cases—chosen to understand *ʿilla* as 'illness.' However, in this specific passage, *ʿilla* is understood as 'reason,' since there is a logical thought process going on. As to the term 'cause,' it seems that the words 'cause' and 'disease' for Galen are somewhat interchangeable, cf. Galen: "Thus at all events

---

221 Al-Rāzī, *Kitāb al-Iklīl*, p. 145 (f. 31[a]).

222 Dozy, *Supplément aux dictionnaires arabes*, p. 253.

223 Maimonides, *Aphorisms 23*, 33, p. 37 (In *Hippocratis De acutorum morborum* [*victu et*] *Galeni commentarius 2*.)

224 Albucasis, *Albucasis on Surgery and Instruments*, p. 642.

you will either say that the disease itself is the cause$_A$, or if the damage to the activity is actually the disease$_E$, the disposition which damages it will be the cause$_A$ of the disease."[225] For more examples on this, see Galen, *Meth. Med. I*, book II (LCL 516).

7:4 **The one who led to this [conclusion] …:** Corresponds to Galen, *Meth. Med. I*, in which Galen refers to Hippocrates in his work *On Wounds* (*Ulcers*): "In every recent wound, other than in a body cavity, it is of benefit for blood to flow immediately from the wound more rather than less, for the wound itself and the surrounding parts become less inflamed. […] Because of this, he was right to also add [the recommendation] to withdraw blood from chronic wounds. But if we have learned that from him in general—that is, when fluxes are beginning it is appropriate to draw them in the opposite direction, whereas when they are fixed in the affected part, it is appropriate to make the evacuation from the affected part itself, or those parts particularly close to it—we are now ready to draw a conclusion about the removal of blood. [This is that], in the beginning, it is appropriate to make the removal of blood from what is distant, but later from the wounded [parts] themselves."[226]

Deflection away from the affected site: this is what is called revulsion or diversion. Galen: "Thus [the blood] is diverted to places nearby and is held back in places lying opposite—for example, diversion is through the nose for what is emptying out via the palate, while revulsion is downward, just as in fact for an emptying out via the anus, diversion is through the uterus whereas revulsion is upward."[227] Brain uses the term 'derivation' instead of diversion: "If bleeding from the mouth is brought to an end by a haemorrhage from the nose, this is derivation, since the flow is diverted to a nearby part; but if the haemorrhage that stops it is from the lower part of the body it is revulsion, since the part to which the blood is attracted is far from the site of the haemorrhage."[228]

7:5 **Many disagreements:** Understood as physicians have differing opinions on how this should be done.

---

225 Galen, *Meth. Med. Hankinson*, 1.7.1., p. 26—$_A$ stands for aition / aitia, $_E$ for energeia / energesthai / energēma (ibid., p. xii).

226 Galen, *Meth. Med. I*, IV, 293K–294K (LCL 516: 444–447).

227 Galen, *Meth. Med. II*, V, 16. (LCL 517: 16–17).

228 Brain, *Galen on Bloodletting*, pp. 129–130.

7:6 **… so that the matter is drawn correctly**: كي تتجذب المادة على استقامة *kay tataǧaḏḏab al-mādda ʿalā istiqāma*, could also be understood as 'so that the matter is drawn in an upright position.'

7:8 **Leeches**: Albucasis: "Leeches are mostly used on those parts of the body to which application of cupping-vessels is impossible, either because of their smallness, such as the lips, the gums, and so on; or because the part is bare of flesh, like the finger, the nose, and so on."[229] Several kinds of leeches described by Indian authors in Sanskrit sources in Rhazes' *Comprehensive Book*.[230] As to the application of leeches, see *Albucasis on Surgery and Instruments*, chapter 97 'On the application of leeches.'[231]

7:9 **The drugs that are put in the nose**: Apparently al-Rāzī both treated the patient with these drugs, despite them being recognised as useless, and also phlebotomised her. It seems to be a general view that these drugs are of little worth. Galen: "When we do this, as you know, we invariably check the haemorrhage from the nostrils, in spite of having previously tried the drugs recommended in the literature for stuffing up the nose and rubbing on the forehead, and found them all ineffective."[232] A few prescriptions for drugs used for treating epistaxis are presented in the *index of prescriptions* in this book.

The cephalic vein on both sides: Corresponds to Galen: "You ought not to despise phlebotomy as a revulsive remedy, since you have often seen me, when there is a copious haemorrhage from the nostrils, making use of the remedy and stanching the flow forthwith. It is expedient, then, as you have seen, not to delay until the patient's strength has reached the last stages of collapse, but, when it appears that the appropriate amount has been evacuated, and the force of the rush of blood continues strong, to cut a vein at the elbow, in the right arm if the right nostril is bleeding, in the other side for the left one."[233] The same thought features even in Galen's *Meth. Med. 11*: "If the patient is still not relieved, it is necessary to cut a vein in the antecubital fossa on the side of the hemorrhage, drawing off a little blood, and then, after an interval of one hour, drawing it again, then repeatedly, according to the capacity of the patient."[234]

229 Albucasis, *Albucasis on Surgery and Instruments*, p. 674.
230 Kahl, *The Sanskrit, Syriac and Persian Sources in the Comprehensive Book of Rhazes*, pp. 78–83.
231 Albucasis, *Albucasis on Surgery and Instruments*, p. 674.
232 Galen, *Cur. Rat. Ven. Sect.*, p. 84.
233 Galen, *Cur. Rat. Ven. Sect.*, p. 84.
234 Galen, *Meth. Med. 11*, V, 316K (LCL 517: 16–19).

8:2 **The best time for extracting blood is the spring**: See commentary for § 1:2.

8:3 **Hot disposition… hurry up to phlebotomise him**: This logic may be related to what al-Rāzī, according to Ibn Abī Uṣaybiʿa, has said about hot illnesses: "Hot illnesses are deadlier than the cold ones due to the speed of the movement of fire."[235]

8:4 **In its proper place**: i.e., chapters 10 and 11 in Ms. Escorial.

8:5 **Whoever is cautious**: understood as someone who is cautious about keeping a strict diet.

8:7 … **[when a surplus of semen] has collected**: Most likely something is missing in this passage. Ms. Parma supports a different reading, as it says: וימנע מהמשגל רק בעת התשוקה החזקה כי הוא יתרון הזרע המקובץ ויציאתו יותר טובה מהנחתו הרבה, "One should abstain from sexual intercourse, except during strong desire, for the accumulation of semen is beneficial, and releasing it is better than its prolonged retention." Allowing the semen to exit the body will bring relief, concisely concluded as "Comfort comes from ejaculation."[236] Already Aristotle dealt with this matter: "Why are the melancholic highly sexual? Is it because they are full of *pneuma*, and the seed is an exiting of *pneuma*? Therefore, those in whom there is a lot of this material must necessarily often desire to purge themselves; for they are thereby relieved."[237] The topic is discussed in Galen, *De locis affectis*.[238]

Coitus: For more on al-Rāzī on sex, see e.g., *The Spiritual Physick of Rhazes*, pp. 83–84; and Pormann, *Al-Rāzī (d. 925) on the Benefits of Sex: A Clinician Caught between Philosophy and Medicine*, in A. Vrolijk, & J.P. Hogendijk (Eds.), O Ye Gentlemen: Arabic Studies on Science and Literary Culture, in Honour of Remke Kruk (pp. 134–145), Brill.

Hotter or colder than customary: Qusṭā ibn Lūqā mentions that the parts can become hot or cold either due to the increase of hot or cold humours, or due to dyscrasia.[239]

235 Ibn Abī Uṣaybiʿa, *Ṭabaqāt*, p. 761, my translation.
236 Swain, *Social Stress and Political Pressure: On Melancholy in Context*, p. 120.
237 Aristotle, *Problems* IV, 30 (LCL 316: 172–173).
238 Galen, *De locis affectis*, Book VI, 417–421, pp. 184–185.
239 Qusṭā ibn Lūqā, *Kitāb fī l-Faṣd*, p. 299.

Drunk: "Drunken and intemperate people, however, accumulate an excess of undigested humours, and do not benefit from such treatment [i.e. venesection or purgation]; the physician should not undertake the management of such patients."[240]

Full of food: Cf. Maimonides, *Aphorisms 12*: "Beware of letting blood while food is still present in the stomach and as long as the humors in the stomach and first [nonpulsatile] vessels are not [completely] cocted."[241]

Raw humours: Cf. Maimonides, *Rules*: "If the body contains a very raw humor, do not even consider bleeding, lest the innate heat become too weak to concoct [the humor]."[242]

8:8: **Day or night**: Corresponds to Galen: "you will not shrink from sometimes opening a vein even during the night."[243]

8:9 **If you see the blood black and slightly foamy**: Corresponds to Galen talking about quartan fevers: "And if, when you open a vein, the flow is black and thick, which is the kind of thing you find particularly in those who are splenetic, be confident about the purging. However, if it appears yellow and thin, stop immediately."[244]

8:10 **Hippocrates … eighth day of his illness**: Corresponds to Hippocrates in *Epidemics III*, in which he talks about a patient with acute fever: "Eighth day. I bled him in the elbow. There was an abundant, proper flow of blood: the pains were relieved, although the dry coughing persisted."[245]

Galen says: Corresponds to Galen: "For on whatever day you observe the indications for phlebotomy in the patient, on that day you will apply the remedy, even if it is the twentieth day from the onset. And what are the indications? The disease severe; strength of the faculties; except in the stage of childhood, and when the ambient air is very hot. Since, in most diseases, the patient's strength will already have been diminished with the passage of time, the oppor-

240 Brain, *Galen on Bloodletting*, p. 132.
241 Maimonides, *Aphorisms* 12, 25, p. 34.
242 Maimonides, *Rules*, 23, p. 10.
243 Galen, *Cur. Rat. Ven. Sect.*, p. 86.
244 Galen, *Meth. Med. G*, Book I, 12, 38K (LCL 523: 392–393).
245 Hippocrates, *Epidemics III*, 8 (LCL 147: 268–269).

tunity for phlebotomy is lost because of the number of days that have elapsed; this, however, is not a primary effect, but is due to the intervention of another factor, namely the antecedent dissolution of the faculties. Hence, if even on the second day after the onset the powers should appear to be dissolved, we shall refrain from phlebotomy."[246]

9:2 **Whoever is phlebotomised …**: The principles of epaphairesis confirmed by Galen: "As for the time for epaphairesis, in those patients in whom we decide simply to evacuate, this should take place on the same day; but for those who are revulsed, it is better that it should be done on two successive days. You should monitor the strength of the patient in all such cases, by feeling his pulse, since some patients are sensitive where strength is concerned, so that they cannot bear copious evacuation. In such cases, the patient should be allowed to recover on the first day, and epaphairesis should be performed on the second."[247]

9:6 ***Madīnat al-Salām***: مدينة السلام, a sobriquet for Baghdad.[248]

9:7 **Al-Ma'mūn**: Al-Ma'mūn, ʿAbdullāh bin Hārūn al-Rašīd (d. 833), who was an Abbasid Caliph.[249]

9:9 **Pulse**: Usually in this edition I have translated the word ضربة *ḍarba*, as 'blow,' a physical affection, but in this case the word is understood as beat, i.e., heartbeat. How does Galen see physical affections? Galen: "Sometimes the term *helkos* (wound, ulcer) is used, sometimes *trauma* (wound, trauma), and sometimes *rhexis* (rupture). But what I have often said is that we must give little thought to names so that we may hasten to discover the knowledge of the matters themselves. Let us press toward this, paying scant attention to names because patients are benefited not by the precise application of names, but by the appropriate remedies."[250]

10:2 **High ceiling**: The unclear Arabic word in Ms. Escorial looks like السمط, understood as نمط, *namaṭ*, 'shape, form.' Ms Parma reads עליון התקרה *ʿelion ha-tiqra*, 'high ceiling.' The expected Arabic words, *saqf* and *saṭḥ*, do not match the writing.

246 Galen, *Cur. Rat. Ven. Sect.*, p. 96.
247 Galen, *Cur. Rat. Ven. Sect.*, p. 97.
248 Wehr, *A Dictionary of Modern Written Arabic*, p. 496.
249 Nasrallah, *Annals of the Caliphs' Kitchens*, p. 534.
250 Galen, *Meth. Med. II*, VI, 385K (LCL 517: 120–121).

Fragrant herbs: Cf. Albucasis: "There should also be in the place where he is sitting such things as are customary for men to enjoy, such as various perfumes, aromatics, and music, and the like, as each one may."[251] In general, the atmosphere should be pleasant and relaxed, as discussed in chapter 95 in *Albucasis on Surgery and Instruments*.[252]

10:3 **Oxymel:** A syrup prepared of vinegar and honey or sugar, beneficial for its cooling effects.[253] For its uses, see e.g., Hippocrates, *Regimen in Acute Diseases* (LCL 148), LVIII. ff. (p. 112 ff.). For more, see list of prescriptions and index of *materia medica*.

Julep: A syrup prepared of rose water and sugar or honey, served as a refreshing drink either diluted in water or served on ice, known for its cooling effects.[254] For more, see list of prescriptions and index of *materia medica*.

Soft-boiled eggs: The Arabic term for soft-cooked eggs is *al-bayḍ al-nīmbarišt*.[255] According to Galen, soft-boiled eggs provide the best nutriment to the body, compared to other means of preparation.[256]

The food should consist of dishes made from goat, mutton, or soured pullets: Galen regards the meat of both goats and sheep as unwholesome due to the humours and residues they produce, but, when they grow up eating food from the soil or trees, they become more suitable for human consumption. Hence, sheep are the best during early and mid-spring, and goats in the early and mid-summer. Galen sees pork meat as the superior, most nutritious of all foods.[257] It is understandable that pork is not included in Ms. Escorial due to the influence of Islam. As to pullets, al-Isrāʾīlī states that their meat is the finest among domesticated birds, as it is compatible with all temperaments, digests quickly, and generates good humours.[258] However, Galen regards all winged animals as poorly nutritious, especially when compared to pigs, yet their meat is easier to

251 Albucasis, *Albucasis on Surgery and Instruments*, p. 642.
252 Albucasis, *Albucasis on Surgery and Instruments*, p. 642.
253 Nasrallah, *Annals of the Caliphs' Kitchens*, p. 555.
254 Nasrallah, *Annals of the Caliphs' Kitchens*, p. 552.
255 Nasrallah, *Annals of the Caliphs' Kitchens*, p. 830.
256 Galen, *Alim. Fac.*, III:21 (p. 134).
257 Galen, *Alim. Fac.*, III:1 (pp. 114–115).
258 Nasrallah, *Annals of the Caliphs' Kitchens*, p. 724.

concoct.[259] For more on the meat of terrestrial animals, see Galen, *Alim. Fac.*, III, entries 1–13 (pp. 114–123).

***Sikbāǧ, ḥiṣrimiyya, rummāniyya, zīrbāǧa, and isfīḏbāǧ*:** The dishes mentioned in this paragraph are all sour. Sour stews are generally considered appropriate for people with hot temperaments, while those who have a cold temperament are recommended to consume white, simple stews, such as *isfīḏbāǧ*, and desserts prepared with honey after consuming sour stews, in order to balance their cold properties.[260] *Sikbāǧ* is a stew mainly cooked with beef, soured with vinegar;[261] *ḥiṣrimiyya* a stew that is soured with juice of unripe grapes;[262] *rummāniyya* a stew made of pomegranate and chicken;[263] *zīrbāǧa* a delicate stew made of birds, lightly seasoned, and soured with vinegar and balanced with sugar, praised by many for its perfectly balanced properties;[264] and *isfīḏbāǧ* a white dish, notorious for being a balanced dish fit for all.[265]

10:5 **Melicratum:** Cf. Riddle, *Dio. Pharm. Med.*: "Very popular as a drink and as a medicine in antiquity was melicraton, or water mead (V. 9). This was a mixture of honey and water allowed to ferment. Among its usages was one for coughs."[266] It is synonymous to hydromel, a mixture of honey and water.[267] For Hippocrates on hydromel, see Hippocrates, *Regimen in Acute Diseases* (LCL 148), LIII. ff. (p. 108 ff.).

10:6 **Animal faculty:** One of the three central faculties. "There are three basic faculties: 1) the natural faculties (*al-quwā aṭ-ṭabīʿiyya*) are the effects of nature which manifest themselves in conception, growth and nourishment; 2) the animal faculties (*al-quwā al-ḥayawāniyya*) ensure life; they manifest themselves in the systole and diastole of the heart and arteries; 3) the psychical faculties determine the reason, the power of discernment, emotion and voluntary movement."[268]

---

259 Galen, *Alim. Fac.*, III:18 (pp. 131–132).
260 Nasrallah, *Annals of the Caliphs' Kitchens*, p. 607.
261 Nasrallah, *Annals of the Caliphs' Kitchens*, p. 617.
262 Nasrallah, *Annals of the Caliphs' Kitchens*, p. 607.
263 Nasrallah, *Annals of the Caliphs' Kitchens*, p. 614.
264 Nasrallah, *Annals of the Caliphs' Kitchens*, p. 620.
265 Nasrallah, *Annals of the Caliphs' Kitchens*, p. 608.
266 Riddle, *Dio. Pharm. Med.*, p. 144.
267 Montanari, *The Brill Dictionary of Ancient Greek*, p. 1305.
268 Ullmann, *Islamic Medicine*, p. 60.

A humour has flowed into the stomach: This seems to be what Galen calls *dyskrasia* of the stomach, and its treatment is discussed in detail for example in Galen, *Meth. Med. II, VII*, Chapters 8–10, 503K–511K (LCL 517: 306–317).

10:11 **But if not**: Treatment with fragrances and musical instruments, that are used to strengthen the animal faculty, are described in detail in Maimonides, *On the Regimen of Health*.[269]

Ġāliya: A men's perfume that comes in various types, the basic components of which are musk, ambergris, and balsam oil.[270] For its preparation, see al-Kindī, *Kitāb kīmiyā al-ʿiṭr wat-taṣʿīdāt*, pp. 56–57.

Mudaqqaqāt, ṭabāhiǧāt, muṭaǧǧanāt, laqāniq: *Mudaqqaqāt* is spicy, ground meat cooked into casserole-like dishes;[271] *ṭabāhiǧāt*, a dish made of red meat, seasoned with spices and herbs;[272] *muṭaǧǧanāt*, dish made of poultry, seasoned with spices and herbs;[273] and *laqāniq*, small, spicy sausages.[274]

Spices: The Arabic term بزور *buzūr*, in singular *bizr*, can stand for seed, or even oil made of seeds,[275] alternatively spices.[276] In the context of this passage, most likely spices are meant.

10:9 **Iron pot**: Ms. Escorial reads قدر جديد, *qidr ǧadīd*. What possibly is meant is *qidr ḥadīd* (قدر حديد), an iron pot, in which case the gender of the noun would match too. However, in the following passage, Ms. Escorial reads قدر نظيفة جديدة, *qidr naẓīfa ǧadīda*, a clean, new pot.

10:10 **Grape jelly**: The Arabic term, *ʿaqīd al-ʿinab*, is most likely an arabicised version of what Galen refers to as 'inpissated must' or 'grape jelly.'[277]

---

269 Maimonides, *RH*, p. 84.
270 Nasrallah, *Annals of the Caliphs' Kitchens*, p. 770.
271 Nasrallah, *Annals of the Caliphs' Kitchens*, p. 611.
272 Nasrallah, *Annals of the Caliphs' Kitchens*, pp. 617–618.
273 Nasrallah, *Annals of the Caliphs' Kitchens*, p. 612.
274 Nasrallah, *Annals of the Caliphs' Kitchens*, p. 610.
275 Ibn Ǧanāḥ I, p. 338.
276 Dozy, *Supplément aux dictionnaires arabes*, p. 81.
277 Ibn Ǧanāḥ I, no. 566 (p. 429). The Arabic word *ʿaqīd* stands for a beverage prepared by evaporating the serous part of milk; the residue is formed into cakes or pieces with the hand, and spread on a horsehair sack to dry (Dozy, *Supplément aux dictionnaires arabes*, p. 151).

11:1 **Foods**: In general, al-Rāzī reckons the role of food and diet important. He said: "If a wise man is able to treat [a patient] with foods, without drugs, he achieves bliss."[278]

11:2 **Fatigue**: Cf. Maimonides, *Rules*: "When the body of the patient is weak, when he suffers from indigestion, or when his body contains a crude humor that has not concocted, one should not bleed [that patient]."[279]

11:3 **Qūqāyā pill**: In *Meth. Med. II*, Galen describes this as "our own little pills compounded from aloes, scammony, colocynth, agaric, bdellium and gum arabic",[280] while in *Meth. Med. III*, where the story of the man with the swollen tongue can be found as well, Galen refers to "the customary little pills which I compound from aloes, scammony and colocynth".[281] For a full prescription, see the *index of prescriptions*.

… thus, I purged him with a *qūqāyā* pill in the evening: According to Galen himself, he advised to use a cooling agent as the first measure, while purgative pills (in Ms. Escorial: a *qūqāyā* pill) given towards the evening was a secondary measure, but the other physician wanted to use purgative pills instead. Galen's preferred treatment was later supported by a dream that the other physician had, and the patient was successfully treated with lettuce juice. Cf. Galen:

> I have in fact seen a tongue so swollen that it could not be contained in the mouth of the person—someone aged sixty who had never been phlebotomized. It was almost the tenth hour of the day when I first saw him, and he seemed to me to be someone who must be purged with the customary little pills which I compound from aloes, scammony and colocynth, the medication being given toward evening. However, I advised that one of the cooling [agents] be placed on the affected part itself as the first measure. Later, I said, we will adapt according to what happens. But to one of the doctors this did not seem good and because of this, the patient took some of the little pills. Consideration of the topical medication was put off to the next day when he hoped something which was tried might be effective after prior evacuation of the whole body and a revulsion down-

278 Ibn Abī Uṣaybiʿa, *Ṭabaqāt*, p. 774, my translation.
279 Maimonides, *Rules*, 38, p. 17.
280 Galen, *Meth. Med. II*, V, 15, 374K (LCL 517: 104–105).
281 Galen, *Meth. Med. III*, XIV, 8, 971K (LCL 518: 464–465).

> ward had occurred. However, during the night, a very clear dream appeared to him, which approved my advice and determined the material of the medication, ordering a thorough washing with the juice of lettuce. And certainly, when he used this alone, the man benefited completely so as to no longer need anything else.[282]

Misunderstanding may also be caused by Galen's verbosity and long-windedness; that, combined with the depth of the thought and uncertainty of the text, may have led to misinterpretations.[283] Being criticised for his verbosity, Galen seemingly replied by writing: "I should not be accused of the fact that my lectures are too long. It is the fault of those who write books full of erroneous arguments."[284]

11:4 **Sucking the honey-like, glossy pod of cassia fistula**: Ms. Escorial reads امتصاص فلوس الخيارشنبر العسلي البراق, *imtiṣāṣ fulūs al-ḫiyāršanbar al-ʿasalī al-barrāq*, lit. 'sucking the honey-coloured, glossy coins/scales of cassia fistula.' According to Alam (1990), the Arabic term *folūs* refers to thin, woody partitions of the pod. The term *folūs*, from *folūs-e ḫiyār*(-*e*) *čanbar*, 'the septa of the cassia fistula' has replaced the term for cassia fistula in Persian. *Folūs* can even mean the pod of cassia fistula, and *maġz-e folūs* 'the pith of *folūs*,' meaning the pulp. Alam also mentions that a cassia fistula with a thinner peel, with a thick, dark and glossy pod has the best medical properties.[285] It could also be that the cassia fistula should be soaked in one of the previously mentioned syrups.

11:5 ***Muzawwarāt***: vegetarian dishes, lighter than meat dishes and easier to digest.[286] The dishes listed here, *ʿadasiyya*, *ḥiṣrimiyya*, *summāqiyya*, and *rummāniyya*, are known as dishes containing meat. As we are talking about *muzawwarāt*, vegetarian dishes, most likely these are vegetarian versions of the dishes known as dishes with meat. With *sikbāǧ*, that also is a dish containing beef, this is evident, as Ms. Escorial reads "of fresh fish the small prepared as *sikbāǧ*."

---

282 Galen, *Meth. Med. III*, XIV, 8. 971K–972K (LCL 518: 462–465).

283 Temkin, *Galenism*, p. 67.

284 Siegel, *Galen's System of Physiology and Medicine*, p. 11.

285 Alam, Houshang, 'Cassia', in *Encyclopædia Iranica*, https://iranicaonline.org/articles/cassia-a-genus-of-shrubs-and-trees-of-the-family-leguminosae, accessed on June 22nd, 2022.

286 Nasrallah, *Annals of the Caliphs' Kitchens*, p. 433.

Sandalwood and rose water: Sandalwood and roses appear as common ingredients in poultices for liver and spleen in al-Kindī, *Aqrābāḏīn*.[287]

11:7 **Tamarind**: Maimonides in *On the Regimen of Health*: "Abū Marwān ibn Zuhr—may God have mercy with him—has said that the best thing for softening the stools is an infusion of rhubarb with tamarind."[288] As to rhubarb, see commentary for § 11:12.

Half a *raṭl* of clear water: The prescription does not mention more than half a *raṭl* of water as a part of the decoction. Most likely the ingredients should be cooked in a larger amount of water as the water is supposed to turn red and the decoction thicker before adding the additional half a *raṭl* of water.

11:8 **Pith of cassia fistula**: Ms. Escorial reads لب خيارشنبر فارسي قصبي *lubb ḫiyāršanbar fārisī qaṣabī*, 'stalky kernel of Persian cassia fistula.' Possibly the author, or al-Rāzī while dictating, has simply added that *ḫiyāršanbar* is a Persian name, as the Arabic term is derived from the Persian *ḫiyār-chanbar: ḫiyār*, 'cucumber,' and *čanbar*, 'circle,' 'collar,' 'necklace,' since, according to Alam (1990), the plant does not grow in Persia.[289] See also commentary for § 11:4.

11:9 **Barley broth cooked with peeled lentils**: Galen: "barley is not only far from warming (such as some foods are betwixt warming and cooling, such as starch and light bread) but it actually seems to be cooling in every way it is used".[290] As to lentils cooked with barley, Galen says it is best to mix lentils with less ptisane (i.e., barley gruel) for the best result.[291]

11:10 **The prescription of barley broth**: The prescription of barley broth, as it appears in the manuscript, seems to be incomplete. For a suggestion of a prescription of barley broth, see the *index of prescriptions*.

11:11 **Seedless raisins**: could refer to *kišmiš*, a variety of seedless raisins (or grapes).[292]

287 Al-Kindī, *Aqrābāḏīn*.
288 Maimonides, *RH*, p. 88.
289 Alam, Houshang, 'Cassia', in *Encyclopædia Iranica*, https://iranicaonline.org/articles/cassia-a-genus-of-shrubs-and-trees-of-the-family-leguminosae, accessed on June 22nd, 2022.
290 Galen, *Alim. Fac.*, I, 9, 501 (p. 47).
291 Galen, *Alim. Fac.*, I, 18, 526–527, (p. 58).
292 Ibn Ǧanāḥ I, 488 (p. 368).

11:12 **Chinese rhubarb**: Chinese rhubarb, *Da huang*, has been used in Chinese medicine for over two thousand years. It was first documented around 200 A.D.. Through trade it reached the rest of the world, and herbalists in Europe recommended it for gastrointestinal issues, in large doses as a laxative, and small doses for diarrhoea. Thus, it was used both as a laxative and as a diuretic. It was also used to treat liver diseases, kidney stones, and gout. Three varieties of the species, *Rheum officinale, Rheum palmatum*, and *Rheum tanguticum*, are still widely cultivated and used as medicinal plants in China. It is a powerful, yet mild laxative that evacuates the intestines and purges the bowels efficiently. As the leaves are poisonous, the roots and the stalks are consumed.[293] The rhubarb root, Radix et Rhizoma Rhei, is among the earliest and most recognised Chinese herbal medicines.[294]

12:1 **Illnesses:** For how several of these illnesses are created, and for their treatment through means other than phlebotomy, see *Zād al-musāfir wa-qūt al-ḥāḍir by* Ibn al-Ǧazzār.

12:3 **Phlebotomising the frontal vein** Galen: "Similarly when a vein in the forehead is cut, heaviness of the head and pains that have become chronic as a result of plethos are usually relieved."[295]

12:3 **Callous hardenings of the face:** النخيلات *al-naḫīlāt*, 'callous hardenings on the face.'[296]

Polyps: See commentary for § 5:10.

12:4 **Phlebotomising the cephalic vein and its benefits:**

Eyes: Galen: "When the eyes are affected, cutting the vein called the humeral, or the one branching from it at the elbow, quickly brings clear benefit."[297] For Galen, the humeral vein is the cephalic vein.[298]

293 Clementi & Misiti, *Potential Health Benefits of Rhubarb*, pp. 407–423.
294 Tang & Eisenbrand, *Chinese Drugs of Plant Origin*, p. 855.
295 Galen, *Cur. Rat. Ven. Sect.*, p. 94.
296 *Maimonides, Aphorisms 23*, 72, p. 55.
297 Galen, *Cur. Rat. Ven. Sect.*, p. 90.
298 Galen, *Cur. Rat. Ven. Sect.*, p. 91, footnote 69.

Throat: Galen: "Parts in the region of the throat and trachea which are much inflamed are greatly benefited at the beginning by venesection at the elbow, but after the beginning by letting blood from the tongue; both the veins in it are cut."[299]

⟨the eye combined with pain, throbbing pain and itching⟩: This part is written in the margin. Where it belongs is not marked in the Ms., but it is likely to be a description of *qurūḥ al-ʿayn al-mutašaqqiqa*.

Ptilosis: Cf. Maimonides, *Aphorisms 23*: "The eyelids that become thick and hard and whose color turns red and whose hairs fall off is an illness that is called sulāq [ptilosis]."[300] The term features in Galen's *Meth. Med. III* as *ptili*, which, according to Galen, "destroy the eyelashes".[301]

Lining of the mouth: Ms. Escorial reads literally 'interior oblong covering,' الغشاء المستطيل المستبطن *al-ġišāʾ al-mustaṭīl al-mustabṭin*. Possible emendation marks above the word *al-mustaṭīl*.

Prolapse of the uvula: Cf. Maimonides, *Aphorisms 15*: "The uvula can be affected by the illness of extreme relaxation without an inflammation, in which case we generally cut it off. But when the uvula is affected by this illness, remedies that heat and that cleanse the phlegm are really beneficial for it, because, at that time, the uvula mostly tends to turn white, as if it were lacking blood."[302]

12:5 **Pleurisy**: ذات الجنب *ḏāt al-ǧanb*, sometimes only الجنب *al-ǧanb*, is pleurisy, "a severe disease, being an inflammatory tumour in the [pleura, or] membrane within the ribs".[303]

Pleuritis: الشوصة *al-šawṣa*. Synonymous to *barsam*, which is a swelling inside the ribs.[304]

---

299 Galen, *Cur. Rat. Ven. Sect.*, p. 94.
300 Maimonides, *Aphorisms 23*, 71, p. 55.
301 Galen, *Meth. Med. III, XIV*, 1017K (LCL 518: 532–533).
302 Maimonides, *Aphorisms 15*, 27, pp. 61–62.
303 Lane, *An Arabic-English Lexicon*, p. 465.
304 Kahl, *The Sanskrit, Syriac and Persian Sources in the Comprehensive Book of Rhazes*, p. 208.

12:6 **Phlebotomising the basilic vein:**

Fleshy-dropsy: The term in Ms. Escorial is *istisqāʾ laḥmī*. *Istisqāʾ* is one of the Arabic translations of the Greek word for dropsy, ὕδρωψ, that is a general term for oedemas and accumulations of fluids in the belly.[305]

Haemorrhoids: Galen: "If you have recourse to phlebotomy because of suppression of a haemorrhoid, and wish to restrain the bleeding further, you should cut the veins in the arms; but to urge it on, those in the legs."[306]

Melancholy: the term for melancholy, in Greek μελαγχολία,[307] signifies "a condition due to an excess amount of black bile".[308] The term features in Ms. Escorial as مالنخونيا *mālinḫūniyā*, instead of the more expected مالنخوليا *mālinḫūliyā*, throughout the manuscript. According to Dozy they both are attested forms,[309] and thus, the spelling is not altered in this edition.

Colic: In the era of al-Rāzī, colic signified abdominal pain arising from intestinal obstruction.[310] According to Ibn Sīnā, it is a disease that causes abnormal retention in the large intestine.[311]

Ileus, which means 'Lord, have mercy': Ms. Escorial states that ileus (*īlāwus*), in Greek *εἴλεός*, signifies '*rabbi irḥam*,' 'Lord, have mercy,' which corresponds to what he states in *al-Taqsīm wa-l-Tašǧīr*.[312] According to Ibn Sīnā, ileus means *al-mustaʿāḏ bi-Allāh minhu*.[313] According to the editors of Ibn Ǧanāḥ, it has been defined as 'that from which one seeks protection,' by Hippocrates, and as 'stinking colic' that causes its sufferer to vomit faeces, by al-Rāzī.[314] Cf. Ibn Ǧanāḥ: "The author of this explanation erroneously assumed that the term is derived from the verb ἐλεέω 'to show mercy'. In fact it originates from another verb, namely εἰλέω 'to shut it'."[315] Maimonides, *Aphorisms 23*: "If the small intest-

305 Ibn Ǧanāḥ, I, no. 402, p. 570.
306 Galen, *Cur. Rat. Ven. Sect.*, pp. 94–95.
307 Montanari, *The Brill Dictionary of Ancient Greek*, p. 1300.
308 Brain, *Galen on Bloodletting*, p. 179.
309 Dozy, *Supplément aux dictionnaires arabes*, p. 565.
310 Al-Rāzī, *Kitāb al-Qawlanǧ*, p. 14.
311 Ibn Sīnā, *Risāla fī l-Qawlanǧ*, p. 157.
312 Ibn Ǧanāḥ I, no. 98, p. 294.
313 Ibn Sīnā, *Risāla fī l-Qawlanǧ*, p. 157.
314 Ibn Ǧanāḥ I, no. 98, p. 295.
315 Ibn Ǧanāḥ I, no. 98, p. 295.

ines are affected by a hard tumor or by a severe obstruction of feces so that the patient vomits his feces, that illness is called "ileus", and hardly anyone can be saved from it."[316] The case features even in Galen, *Nat. Fac.*: "And when the animal becomes sick, this means that the stomach is striving to be evacuated by vomiting. And the expulsive faculty has in it so violent and forcible an element that in cases of ileus [volvulus], when the lower exit is completely closed, vomiting of faeces occurs".[317] For more on ileus, see, e.g., Buḫtīšūʿ in Kahl, *The Sanskrit, Syriac and Persian Sources in the Comprehensive Book of Rhazes*, p. 191ff., and Maimonides, *Aphorisms 23*, 93, p. 63.

Gout: Ms. Escorial reads that gout appears especially in the joints of a man في مفاصل الرجل *fī mafāṣil al-rağul.* Statement supported by al-Rāzī himself in his *Maqāla fī l-Naqras* ('Treatise on Gout'), in which he explains that women do not suffer from gout since their excess blood is discharged during menstruation instead of flowing to the feet, and their disposition is naturally moist and thus, the blood will not turn to the sort that would cause gout.[318] As to phlebotomising for gout, in this treatise al-Rāzī suggests phlebotomising the median cubital vein "provided it is wide and thin-walled; otherwise, blood may be let through the basilic vein."[319]

Varicose veins: Ms. Escorial offers the word حمالين *ḥammālīn*, 'carriers' or 'porters.' It is also possible that the word pregnant, حامل *ḥāmil*, is intended.

Elephantiasis: It is worth discussing the terms 'leprosy' and 'elephantiasis.' Ullmann defines the term الجذام *al-ğuḏām* as both leprosy and elephantiasis,[320] yet Ms. Escorial also includes a term that more specifically refers to elephantiasis, namely داء الفيل *dāʾ al-fīl*, i.e., 'elephant illness.' According to Johnston (2006) the term 'elephantiasis' in the Antiquities was not used in the modern sense, but possibly for leprosy,[321] and presents the term 'alphos' a "dull-white leprosy, esp. on the face"[322] that does not correspond to leprosy as today, but as a skin disease causing the loss of pigmentation.[323] Since the Arabic term *ğuḏām*

316 Maimonides, *Aphorisms 23*, p. 63.
317 Galen, *Nat. Fac.*, III. XIII, 193 (LCL 71: 299).
318 Rhazes, *Naqras*, p. 20.
319 Rhazes, *Naqras*, p. 35.
320 Ullmann, *Islamic Medicine*, p. 88.
321 Galen, *Dis.*, p. 54.
322 Galen, *Dis.*, p. 50.
323 Galen, *Dis.*, pp. 50–51.

for 'leprosy' features in the manuscript in the context of illnesses that occur in the head, it is likely that it refers to the aforementioned condition. Galen mentions lepra, i.e., "leprosy which makes the skin scaly [...] a skin disease characterized by eruptions and loss of skin pigmentation."[324] As to elephantiasis, Ms. Escorial specifies that it is an illness that causes the skin pigmentation to change and the lower body parts to become enormous, which could suggest the more modern idea of the illness today known by this name. Cf. Galen:

> When I speak of opposites to those things mentioned, I refer to the liver being adapted to the generation of such a superfluity, a diet consisting of those foods which by nature generate blood that is thick and muddy, and a spleen that is weaker in nature and more unable to draw all that is generated to itself. In such a body, the blood becomes turbid and thickened in the veins. But sometimes the veins themselves are provided with a separative capacity for getting rid of what is abnormal, just as all other parts are, and pour this humor out through hemorrhoids. Often it rushes down to dilated (varicose) veins and is sometimes thrust toward the skin as a whole. This is the genesis of the affection people call *elephas/elephantiasis*.[325]

In *Meth. Med. G*, Galen recommends purging the melancholic humour and phlebotomy for treating elephantiasis;[326] and Išlimūn notes: "Useful against elephantiasis is to bleed the (small) saphenous vein in both shanks, and to keep shaking off (matter) by (using) that which purges the black bile."[327]

12:7 **Galen phlebotomised in putrid blood fever...**: In *Meth. Med. III*, Galen talks about "evacuating the abundance"[328] in order to cure the fever and stop the putrefaction. He also says: "It is best, then, as I said, to open a vein, not only in the continuous fevers but also in all the other fevers due to putrefaction of humors, at least whenever the factors of age and capacity do not prevent this."[329]

---

324 Galen, *Dis.*, p. 56.
325 Galen, *Meth. Med. G*, Book II, 140K (LCL 523: 550–551).
326 Galen, *Meth. Med. G*, 12 (LCL 523: 335).
327 Kahl, *The Sanskrit, Syriac and Persian Sources in the Comprehensive Book of Rhazes*, p. 169.
328 Galen, *Meth. Med. III, XI*, chapter 10 (LCL 518).
329 Galen, *Meth. Med. III, XI*, chapter 15, 785K (LCL 518).

Bad smell of urine: Hippocrates: "If the urine contain blood, pus and scales, and its odour be strong, it means ulceration of the bladder."[330] See also commentary for § 3:3.

Small particles in the urine: Ms. Escorial reads something that looks like بوره which could be بثوره 'its pustules, pustules in it,' yet the word نثرة *naṯra*, 'tiny particle' is more likely to be meant.

Lassitude: Ms. Escorial offers an uncertain reading of فورة, in this case understood as فتور *futūr*, lassitude: "In patients suffering from lassitude, says Galen, there is not much good blood, but an abundance of crude or uncocted humours; if peripheral blood is taken away by venesection, it will only be replaced by worse blood spreading outwards from the first veins to take its place."[331]

12:9 **Phlebotomising the popliteal fossa and the saphenous vein:** Galen: "You should always evacuate women who suffer from suppression of the menses from the legs, either by opening a vein or by scarifying."[332]

13:2 & 13:3 **Galen's preparation:** This prescription and the instructions of its usage correspond to Galen in *Meth. Med. 11.* Galen:

> the best of all the medications I know, and the one which is safer to use for hemorrhages from the meninges, is the one I shall speak of. Mix one part of frankincense with half a part of aloes, and then, when it comes to the time for use, mix in the white of an egg to such a degree that the whole has a honeylike consistency. Next, let this be taken up by the softest hairs of a hare, and then let it be applied in abundance to the vessel and to the whole wound. Bind externally with a linen cloth in an underbandage, making the first four or five turns on the hemorrhaging vein itself, and from that point, distribute it to the root of the vessel in those parts where it is possible to distribute to the root, which is almost all parts except for the meninges. Then, when you release it on the third day, if the medication is still adhering safely to the wound, apply another encircling bandage, moistening the tampon from the hairs, as you bound it initially. If the first tampon should fall

330 Hippocrates, *Aphorisms* IV, LXXXI (LCL 150: 156–157).
331 Brain, *Galen on Bloodletting*, p. 123.
332 Galen, *Cur. Rat. Ven. Sect.*, p. 83.

> off spontaneously, gently compress the root of the vessel with your finger until there is no further flow, then remove your finger carefully and apply another tampon.[333]

See also Maimonides, *Rules*:

> If you want to stop a hemorrhage, you should first of all put a medicine on it that stops the bleeding; then apply a bandage and observe: if it still bleeds a little bit, you should not untie the bandage; but if it bleeds a lot, you should untie the first bandage and repeat this procedure after you let the patient rest for a little while. You should leave on the bandage until the third day, then untie it gently, and if you find the medicine [still] adhering to the wound, you should add [some more medicine] to it and put a [new] bandage on it. And if you find that [the wound] has healed, you should remove it [the bandage] gently and do the same thing again.[334]

More aloe for the bodies that are dominated by dryness: Galen in *Meth. Med. II*: "Obviously, we must apply aloes more to hard bodies".[335]

Processed cotton: Ms. Escorial reads قطن لين مدبر, understood as processed cotton. What most probably is meant is what Galen above has stated, i.e., a linen cloth in an underbandage.

13:4 **And if he develops fever:** This could be understood in two ways: either as 'if he [i.e., the patient] develops a fever,' alternatively as 'if it [i.e., the phlebotomised site] becomes warm'. The first reading is deemed more plausible, suggested in Ms. Parma: "נתחדשה בו קדחת או שנפחד מזה יזה עליו פעם אחר פעם עם מי ורודים ולא יתיר", "If the patient develops fever, or if one is afraid that it could happen, one sprinkles rose water time after time on it [i.e., the wound], and does not untie it."

13:5 **Burned chalcitis:** According to Galen, chalcitis is a very strong medication to cicatrise wounds.[336] For more on the topic of healing wounds, see Galen, *Meth. Med. III* and *IV*.

---

333 Galen, *Meth. Med. II*, V, 320K–321K (LCL: 517: 22–25).
334 Maimonides, *Rules*, 75, p. 28.
335 Galen, *Meth. Med. II*, V, 322K (LCL 517: 26–27).
336 Galen, *Meth. Med. I*, III (LCL 516: 304–305).

Its prescription: In al-Rāzī's work on alchemy, *Kitāb al-Asrār*, the prescription is as follows: "You take vitriol, purify it, add the liquid of a distilled egg yolk in the amount of a quarter of the vitriol and let it solidify."[337]

The three vitriols: In Ms. Escorial al-Rāzī states that there are three vitriols. In his book on alchemy, al-Rāzī lists five vitriols: black, white, yellow, red, and green vitriol.[338] For producing vitriols artificially, see al-Rāzī, *Asrār*, pp. 107–108.

13:8 **Roman earth**: Another name for *terra sigillata*.[339]

Red and white sandalwood: The term صندلين *ṣandalayn* can be understood as a designation for the two common types of sandalwood, i.e., red sandalwood and white sandalwood, as they often are mentioned side by side.[340]

14:2 **The lateral parts of the neck**: Fonahn defines the term الأخدعان *al-aḫdaʿān* as 'the lateral parts of the neck.'[341]

14:3 **Cupping takes the blood from small veins**: Cf. Qusṭā ibn Lūqā, *Numbness*: "by cupping, the blood is extracted from narrow, invisible passages."[342]

14:5 **It relieves the head:** possibly what is meant is that cupping relieves the pain in the head and the other mentioned parts. Galen: "use a cupping glass affixed to the occiput to drive [the blood] back."[343]

14:9 … **it also makes the menstruation flow**: Galen: "You know that I have the same opinion concerning women whose menstrual purgation has been suppressed. Evacuation should not be deferred in these patients either; it is not essential, however, to open a vein, for in fact scarifications of the ankles are sufficient to eliminate the excess, since they possess some other power to urge on the menstrual changes, just as venesections at the ankles and hams do. You should always evacuate women who suffer from suppression of the menses

337 Al-Rāzī, *Asrār*, p. 108.
338 Al-Rāzī, *Asrār*, p. 102.
339 Käs, *Mineralien II*, pp. 845–847.
340 Schmucker, *Firdaws*, no. 461.
341 Fonahn, *Arabic and Latin Anatomical Terminology: Chiefly from the Middle Ages*, p. 6.
342 Qusṭā ibn Lūqā, *Numbness*, p. 59.
343 Galen, *Meth. Med. II*, V, 332K (LCL 517: 40–41).

from the legs, either by opening a vein or by scarifying."[344] In *Meth. Med.* II, XIII, Galen writes: "And if we wish to set in motion the menstrual flow, we place the cupping glass on the pubes and the inguinal glands."[345]

For women …: Ms. Escorial reads: "whoever is of the women, the appearance of her face is beautiful, and her colour is white". Qusṭā ibn Lūqā also refers to women in similar words: "who was of women, her colour white."[346] This, according to Galen, is because "Those of them who are of fairer complexion collect thinner blood, and hence derive the greatest benefit from scarification at the ankles. But treat those who are darker by phlebotomy, since they accumulate thicker and more melancholic blood, particularly if they appear to have large veins; these are found in the more slender and darker women, while smallness of the veins is characteristic of those who are plump and fair, and in these it is better to scarify the ankles than to cut a vein. And indeed these women have small veins in their legs, so that the right amount does not escape even if they are well phlebotomised."[347]

14:10 **Gradually**: Understood as increasing the strength of the suction gradually. It is the vacuum caused by the heat that causes the cup to adhere, and this could be controlled by the degree of heating the cup.[348]

14:15 **These cupping vessels may be made of copper or silver**: For more on cupping vessels, see Bliquez, *The Tools of Asclepius*, p. 56 ff.

14:16 **When they are fastened … they stanch epistaxis**: Galen: "On the same basis too, very large cupping glasses, when applied to the hypochondrium, stop hemorrhages from the nose. However, when [blood] flows from the right nostril, it is necessary to place [the cupping glass] over the liver, while when it flows from the left nostril, it is necessary to place it over the spleen, and when it flows from both nostrils, over both viscera."[349] Qusṭā ibn Lūqā confirms that cupping the false ribs is beneficial for ending epistaxis, adding that it should be conducted on the same side as the bleeding nostril.[350]

---

344 Galen, *Cur. Rat. Ven. Sect.*, p. 83.
345 Galen, *Meth. Med.* III, XIII, 971K (LCL 518: 396–397).
346 Qusṭā ibn Lūqā, *Kitāb fī l-Faṣd*, p. 339.
347 Galen, *Cur. Rat. Ven. Sect.*, pp. 83–84.
348 Bliquez, *The Tools of Asclepius*, p. 59.
349 Galen, *Meth. Med.* II, V, 316K (LCL 517: 16–17).
350 Qusṭā ibn Lūqā, *Kitāb fī l-Faṣd*, p. 342.

14:17 **If they are fastened on the breasts**: Hippocrates: "To restrain menstruation in women, apply a very large cupping instrument to the breast."[351]

14:20 †…………………†: The text is corrupt beginning from the words والحمد لله رب which are still possible to be identified somewhat clearly. Being aware of the context, the continuation most probably contains at least والحمد لله رب العالمين, of which fragments can be observed, but the last line of the text is completely erased. See commentary for § 0:1.

351 Hippocrates, *Epidemics* II, 16 (LCL 477: 80–81).

Indices

1 Index of *materia medica*

Including foodstuffs and compound drugs. Arranged in Latin alphabetical order according to the transliterated Arabic form. The vowels here are not the only possible, as there are sometimes several variant readings. The references are given in an abbreviated form. See the *key to index of materia medica* for English-Arabic.

ās آس myrtle: Cf. Ibn Ǧanāḥ II, no. 520 (p. 695): the common name for Myrtus communis L. (Myrtaceae).

afāwīh أفاويه aromatic substances: Cf. Schmucker, *Firdaws*, no. 53 (p. 78): "perfume or odoriferous substance or a thing, or substance, with which a perfume, or odoriferous substance, is compounded or prepared"; spices, fragrant flowers. All kinds of aromatic additions to drugs, food, incense and the like. Ibn Māsawayh (p. 6) divides simple aromatic substances into two categories: *al-uṣūl*, the five principal aromatic substances, that include musk, ambergris, aloeswood, camphor, and saffron, and *al-afāwīh*, 24 other aromatic substances, that include nard, cloves, sandalwood, nutmeg and mace, rose, Indian plum, cinnamon, agarwood seed, black cardamom, cubeb, cardamom, Sichuan pepper, flemingia, costus, unguis odoratus, bunk, mastic, styrax, ladanum, and kamala, while the remaining are difficult to verify, yet are given in Arabic and French: *zarnab* (l'if commun), *ḥabb al-mīsam* (le ben oléifère), *maḥlab* (le mahaleb). Cf. Ibn Ǧanāḥ I, No. 143: Ibn Māsawayh (p. 21) describes *ḥabb al-mīsam* by saying it is similar to *ḥabba ḫaḍrā'*, i.e., terebinth.

'adas عدس lentils: Cf. DTr II, no. 91 (pp. 255–256): Lens culinaris Medik. Considered difficult to digest if consumed continuously, causing several issues. Cf. Galen, *Alim. Fac.*, 1:18, p. 58: "Their juice, as stated previously, is the reverse of astringent. This is why if, after boiling them in water, one were to drink it seasoned with salt or fish sauce, and oil as well, the draught is aperient. But on boiling it twice, as described, the soup prepared from these lentils has the opposite property to the juice—drying up gastric fluxes and increasing the tone in the oesophagus, intestines and the stomach as a whole. This is why it is an appropriate food for those with gastric or dysenteric complaints."

'adasiyya عدسية 'adasiyya: Cf. Nasrallah, p. 293: A lentil dish with several varieties.

aqāqiyā أقاقيا acacia gum: Cf. Ibn Ǧanāḥ I, no. 51 (pp. 256–257): acacia gum, also Senegal gum, clearly distinguished from gum Arabic by the Arabs. Acacia gum comes from the acacia tree (Acacia nilotica (L.) Delile, Leguminosae), in Greek ἀκακία, denoting both the tree and the gum, in Arabic *aqāqiyā*, which is used only for the gum.

ʿaqīd al-ʿinab عقيد العنب grape jelly: Cf. Ibn Ǧanāḥ II, no. 566 (p. 737): grape jelly, the inpissated must of grapes.

ʿasal عسل honey: Cf. DTr II, no. 64 (p. 238): Mel commune, honey, praised as a medicine since the ancient times and used in electuaries, syrups, herbal and sour honeys, ointments, suppositories and enemas.

banafsaǧ بنفسج violet: Cf. DTr IV, no. 110 (pp. 623–624): Viola odorata L., the leaves, flowers, seeds and roots of which were used as emetics and laxatives.

bāqillāʾ باقلاء fava beans: Cf. Nasrallah, p. 796: *bāqilāʾ*, a term for fava beans used in Iraq. Cf. DTr II, no. 89 (p. 253): *al-bāqillā*, bean. Vicia faba L. and Bastarde, Leguminosae. Cf. Ibn Ǧanāḥ I, no. 184 (p. 373): *Bāqillā* (باقلّى), common name for the broad bean.

baqla ḥamqāʾ بقلة حمقاء purslane: Cf. Ibn Ǧanāḥ II, no. 751 (pp. 892–893): common purslane, Portulaca oleracea L., Portulacaceae.

barbārīs برباريس barberry, berberis: Cf. DTr I, no. 62 (pp. 145–146): *barbārīs* usually refers to Berberis vulgaris L., barberry. Dioscurides did not describe the barberry, which was unknown to the Greeks, but a rose plant, which most authors consider Crataegus oxyacantha L., hawthorn. The confusion may have arisen from the Arabs who understood barberry and hawthorn to be the same plant.

bayāḍ al-bayḍ بياض البيض egg white: in Ms. Escorial used in dressings to treat wounds.

al-bayḍ al-nīmbarišt البيض النيمبرشت soft-cooked eggs: Cf. Nasrallah, p. 830: The Arabic term for soft-cooked eggs is *al-bayḍ al-nīmbarišt*. Cf. Ibn Ǧanāḥ II, no. 626 (p. 783): *nīmbirišt*, Persian for half boiled, poached egg, as in Ḥunayn's translation of Galen's *Simple Drugs*.

biṭṭīḫ بطيخ melon: Cf. DTr II, no. 118 (p. 283): Cucumis melo L. et. al. Cucurbitaceae; Citrullus vulgaris. Cf. Ibn Ǧanāḥ I, no. 122 (p. 319): "*Biṭṭīkh Shaʾmī wa-Filasṭīnī* (Syrian and Palestinian melon). According to al-Isrāʾīlī this is the watermelon (*dullāʿ*), which is the Sindhian (*Sindī*) variety." Commentary: "*Dullāʿ* and *biṭṭīkh* are names of the common melon, Cucumis melo L., and of the watermelon, Citrullus lanatus (Thunb.) Matsum. & Nakai (synonym of Citrullis lanatus var. lanatus and Vitrullus vulgaris Schrad.; Cucurbitaceae)." Thus, *biṭṭīḫ* seems to be the term for watermelon.

bizr, pl. ***buzūr*** بزر ج. بزور Seed; spices: Cf. Ibn Ǧanāḥ I, no. 145 (p. 338): *Bizr* or *bazr*, seed; oil made of seeds. Cf. Dozy, *Supplément aux dictionnaires arabes*, p. 81: In plural it can also mean spices.

dam al-aḫawayn دم الأخوين dragon's blood: Cf. Ibn Ǧanāḥ I, no. 72 (p. 275): "the resin of Dracaena cinnabari Balf.f. (Asparagaceae), a tree found on the island of Socotra in the Arabian Sea."

dārfulful دارفلفل long pepper: Cf. DTr III, no. 134 (p. 498): Piper longum L., Piperaceae. Cf. Dioscorides, *GHD*, Book II, no. 189 (p. 199): All types of pepper generally have warming, diuretic, digestive, and dissolving properties. Cf. Nasrallah (p. 648): long pepper is beneficial for treating cold-related illnesses, strengthening the stomach, and for aiding digestion.

dārṣīnī دارصيني cinnamon: Cf. Ibn Ǧanāḥ I, no. 239 (p. 431): "*Dārṣīnī*, derived from the Persian *dār chīnī* ('Chinese wood'), is the common Arabic name of cinnamon (Cinnamomum verum J.Presl; Lauraceae [...])".

dawāʾ دواء drug, remedy: Cf. Fellmann, *Qalānisī*, no. 3. 12. (p. 183): A generic term for drugs, designating both simple and compound drugs.

dawāʾ mushil دواء مسهل purgative drug: Cf. Fellmann, *Qalānisī*, no. 3. 64. (p. 250): laxative, purgative drug, either for oral or rectal use. *Mushil* designates all drugs that have a purgative effect in the sense of humoral pathology: treating diseases equals balancing out the imbalance in body fluids which was seen as the cause of diseases. The term mostly applies to purgative drugs, but also expectorant and sweat-inducing agents come under this term.

duhn دهن oil: Cf. Fellmann, *Qalānisī*, no. 3. 13. (p. 183): pure oil, or medicinal oil.

dullāʿ دلاع common melon: Ibn Ǧanāḥ I, no. 122 (p. 319): "*Dullāʿ* and *biṭṭīkh* are names of the common melon, Cucumis melo L., and of the watermelon, Citrullus lanatus (Thunb.) Matsum. & Nakai (synonym of Citrullis lanatus var. lanatus and Vitrullus vulgaris Schrad.; Cucurbitaceae)." See also *biṭṭīḫ* above.

fawākih فواكه fruit: Cf. Galen, *Alim. Fac. II*, 7 (p. 76): "pears, apples, figs, peaches and pomegranates, and all such fruits that are useful to people as food".

ġāliya الغالية al-ġāliya: Cf. Fellmann, *Qalānisī*, no. 3. 22. (p. 196): A perfume blend that comes in various types, the basic components of which are musk and ambergris that are mixed with ben oil. Various other fragrances may be added.

ǧullāb جلاب julep, rose water syrup: Cf. Fellmann, *Qalānisī*, no. 3. 27. (p. 201): A syrup made of rose water, sugar, and perhaps other ingredients. It is used both as a cooling drink and as a purgative. For a simple julep one takes two parts of sugar mixed with six parts of rose water, boils it until half of it remains and removes the foam. Powdered saffron is added, and the drink may be dissolved with ice.

ḫall خل vinegar: Cf. Fellmann, *Qalānisī*, no. 3. 33. (pp. 210–211): Vinegar itself was regarded as a medicine, as it was thought to have a cooling effect. Vinegar also serves as a solubiliser. Cf. *Qalānisī*, no. 3. 84. (pp. 267–268): Alkaloids can be extracted from the drugs better with vinegar than with water, because they form a soluble compound with it. Thus, vinegar extracts are usually stronger than decoctions made with water. Although this chemical process naturally was unknown, the increased effect was most evidently noticed.

halīlaǧ هليلج myrobalan: Cf. Ibn Ǧulǧul, *Dio.*, no. 1 (p. 27): the fruit of Terminalia chebula tree. Cf. Ibn Ǧanāḥ II, no. 1028 (p. 1141): three kinds of myrobalan: *halīlaǧ*, chebulic myrobalan; *balīlaǧ*, myrobalan; and *amlaǧ*, emblic myrobalan.

ḥalwāʾ حلواء confection: Cf. Lane, *An Arabic-English Lexicon*, p. 634: sweetmeat; could also mean sweet fruit, or more specifically, *maǧīʿ*, a confection prepared of dates kneaded with milk.

ḫass خس lettuce: Either *ḫass barrī* (DTr IV, no. 18, p. 530) or *ḫass bustānī*, Lactuca sativa L. (DTr II, no. 119, p. 284).

ḫawlān خولان buckthorn: Cf. Ibn Ǧanāḥ, I, no. 345 (p. 524): *kuḥl Ḫawlān*, i.e., 'collyrium of the Ḫawlān,' synonymous to *ḥuḍaḍ*, which is the Arabic equivalent of varieties of buckthorn, e.g., Mediterranean buckthorn (Rhamnus lycioides L.; Rhamnaceae), and rock buckthorn (Rhamnus saxatilis Jacq.).

hindibāʾ هندباء endive: Cf. Ibn Ǧanāḥ I, no. 275 (pp. 460–461): endive, Cichorium endivia L. There are two types of *hindibāʾ*, *al-sarīs*, from the Greek σέρις, that grows in gardens, and another that grows in the wild that comes in two varieties. Like the Greek term σέρις, the Arabic *hindibāʾ* can also mean chicory (Cichorum intybus L.; Compositae). Cf. DTr II, no. 114 (p. 280): *hindibāʾ*, endive, that is *al-sarīs*, from the Greek σέρις. There are three varieties of *al-sarīs:* two wild, and one tame. The species are Cichorum intybus L., and Cichorum endivia L., endive, Compositae, and Lactuca serriola, of which endive is probably the latter.

ḥiṣrim حصرم verjuice: Cf. Schmucker, *Firdaws*, no. 245 (p. 167): juice of unripe grapes. Cf. Liddell/Scott, p. 1229a: "An acidic juice obtained by pressing unripe grapes, or a juice of other unripe fruits". Lane (*An Arabic-English Lexicon*, p. 584) mentions that crude and sour grapes (ḥiṣrim), when rubbed on the body in the bath, either bruised or pulverised, strengthens and cools the body.

ḥiṣrimiyya حصرمية ḥiṣrimiyya: Cf. Nasrallah, p. 607: a stew that is soured with the juice of unripe grapes.

ḫiyār خيار cucumber: Cf. Ibn Ǧanāḥ I, no. 190 (p. 377): Common name for cucumber (Cucumus sativus L., Cucurbitaceae).

ḫiyāršanbar خيارشنبر cassia fistula: Cf. Ibn Ǧanāḥ II, no. 875 (p. 1010): "The loanword *khiyārshanbar* refers to purging cassia, also known as 'Indian laburnum,' 'golden rain,' or 'golden shower tree' (Cassia fistula L., Leguminosae). The Arabic term is derived from the Persian form *khiyār-chanbar* composed of *khiyār* ('cucumber') and *chanbar* ('circle, collar, necklace')."

lubb ḫiyāršanbar لب خيارشنبر pulp of cassia fistula: Cf. Ibn Ǧulǧul, *Dio.*, no. 4 (p. 29): The black, slightly laxative pulp contained in the fruit of cassia fistula.

ḫubbayzā خبيزى mallow: Cf. DTr II, no. 101 (p. 266): *al-ḫubbāzā*, mallow, Malva silvestris L.; the leaves and flowers have been prescribed since the ancient times because their mucilage serves as an astringent, expectorant and soothing agent in cough medicines and gargles. The leaves are eaten as a vegetable.

ḥuqna, ḥuqan حقنة ج. حقن enema: Cf. Fellmann, *Qalānisī*, no. 3. 32. (p. 209): Enemas are water and the like boiled with drugs and oil, thereafter poured into the rectum. The composition of laxative enemas is similar to the composition of laxative decoctions, since they are both composed of laxative and diluting drugs.

ihlīlağ إهليلج myrobalan: see *halīlağ* above.

ihlīlağ aṣfar إهليلج أصفر yellow myrobalan: Cf. Ibn Ǧulǧul, *Dio.* no. 1 (p. 28): Terminalia citrina, Combretaceae.

iǧǧāṣ إجاص plum: Cf. DTr I, no. 97. (p. 184): Prunus domestica and its varieties in the Rosaceae family. Cf. Galen, *Alim. Fac.*, II:31 (p. 94): According to Galen, plums are laxative due to their moisture and viscidity, and beneficial for moistening and cooling the stomach.

ʿinab عنب grape (Schmucker, *Firdaws*, no. 500). Cf. Ibn Ǧanāḥ I, no. 65 (pp. 267–268): grapevine, Vitis vinifera L., Vitaceae. Galen regards grapes as more nutritious than other seasonal fruits (Galen, *Alim. Fac.*, II:9, pp. 77–78).

ʿinab al-ṯaʿlab عنب الثعلب nightshade: Cf. DTr IV, no. 63 (p. 573f.): Several species of nightshade plants from the Solanaceae family, including e.g., Solanum nigrum L., Solanum villosum L., Solanum dulcamara L., Solanum alkekengi L., Atropa belladonna L. They have a soporific effect that can lead to death.

isfānāḫ إسفاناخ spinach: Cf. Schmucker, *Firdaws*, no. 30 (p. 67): Spinacia oleracea L., spinach.

isfīdāǧ إسفيداج ceruse: Cf. Ibn Ǧanāḥ I, no. 76 (p. 278): ceruse, white lead.

isfīḏbāǧ إسفيذباج isfīḏbāǧ: Cf. Nasrallah, p. 608: A white dish, notorious for being a balanced dish fit for all. Cf. Fellmann, *Qalānisī*, no. 3. 67. (p. 252): *isfīḏbāǧa*, a dish, perhaps a soup, made of meat, onions, oil and cottage cheese.

iyāraǧ al-fīqrā ايارج الفيقرا hiera picra, bitter hiera: Cf. Fellmann, *Qalānisī*, no. 3. 38. (p. 216): *iyāraǧ fīqrā*, from the Greek ἱερὰ πικρά = bitteres Heiligmittel, i.e., 'divine bitter'; Cf. Kahl, *Sābūr ibn Sahl; The Small Dispensatory*, p. 72; ἱερά, a name for several medicines in the Greek pharmacological tradition.

kāfūr كافور camphor: Cf. DTr III, no. 24 (p. 370): The white, translucent mass obtained from Cinnamomum camphora [L.], or Drybalanops aromatica,

Dipterocarpaceae. Cf. Ibn Ǧanāḥ I, no. 211 (p. 398): "the bract (*qishr*) of the inflorescence of the date palm".

kaṯīrā' كثيراء tragacanth: Cf. DTr III, no. 21 (p. 366): the gum resin that forms in the root and stem of several species of Astragalus gummifer Labill et. al.

kummaṯrā كمثرى pear: Cf. DTr I, no. 91 (p. 179): Pyrus communis L., Rosaceae. The word comes originally from Akkadian.

kundur كندر frankincense: Cf. DTr I, no. 30 (p. 113): *al-kundur*, synonymous with *al-lubān* or *al-lūbān*, is frankincense, the dried gum resin of Boswellia species, particularly Boswellia Carteri Birdw., Burseraceae. It originates from Southern Arabia and Somalia, especially Šiḥr in Oman, as mentioned by Dioscorides.

kuzbura كزبرة coriander: DTr III, no. 60 (p. 411): Coriandrum sativum L., used both medically and as a spice. The name originates from Akkadian.

laqāniq لقانق laqāniq: Cf. Nasrallah, p. 610: Small, spicy sausages.

liḥyat al-tays لحية التيس goatsbeard: Cf. DTr II, no. 126 (p. 292): *liḥyat al-tays*, lit. goatsbeard, from the Greek τραγοπώγων, which is either Tragopogon pratensis L. or Tragopogon porrifolious L. The fresh plant provides good fodder and vegetables. In medicine especially its milky juice, *ʿuṣāra*, is used.

lubāb al-ḫubz لباب الخبز bread pith (Nasrallah, p. 570).

mā' ماء water: Cf. Fellmann, *Qalānisī*, no. 3. 53. (p. 239): Water, *mā'*, usually refers to a drug extract that is made with water.

mā' al-šaʿīr ماء الشعير barley broth: Cf. Nasrallah, p. 448: A decoction of barley with water. Literally barley water, also known as barley broth, barley gruel, or ptisane.

maḥmūda محمودة scammony: Cf. DTr IV, no. 160 (p. 674): المحمودة, *al-maḥmūda*, is a synonym for السقمونيا, *al-saqmūniyā*, convolvulus scammonia. The resin of the dried, milky sap extracted from its living roots has a strong laxative effect.

māmīṯā ماميثا glaucium: Cf. DTr III, no. 81 (p. 437): Glaucium, arabicised as *ġalawqiyūn* from the Greek γλαύκιον, *šiyāf māmiṯā*, or simply *māmiṯā*. The drug is the juice of Glaucium corniculatum L. a variety of red-horned poppy, and Glaucium flavum, yellow-horned poppy, Papaveraceae. The root of the red-horned poppy is said to have a smell similar to opium, and the crushed seeds were used as an eye remedy.

martak مرتك litharge: Cf. Ibn Ǧanāḥ II, no. 543 (p. 716): synonymous with *murdāsanǧ*, both denoting litharge, lead oxide. Both terms appear in Ms. Escorial.

maṣṭakā مصطكى mastic: Cf. Ibn Ǧanāḥ II, no. 562 (p. 733): mastic, resin of Pistacia lentiscus L. (Anacardiaceae).

maṭbūḫ مطبوخ decoction: Cf. Fellmann, *Qalānisī*, no. 3. 63. (pp. 245–246): decoctions are juices of drugs when cooked in water. Boiling on light to medium fire allows the powers of the drugs to release without being destroyed. The purpose of decoctions is to soften the nature and to purify it.

mayba ميبة mayba: Cf. Fellmann, *Qalānisī*, no. 3. 53 (p. 238): Mayba is a composite drink made from quince juice and wine. Quince juice is boiled with honey until the mixture defoams and thickens, and sugar and various spices are added.

milḥ ملح salt: Cf. Schmucker, *Firdaws*, no. 737: salt.

misk مسك musk: Cf. Ibn Ǧulǧul, *Dio.*, no. 33 (p. 51): Musk, the glandular secretion of the male musk deer (Moschus moschiferus L., Cervidae), obtained from the preputial sac near the navel of the animal.

mudaqqaqāt مدققات mudaqqaqāt: Cf. Nasrallah, p. 611: Spicy, ground meat cooked into casserole-like dishes.

murr مر myrrh: Cf. DTr I, no. 27 (p. 110): The gum resin obtained from the bark of several species of Commiphora abyssinica Burseraceae. Cf. Lane, *An Arabic-English Lexicon*, p. 2701: Myrrh, a certain medicine, used orally for cough and intestinal worms, and on a plaster for scorpion stings.

murdāsanǧ مرداسنج litharge: see *martak* above.

muṭaǧǧanāt مطجنات muṭaǧǧanāt: Cf. Nasrallah, p. 612: A dish made of poultry, seasoned with spices and herbs.

muzawwarāt مزورات muzawwarāt: Cf. Nasrallah, p. 433: Vegetarian dishes, lighter than meat dishes and easier to digest.

nabīḏ نبيذ wine: Cf. Nasrallah, pp. 468–470: wine made by using either dates, *dāḏī* (strong date wine), or grapes, or a combination of these. Cf. Galen, *Alim. Fac.* III:39 (pp. 149–150): "The thick, red ones are the most useful of all wines for the production of blood, since they require the least change into it".

nasǧ al-ʿankabūt نسج العنكبوت cobweb: (Dozy, *Supplément aux dictionnaires arabes*, p. 666). Cf. Riddle, *Dio. Pharm. Med.* (Book II, 68, p. 107): According to Dioscorides, when cobweb is applied, it stops bleeding and prevents the occurrences of ulcers that emerge on the surface of the skin due to inflammation.

našāʾ نشاء starch: Cf. Schmucker, *Firdaws*, no. 769 (p. 509): starch, starch paste, amylum. The best kind is made from good wheat.

qāqulla قاقلة black cardamom: Cf. Ibn Ǧanāḥ I, no. 280 (pp. 467–468): *qāqulla*, *hāl* and *hīl* all denote cardamom. Whereas *hāl*, *hīl* and *hīl bū* stand for the smaller variety, *qāqulla* is the larger variety, i.e., black cardamom. Cf. Ibn Ǧulǧul, *Dio.*, no. 9 (p. 33): *qāqulla* is Elettaria cardamum maior, Zingiberaceae.

qarʿ قرع gourd, pumpkin: Cf. DTr II, no. 116 (p. 282): Three different plants from the cucurbitaceae family: Cucurbita maxima, Cucurbita pepo, Lagenaria vulgaris.

qarāsiyā قراسيا cherry: Cf. DTr I, no. 84 (p. 174): Prunus avium L. et. al., Rosaceae, and Prunus mahaleb L., et. al. Cf. Ibn Ǧanāḥ II, no. 869 (p. 1004): *al-qarāsiyā*, from the Greek κεράσια, cherry.

qaranful قرنفل cloves: Cf. Ibn Ǧulǧul, *Dio.*, no. 19 (p. 34): cloves, "Syzygium aromaticum [L.] Merr. et L.M. Perry, Myrtaceae (Caryophyllus aromaticus L.)."

qaṭaf قطف orach: Cf. Ibn Ǧanāḥ I, no. 124 (p. 322): *Qaṭaf*, the Arabic name for garden orach (Atriplex hortensis L., Amaranthaceae). Other names for it are *al-baqla al-ḏahabiyya*, 'the golden vegetable,' and *baql al-Rūm*, 'vegetable of the Romans.'

qiṯṯāʾ قثاء cucumber: Cf. Ibn Ǧulǧul, *Dio.*, no. 43 (p. 57): often treated as synonymous to *ḫiyār*, Cucumis sativus L. and Var. Cf. DTr IV, no. 139 (pp. 655–656): *al-qiṯṯāʾ al-barrī*, also known as *qiṯṯāʾ al-ḥimār*, i.e., Ecballium elaterium, squirting cucumber.

qulquṭār قلقطار chalcitis: Cf. Ibn Ǧanāḥ II, no. 817 (pp. 952–953): *qulquṭār* is chalcitis, a variety of vitriol.

qūqāyā قوقايا qūqāyā: Cf. Galen, *Meth. Med.* III, XIV (p. 971:8): a compound drug composed of aloes, scammony and colocynth. Cf. Fellmann, *Qalānisī*, no. 3. 29. 1. (pp. 205–206): *Qūqāyā* cleanses the head, hence the name, as al-Qalānisī traces the name back to the Greek and the Syriac word for 'head.' The name *ḥabb al-qūqāyā* is a tautology, as the Greek word *qūqāyā* means berry, grain, the same as the Arabic *ḥabb*.

qurṣ, aqrāṣ قرص ج. أقراص pastille: Cf. Fellmann, *Qalānisī*, no. 3. 75: pastille.

rāwand ṣīnī راوند صيني Chinese rhubarb: Cf. DTr III, 2 (p. 344): Chinese rhubarb, Rheum palmatum var. tanguticum, Polygonaceae, used as a laxative and astringent for gastrointestinal ailments. Cf. Schmucker, *Firdaws*, no. 321 (pp. 205–206): *rāwand ṣīnī* at times designates a separate species, at times a synonym for *rāwand*, for which it is representative as the most well-known species: Chinese rhubarb, usually called Rheum palmatum var. tanguticum, medicinal rhubarb, native to high Asia (Tibet and the Chinese provinces of Kansu and Shensi). Cf. Clementi & Misiti, *Potential Health Benefits of Rhubarb*, p. 407 ff.: *Da huang*. Chinese rhubarb has been used as a purgative drug in Chinese herbal medicine for over two thousand years. The root and the stalk are used in medicine, while the leaves are poisonous.

rāziyānaǧ aḫḍar رازيانج أخضر green fennel: Cf. DTr III, no. 66 (p. 419): Foeniculum vulgare L. et. al., several varieties of fennel. Both the seeds and the root were used in medicine.

rayāḥīn رياحين fragrant herbs: Cf. Schmucker, *Firdaws*, no. 332 (p. 209): plural of *rayḥān*, a generic name for fragrant herbs that are similar to basil.

riǧla رجلة purslane: Cf. Ibn Ǧanāḥ II, no. 751 (pp. 892–893): common purslane, Portulaca oleracea L., Portulacaceae.

rummān رمان pomegranate: Cf. DTr I, no. 81 (p. 170): The fruit of Punica granatum L. et. al., Punicacaea. Cf. Dioscorides, *GHD*, Book I, 151 (p. 80): Dioscorides identifies three sorts of pomegranates: the sweet, that is the best for the stomach; a sharp one, that helps a burning stomach; and a species that in its taste resembles wine, that is of middle strength. They all are tasty and good for the stomach, yet do not nourish.

rummāniyya رمانية rummāniyya: Cf. Nasrallah, p. 614: a dish prepared with pomegranate and chicken.

sabistān سبستان sebesten: Cf. Ibn Ǧanāḥ II, no. 666 (pp. 825–826): "*sabistān* is a common Arabic name 'sebesten fruits' produced by Cordia myxa L. ('Assyrian plum', Boraginaceae)."

safarǧal سفرجل quince: Cf. DTr I, no. 87 (p. 176): Cydonia oblonga Mill., Rosaceae. Cf. Galen, *Alim. Fac.* II:23 (pp. 89–90): Galen, calling these Cydonian and Strouthian apples, mentions that quinces are more astringent than other apples, thus good for preserving. He refers to his own medication of the Strouthian apple, i.e., quince, containing quince juice, honey, white pepper, ginger, and vinegar, that he used to treat people with anorexia.

sarīs سريس endive: Cf. DTr II, no. 114 (p. 280): Possible species are Cichorium intybus L. et. al., and Cichorium endivia L. et. al., Compositae. See also *hindibāʾ*.

sawīq al-šaʿīr سويق الشعير Barley gruel: Cf. Ibn Ǧanāḥ II, no. 1038 (p. 1153): *sawīq*, gruel. See also *māʾ al-šaʿīr*.

sukkar سكر sugar: Cf. DTr II, no. 65 (p. 238): Saccharum officinarum L., cane sugar, or sugar cane. It is said to have been brought from India to Egypt in the ancient times. Used both for its medicinal effects and for its taste.

sukkar ṭabarzadī سكر طبرزدي Ṭabarzad sugar:: Cf. Nasrallah, p. 602: "*ṭabarzad* (طبرزد) *tabarzan* (تبرزن) *tabarzal* (تبرزل) fine-quality white and refined cane sugar *qand*. It is usually sold in solid molded cone-shaped masses as they take the shape of the clay vessels in which cane sugar is washed and refined. […] The medieval name *ṭabarzad* is not descriptive of the quality of the sugar itself as much as the way it is used: *tabar* is a Persian loan word for hatchet or axe used to chisel the amount needed from the solid mass of sugar." Cf. Ibn Ǧanāḥ II, no. 634 (p. 791): crystalline sugar.

sikanǧubīn سكنجبين Oxymel:, or sour honey: Cf. Fellmann, *Qalānisī*, no. 3. 84. (pp. 267–268): a potion composed of vinegar and honey. For pure oxymel one part of wine vinegar, two parts of fresh water, and three parts of *ṭabar-*

zad sugar are boiled until the liquid becomes consistent. This recipe could be used as a base, and altered by changing the honey to sugar, or the vinegar to quince juice and the like. Alkaloids can be extracted from the drugs better with vinegar than with water, because they form a soluble compound with it. Thus, vinegar extracts are usually stronger than decoctions made with water. Although this chemical process naturally was unknow, the increased effect was most evidently noticed. As for sugar and honey, that generally were considered interchangeable, they were credited for enhancing the moist properties. Thus, oxymel helped to combine the power of drugs with the medicinal effects of vinegar and sugar.

sikbāǧ سكباج sikbāǧ: Cf. Nasrallah, pp. 248–255: a variety of beef stews soured with vinegar.

silq سلق chard: Cf. Ibn Ǧanāḥ II, no. 647 (pp. 807–808): chard, Beta vulgaris L.

summāqiyya سماقية summāqiyya: Cf. Nasrallah, p. 299: a meat dish with strained sumac juice. As for sumac, cf. Ibn Ǧanāḥ II, no. 1003 (p. 1120): tanner's sumach, Rhus coriaria L., and smokebush, Cotinus coggygria Scop.; Anacardiaceae.

sunbul al-ṭīb سنبل الطيب Indian nard: Cf. Schmucker, *Firdaws*, no. 403 (p. 248): Valeriana jatamansi Roxb. (Valerianaceae), Indian nard.

sūs سوس liquorice: Cf. Ibn Ǧanāḥ II, no. 695 (pp. 846–847): "The term *sūs*, derived from a Semitic root, is the common Arabic name of liquorice, the root of Glycyrrhiza glabra L."

šāhasbaram شاهسبرم šāhasbaram: Cf. Nasrallah, p. 671: شاهسبرم also *šāhasfaram*, شاهسفرم, is an aromatic variety of mint with small leaves that also helps to induce sleep and relieve headache. Cf. Ibn Ǧanāḥ II, no. 987 (pp. 1105–1106): one of several variant spellings of *šāh-išbaram*, *rayḥān al-malik*, or *iklīl al-malik*, a variety of basil with small leaves, probably bush basil (Ocimum minimum L., Lamiaceae).

šaḥm شحم fat: Cf. DTr II, no. 63 (p. 237): Fat, lard, tallow, etc.; fatty substances in general are among the oldest medical substances as they are easily obtained and durable. The variety of fatty substances used depends on the number of native, mainly domestic, animals. In Islam, pork fat was not used, and animal fats were replaced by vegetable oils as much as possible. In medicine, fats were used for rubbing in, and as a basis for plasters, ointments, and waxes.

šaʿīr شعير barley: Cf. DTr II, no. 72 (p. 242): parent plant for barley is Hordeum vulgare L, and var., Gramineae.

šamʿ شمع wax (Ibn Ǧanāḥ II, no. 539, p. 713).

šarāb, ašriba شراب ج. أشربة syrup, potion: Cf. Fellmann, *Qalānisī*, no. 3. 87. (p. 269): Syrups prepared of fruit and other juices, boiled with sugar and honey until they have a consistency similar to oxymel or apple syrup. When you squeeze fruit or vegetables, the resulting juice is 'press juice,' i.e., sap (*ʿuṣāra*). When the juice is thickened by boiling, or by leaving it in the sun, it is called 'thickened juice' (*rubb*), and when sugar is added and it is thickened, it is called syrup (*šarāb*). Syrup contains more sugar in relation to fruit.

šarāb al-ʿasal شراب العسل melicratum: Cf. Riddle, *Dio. Pharm. Med.*, p. 144: "Very popular as a drink and as a medicine in antiquity was melicraton, or water mead (V. 9). This was a mixture of honey and water allowed to ferment. Among its usages was one for coughs."

ṣabir صبر aloe:: Cf. Ibn Ǧanāḥ II, no. 522 (pp. 696–697): "*Ṣabir* is the common Arabic name of aloe (Aloe vera (L.) Burm.f.; or Aloe ferox Mill.)."

ṣaʿtar صعتر oregano: Cf. Ibn Ǧanāḥ I, no. 365 (p. 540): "*ṣaʿtar* is an Arabic name of oregano (Origanum vulgare L., Lamiaceae)".

ṣamġ ʿarabī صمغ عربي gum Arabic: Cf. Schmucker, *Firdaws*, no. 460 (p. 282): gum from Acacia gummifera, A. spirocarpa, i.e., Mimosa gummifera, A. vera, i.e., Mimosa nilotica. Cf. Abdelkareem (p. 184): the fluid from Acacia seyal or Acacia senegal trees, used in traditional medicine for pain relief, as a glue, and a number of other ailments.

ṣandal صندل sandalwood: Cf. Schmucker, *Firdaws*, no. 461: white sandalwood, Santalum album L. (Santalaceae); red sandalwood, Pterocarpus santalinus L. (Papilionaceae). The term *ṣandalayn* can be understood as a designation for the two common types, i.e., red sandalwood and white sandalwood, since they often are mentioned side by side. Cf. Dozy, *Supplément aux dictionnaires arabes*, pp. 358–359, on the sobriquet *maqāṣīrī*: white sandalwood, *sandalos cetrinos*, of yellowish colour. This yellow, pale species is called *santalum citrinum* in pharmacies, in Latin *santalum pallidum* or *santalum odoratum*. There are several kinds of sandal: the best is the yellow sandal, that has an aromatic smell, and it is called *maqāṣīrī. Maqāṣīrī* is yellow, *Ǧawrī* is white. Cf. DTr III, no. 38 (p. 385): ʿAbdallāh b. Ṣāliḥ says that even thyme, Thymus serpullum L., Labiatae is called *ṣandal*.

tamr hindī تمر هندي tamarind: Cf. Ibn Ǧulǧul, *Dio.*, no. 5 (p. 30): Tamarindus indica L., Leguminosae.

taranǧubīn ترنجبين manna: Cf. Maimonides, *Glossary*, no. 386: arabicised from the Persian tarangubīn "honey of dew", that corresponds to the Biblical *mān*.

tīn تين fig: Cf. DTr I, no. 107 (p. 192): Ficus carica Moraceae, native to the Near East and highly valued since earliest antiquity.

tuffāḥ تفاح apple: Cf. DTr I, no. 86 (p. 175): understood by most authors as Malus sylvestris [L.] Mill. (Pyrus Malus L.).

ṭabāhiǧāt طباهجات ṭabāhiǧāt: Cf. Nasrallah, (pp. 617–618): A dish made of red meat, seasoned with spices and herbs.

ṭabāšīr طباشير tabasheer, bamboo chalk; Cf. Ibn Ǧanāḥ II, no. 904, (p. 1035): "'Tabasheer' is a white substance obtained from the nodal joints of bamboo (Bambusa bambos (L.) Voss)."

ṭīn maḫtūm طين مختوم terra sigillata; sealed earth: Cf. Ibn Ǧanāḥ II, no. 569, (p. 739): terra sigillata, famous red earth, from the isle of Lemnos. Cf. Riddle, *Dio. Pharm. Med.*, p. 162: "Taking dirt as a medicine appears at first to be 'dirty, ignorant medicine'. Any soil scientist and a few historians of pharmacy will know that dirt is a word that describes a variety of minerals, some of which have medicinal use."

ṭīn rūmī طين رومي Roman earth: Cf. Ibn Ǧanāḥ II, no. 1054, (p. 1166): Roman earth, *ṭīn rūmī*, according to al-Rāzī is the same as *ḫawātim al-buḥayra*, that is listed as equal to terra sigillata in his *Ḥāwī*. Cf. Käs, *Mineralien II*, pp. 845–847: *ṭīn rūmī*, another name for *ṭīn maḫtūm*, terra sigillata.

usṭumāḫīqūn, usṭumāḫīqūnāt اسطماخيقون ج. اسطماخيقونات stomachic: Cf. Fellmann, *Qalānisī*, no. 3. 29. 3. (p. 207): Usṭumaḫīqūn, a stomach pill, a purgative remedy, deriving from the Greek word στομαχικός.

utruǧǧ أترج citron: Cf. DTr I, no. 90 (p. 178): Citrus Limon [L.] Burm. (Citrus medica L.) et. al.

ʿunnāb عناب jujube: Cf. Ibn Ǧanāḥ II, no. 736 (p. 542): Ziziphus jujuba Mill., also called Chinese date. Cf. Galen, *Alim. Fac.* II:32 (p. 95): Galen viewed jujube only as "poorly nutritious and difficult to concoct, and at the same time bad for the stomach".

ʿuṣāra عصارة sap: Cf. Fellmann, *Qalānisī*, no. 3. 53. (p. 239): sap, *ʿuṣāra*, is a juice that is pressed out of the drug without adding water. Ibid. p. 269: When you squeeze fruit or vegetables, the resulting juice is 'press juice,' i.e., sap (*ʿuṣāra*).

wabar al-arnab وبر الأرنب hare's fur: in Ms. Escorial an ingredient in a dressing.

ward ورد rose: Cf. DTr I, no. 68 (p. 155): Genus Rosa, numerous species of the Rosaceae family.

zabīb زبيب raisins: Cf. Ibn Ǧanāḥ I, no. 488 (p. 659): Small, seedless grapes, or raisins, also known as *kišmiš*.

zaʿfarān زعفران saffron: Cf. DTr I, no. 23 (p. 108) Crocus sativus L. et. al., Iridaceae. Cf. Lane, *An Arabic-English Lexicon*, p. 1231: saffron, a perfume and a dye.

zāǧ زاج vitriol: Cf. Schmucker, *Firdaws*, no. 336 (p. 210): vitriol, mostly iron, copper, or zinc sulfate (crystallised and containing water of crystallisation).

zāǧ aḫḍar زاج أخضر green vitriol: Cf. Ibn Ǧanāḥ I, no. 313, (pp. 494–495): Green vitriol (*zāǧ aḫḍar*) is the same as Cyprian vitriol (*zāǧ Qubrusī*). Dozy (*Supplément aux dictionnaires arabes*, p. 610) gives iron sulfate.

zāǧ aṣfar زاج أصفر yellow vitriol: Cf. Ibn Ǧanāḥ I, no. 314, (p. 495): yellow vitriol (*zāǧ aṣfar*) is the vitriol of the shoemakers (*zāǧ al-asākifa*). According to most Arabic sources it is a synonym for *qulquṭār*, chalcitis (χαλκῖτις) for Dioscorides.

zanǧabīl زنجبيل ginger: Cf. DTr II, no. 144 (p. 306): Zingiber officinalis Roscoe, Zingiberaceae.

zīrbāǧa زيرباجة *zīrbāǧa*: Cf. Nasrallah, p. 620: A delicate stew made of birds, lightly seasoned, and soured with vinegar and balanced with sugar, praised by many for its perfectly balanced properties. Cf. Fellmann, *Qalānisī*, no. 3. 67. (p. 252): broth or spoon-meat.

2 Key to Index of *materia medica*

(English–transliterated Arabic form)

aromatic substances	*afāwīh*
ʿadasiyya, a lentil dish	*ʿadasiyya*
acacia gum	*aqāqiyā*
aloe	*ṣabir*
apple	*tuffāḥ*
barberry; berberis	*barbārīs*
barley	*šaʿīr*
barley broth	*māʾ al-šaʿīr*
barley gruel	*sawīq al-šaʿīr*
black cardamom	*qāqulla*
buckthorn	*ḫawlān*
bitter hiera	*iyāraǧ al-fīqrā*
bread pith	*lubāb al-ḫubz*
cassia fistula	*ḫiyāršanbar*
camphor	*kāfūr*
ceruse	*isfīdāǧ*
chalcitis	*qulquṭār*
chard	*silq*
cherry	*qarāsiyā*
Chinese rhubarb	*rāwand ṣīnī*
cinnamon	*dārṣīnī*
citron	*utruǧǧ*
cloves	*qaranful*
cobweb	*nasǧ al-ʿankabūt*
common melon	*dullāʿ*
confection	*ḥalwāʾ*

coriander	*kuzbura*
cucumber	*ḫiyār*
cucumber, squirting	*qiṯṯāʾ*
decoction	*maṭbūḫ*
dragon's blood	*dam al-aḫawayn*
drug	*dawāʾ*
eggwhite	*bayāḍ al-bayḍ*
endive	*hindibāʾ, sarīs*
enema	*ḥuqna*
fat	*šaḥm*
fava beans	*bāqillāʾ*
fennel, green	*rāziyānaǧ aḫḍar*
fig	*tīn*
fragrant herbs	*rayāḥīn*
frankincense	*kundur*
fruit	*fawākih*
ġāliya	*ġāliya*
ginger	*zanǧabīl*
glaucium	*māmīṯā*
goatsbeard	*liḥyat al-tays*
gourd	*qarʿ*
grape	*ʿinab*
grape jelly	*ʿaqīd al-ʿinab*
gum Arabic	*ṣamġ ʿarabī*
hare's fur	*wabar al-arnab*
ḥiṣrimiyya, a dish	*ḥiṣrimiyya*
honey	*ʿasal*
Indian nard	*sunbul al-ṭīb*
isfīḏbāǧ, a dish	*isfīḏbāǧ*
jujube	*ʿunnāb*
julep	*ǧullāb*
laqāniq, a dish	*laqāniq*
lentils	*ʿadas*
litharge	*martak, murdāsanǧ*
liquorice	*sūs*
long pepper	*dārfulful*
manna	*taranǧubīn*
mallow	*ḫubbayzā*
mastic	*maṣṭakā*
mayba: quince wine	*mayba*

melon	*biṭṭīḫ*
melicratum	*šarāb al-ʿasal*
musk	*misk*
mudaqqaqāt, a dish	*mudaqqaqāt*
muṭaǧǧanāt, a dish	*muṭaǧǧanāt*
muzawwarāt, a dish	*muzawwarāt*
myrrh	*murr*
myrobalan	*halīlaǧ, ihlīlaǧ*
myrobalan, yellow	*ihlīlaǧ aṣfar*
myrtle	*ās*
nightshade	*ʿinab al-ṯaʿlab*
oil	*duhn*
orach	*qaṭaf*
oregano	*ṣaʿtar*
oxymel	*sikanǧubīn*
pastille	*qurṣ*
pear	*kummaṯrā*
plum	*iǧǧāṣ*
pomegranate	*rummān*
purgative drug	*dawāʾ mushil*
purslane	*riǧla, baqla ḥamqāʾ*
quince	*safarǧal*
qūqāyā	*qūqāyā*
raisins	*zabīb*
Roman Earth	*ṭīn rūmī*
rose	*ward*
rummāniyya, a dish	*rummāniyya*
saffron	*zaʿfarān*
salt	*milḥ*
sap	*ʿuṣāra*
scammony	*maḥmūda*
sandalwood	*ṣandal*
sebesten	*sabistān*
seed	*bizr*
soft-cooked eggs	*al-bayḍ al-nīmbarišt*
starch	*našāʾ*
stomachic	*usṭumāḫīqūn*
spinach	*isfānāḫ*
sugar	*sukkar*
sugar, crystalline	*sukkar ṭabarzadī*

summāqiyya, a dish	*summāqiyya*
syrup	*šarāb*
šāhasbaram	*šāhasbaram*
tamarind	*tamr hindī*
tragacanth	*kaṯīrāʾ*
ṭabāhiğāt, a dish	*ṭabāhiğāt*
bamboo chalk	*ṭabāšīr*
terra sigillata	*ṭīn maḫtūm*
verjuice	*ḥiṣrim*
violet	*banafsağ*
vinegar	*ḫall*
vitriol	*zāğ*
vitriol, green	*zāğ aḫḍar*
vitriol, yellow	*zāğ aṣfar*
water	*māʾ*
wax	*šamʿ*
wine	*nabīḏ*
zīrbağa, a dish	*zīrbāğa*

3 Index of Weights and Measures

The basis of all Islamic weighting is formed by the *dirham*, deriving from the Greek drachma, and the *miṯqāl*, deriving from the Roman-Byzantine solidus. According to Islamic law, the relation between *miṯqāl* and *dirham* is 10:7, in practice, 3:2. However, a multitude weights in the Islamic world, varying according to time and place, have developed, and they denote somewhat varying weights.[1] In the case of al-Rāzī, one could assume that the values of different weights and measures are the ones that were used in Iraq.

The weights and measures presented below are mentioned in Hinz, *Islamische Masse und Gewichte*, and more specifically for al-Rāzī, in Kahl, *The Sanskrit, Syriac and Persian Sources in the Comprehensive Book of Rhazes*.

3.1 *Dirham* and *miṯqāl*

Hinz suggests that we can assume the standard value of one *dirham* to be of 3.125 grams, unless specified otherwise. By using the standard value of 3.125 g

1 Hinz, *Islamische Masse und Gewichte*, p. 1.

for a *dirham*, applied in the ratio of 7:10 to reach the weight of the canonical *miṯqāl*, the latter weighs 4.464 g.[2] These values seem to be the same for Iraq and Syria, and comparing with data provided by different authors the value of *miṯqāl* and *dirham* safely can be assumed to be as attested above.[3]

A measure called *dirham al-kayl* is mentioned in Ms. Escorial as well.[4] Since one *dirham al-kayl*, 'weight *dirham*,' is 2/3 *miṯqāl*, *dirham al-kayl* is exactly 3.125 g.[5] Hence, it seems to denote the same measure as a regular *dirham*. Kahl suggests that *dirham* and *miṯqāl*, as used by al-Rāzī, correspond to one *dirham* being 3.13 g and one *miṯqāl* 4.46 g.[6]

3.2 *Raṭl*

An Umayyad *raṭl* from Syria from 744 A.D. weighs 337.55 g. It should represent a provincial pound to 72 *miṯqāls*. A *raṭl* from the Fatimid times, the weight of which is 140 *dirhams*, weighs 437.2067 g, confirming the weight of a *dirham* as 3.123 g.[7]

The *raṭl* of Baghdad was canonical: it was stated by one school of law to consist of 128 4/7 *dirhams*, and according to another of 130 *dirhams*. Around the year 1050, the authority of Mar Eliya of Nisib consistently based its value to be 130 *dirhams* (i.e., 406.25 g).[8] Kahl's definition of a *raṭl* is 406 g.[9]

3.3 *Ūqiyya*

The *ūqiyya*, or ounce, is basically 1/12 *raṭls*.[10] The ounce of Baghdad was 10 5/6 *dirhams*, i.e., 33.85 grams.[11] For *ūqiyya*, Kahl suggests the weight of 33 g.[12]

dirham, darāhim	درهم ج. دراهم	*dirham* (3.125 g)
dirham al-kayl	درهم الكيل	*dirham al-kayl* (3.125 g)
ǧuzʾ, aǧzāʾ	جزء ج. أجزاء	part

2 Hinz, *Islamische Masse und Gewichte*, pp. 3–4.
3 Hinz, *Islamische Masse und Gewichte*, p. 5.
4 Spelled in Ms. Escorial as *dirham kaylan*.
5 Hinz, *Islamische Masse und Gewichte*, p. 3.
6 Kahl, *The Sanskrit, Syriac and Persian Sources in the Comprehensive Book of Rhazes*, p. 67.
7 Hinz, *Islamische Masse und Gewichte*, p. 3.
8 Hinz, *Islamische Masse und Gewichte*, p. 31.
9 Kahl, *The Sanskrit, Syriac and Persian Sources in the Comprehensive Book of Rhazes*, p. 67.
10 Hinz, *Islamische Masse und Gewichte*, p. 34.
11 Hinz, *Islamische Masse und Gewichte*, p. 35.
12 Kahl, *The Sanskrit, Syriac and Persian Sources in the Comprehensive Book of Rhazes*, p. 67.

miṯqāl, maṯāqīl	مثقال ج. مثاقيل	*miṯqāl* (4.46 g)
raṭl, arṭāl	رطل ج. أرطال	*raṭl*, pound (406.25 g)
rubʿ, arbāʿ	ربع ج. أرباع	quarter
ūqiyya, -āt	أوقية -ات	*ūqiyya*, ounce (33.85 g)

4 Index of Instruments and Utensils

hāwūn, hawāwīn	هاوون ج. هواوين	mortar
ḫirqa, ḫiraq	خرقة ج. خرق	cloth
ḥuqna, ḥuqan	حقنة ج. حقن	enema
ibra, ibar	إبرة ج. إبر	needle
kūz faḫḫār, akwāz faḫḫār	كوز فخار ج. أكواز فخار	ceramic jug
mibḍaʿ, mabāḍiʿ	مبضع ج. مباضع	scalpel
miḥǧama, maḥāǧim	محجمة ج. محاجم	cupping vessel
qidr, qudūr	قدر ج. قدور	cooking pot
šafra, šifār	شفرة ج. شفار	blade
sinnāra, sanānīr	سنارة ج. سنانير	hook
zuǧāǧa, -āt	زجاجة -ات	bottle
ẓarf zuǧāǧ, ẓurūf zuǧāǧ	ظرف زجاج ج. ظروف زجاج	receptacle of glass

5 Index of Places

6 Index of Personal Names

7 Index of Works Cited

8 Index of Pharmaceutical Forms

ʿiṣāba, ʿaṣāʾib	عصابة ج. عصائب	bandage
ʿuṣāra	عصارة	sap

9 Index of Terms Used in Preparations of Drugs

aḏāba	أذاب	melt
aḍāfa	أضاف	add
ʿaǧana	عجن	knead
aḫaḏa	أخذ	take
alqā ʿalayhi	ألقى عليه	add
anqā	أنقى	cleanse, purify
ʿaṣara	عصر	press, squeeze
ḍamada	ضمد	dress, bandage
daqqa	دقّ	pound
ǧaffafa	جفّف	dry
ǧamaʿa	جمع	bring together
ǧaraša	جرش	crush
ḥalla	حلّ	dissolve
marasa	مرس	soak
naḫala	نخل	sieve
naqaʿa	نقع	soak, infuse, macerate
nazaʿa al-raġwa	نزع الرغوة	skim
nazala ʿan al-nār	نزل عن النار	remove from the fire
qarraṣa	قرّص	form into a pastille
qašara	قشر	peel
rawwaqa	روّق	clarify, filter
ṣabba	صبّ	pour
šadda fī ḫirqa	شدّ في خرقة	tie into a cloth
ṣaffā	صفّى	filter, clarify
saḥaqa	سحق	grind
ṭabaḫa	طبخ	boil, cook
taraka	ترك	leave

10 Index of Prescriptions

This chapter presents the prescriptions described in Ms. Escorial in an edited form. This chapter also contains examples of prescriptions of drugs mentioned, but not explained, in Ms. Escorial.

Chebulic myrobalan pill (§ 2:14)

Seedless chebulic myrobalan fruit

Cover the seedless chebulic myrobalan fruits with water and place it in the sun in high summer for forty days until the water is gone. Stir several times daily. Form it into a pill, and consume with sugar and scammony.

Melicratum (§ 10:9)

clear honey	1 *raṭl*
fresh water	5 *raṭls*
long pepper	
ginger	
cinnamon	
Indian nard	
mastic	
cloves	1 *dirham* each

Take one *raṭl* of honey and pour five *raṭls* of water on it in a new pot. Cook on low fire and skim. When it gets close to the consistency of julep, take one *dirham* of long pepper, ginger, cinnamon, Indian nard, mastic, and cloves, and grind them well. Then, compress them in a linen cloth and suspend the cloth in the pot and cook until the liquid reaches the consistency of julep. Let the cloth soak in the drink. Remove from the fire and let cool down.

Mayba (§ 10:10)

quince juice	20 *raṭls*
grape jelly	10 *raṭls*
skimmed honey	5 *raṭls*
ginger	
mastic	
black cardamom	

small cardamom	
cinnamon	
cloves	
saffron	20 *dirhams* each
musk	1/8 *dirham*

Take fresh, juicy, sour quinces, peel them, clean their inside and grind them in a stone mortar. Squeeze from their juice 20 *raṭls*. Add 10 *raṭl*s of grape jelly and infuse it with the residues of the quince in some quince juice. Filter. Put the juices in a pot, boil gently on embers, and skim until half of the liquid remains. Remove from the fire. Then filter it for three days, a few times every day, in a thick, twofold cloth. After three days, add five *raṭl*s of skimmed honey in the mixture. Then crush and grind 20 *dirhams* of ginger root, mastic, black cardamom, small cardamom, cinnamon, cloves, and saffron, and bind them tightly in a thin linen cloth. Suspend the cloth in the pot and cook it altogether for a second time on low fire. Soak the spices in the liquid time after time until the mixture reaches the consistency of syrup and becomes clear. Then add 1/8 *dirham* of ground musk. Put the syrup in a glass receptacle. Leave the cloth soaking in it for two weeks, after which you remove it. If you want, you can let the spices sink to the bottom of the glass receptacle.

Mayba II (§ 10:11)

quince juice	1 part
clear, skimmed honey*	1 part
(*alt. crystalline sugar)	
very sour vinegar	3/4 part

Cook one part of quince juice and one part of honey (or crystalline sugar for whoever is of hot disposition) gently on embers, skim it, keep boiling until it reaches the consistency of syrup. Whoever wants sourness may add vinegar. This prescription is similar to Galen's plain quince wine, see Kahl, *The Dispensatory of Ibn al-Tilmīḏ*, p. 241.

Decoction I: A decoction that loosens the bowels and prevents the surplus of blood (§ 11:7)

[water]	
tamarind	2 *ūqiyyas*
plum	
jujube	

large sebesten	10 grains of each
dry, red rose	
blue violet leaves	
peeled lentils	
barberry	
endive seed	
purslane seed	3 *dirhams* each
dry coriander	2 *dirhams*
endive leaves	
nightshade leaves	1 part of each
kernel of cassia fistula cane cleaned from its seed	1 *ūqiyya*

Take two *ūqiyyas* tamarind, 10 grains of plum, jujube and sebesten, three *dirhams* of dry, red rose, blue violet leaves, peeled lentils, barberry, endive seeds and purslane seeds, two *dirhams* of dry coriander, and a part of endive and nightshade leaves. Boil on low fire until the water becomes red and thickens. Add half a *raṭl* of clear water and soak the kernel of the cane of cassia fistula in the decoction. Filter for a moment.

Decoction 11: A less cooling decoction that loosens the stomach (§ 11:8)

[water]	
yellow myrobalan	6 *dirhams*
seedless raisins	
tamarind	1 *ūqiyya* each
plum	
jujube	
sebesten	10 grains of each
cassia fistula	1 *ūqiyya*

Boil the ingredients apart from the cassia fistula on low fire until the water thickens a little. Then filter the water, and take half a *raṭl* of the filtered water to dissolve one *ūqiyya* (or more, according to strength) of cassia fistula in it. Use when needed.

Barley broth (§ 11:10)

barley	2 parts
peeled lentils*	1 part
(*alt. plum or jujube)	

Cook the barley and the lentils [in water]—or if you want, you may use plum or jujube.

This prescription is possibly incomplete. According to Ibn Māsawayh's prescription, barley broth is made by washing new or old barley with the husk, after which it is washed clean. It is soaked for a whole hour, drained, and covered with a thick cloth overnight. On the following day the barley is pounded in a mortar, cleaned from the husk, and put in a clean pot. Thereafter it is cooked with water, for each *kayl* of barley 14 *kayls* of water, simmering on low fire until it thickens. It is consumed with or without sugar.[13]

Decoction III: A decoction that loosens the stomach for whoever is afraid of his disposition turning cold (§ 11:11)

[water]	
yellow myrobalan, stoneless	6 *dirhams*
tamarind	1 *ūqiyya*
seedless raisins	1.5 *ūqiyyas*
red rose, dry	
violet leaves	4 *dirhams* of each
plum	
jujube	
sebesten	10 grains of each
fennel seeds, green	a handful
cassia fistula	
manna	3/4 *ūqiyya* of each

Boil the ingredients apart from cassia fistula and manna in water on low fire. Filter. Take half a *raṭl* from the filtered water and soak the cassia fistula and manna in it. Filter another time, and put aside for fourteen days.

Pastille I: A pastille that extinguishes the surplus of blood, cleanses it, strengthens the stomach and opens the obstructions of the liver (§ 11:12)

dry, red rose	10 *dirhams*
purslane seeds	
endive seeds	
barberry	

---

13 Adapted from Nasrallah, *Annals of the Caliphs' Kitchens*, p. 448. Barley broth is mentioned in § 2:5, 11:5, 11:6, 11:19, and 11:10.

gum Arabic	
white tragacanth	2 *dirhams* of each
white sandalwood	
chalk	1.5 *dirham* of each
upper part of peeled liquorice root	3 *dirhams*
Chinese rhubarb	1 *dirham*
saffron	0.5 *dirham*
camphor (optional)	1/4 *dirham*

Pound the ingredients and knead them in boiled, filtered nightshade pulp. Form pastilles à one *dirham* of weight, and let dry in the shade. Take one pastille with every meal with one *ūqiyya* of oxymel. If the patient has coarseness in the chest, consume the pastilles with sweeter syrups, such as cherry syrup or the syrup made of both types of pomegranates.

Pastille II: A pastille that is less cooling than the first one (§ 11:13)

dry, red rose	8 *dirhams*
endive seeds	
barberry seeds	
purslane seeds	
gum Arabic	
tragacanth	
starch	
peeled melon seeds	
Indian nard	
mastic	
manna	2 *dirhams* of each
liquorice root, peeled	4 *dirhams*
chalk	1 *dirham*
Chinese rhubarb	1.5 *dirham*
saffron	0.5 *dirham*

Infuse manna in water and add the rest of the components. Form pastilles à 1.5 *dirhams* of weight. Let dry in the shade. Consume with the described syrups.

Galen's remedy (§ 13:3)

frankincense	1 part
aloe	1/2 part

egg white
hare's fur*
(*alt. cobweb or a soft cotton cloth)

Mix one part of frankincense and 0.5 part of aloe with egg white until it reaches the consistency of honey. Use more aloe for dry bodies. Then add hare's fur, and apply it on the spot. If hare's fur is not available, you may use cobweb or a cotton cloth in its stead.

Dressing I: Prescription of another dressing (§ 13:4)

aloe	
frankincense	
dragon's blood	equal parts of each
egg white	

Knead the ingredients into a firm dough, and do as is described in the previous prescription.

Dressing II: 'A Christian man's dressing' (§ 13:5)

burned chalcitis

Put the chalcitis in a ceramic jug, coat its head with clay, and insert it into the oven. [Burn, and use the burned chalcitis as a dressing.]

Dressing III: Another strong dressing (§ 13:6)

frankincense peels	
green vitriol	
myrrh	
chalcitis	
terra sigillata	
goatsbeard sap	
mastic	
acacia gum	1 part of each
cobweb	
egg white	

Grind the ingredients. Coat the spot with some egg white and the ground drugs. Press some cobweb and egg white on the spot.

Dressing IV: Another dressing to treat a swelling in the muscle, nerve, and flesh (§ 13:8)

buckthorn	
aloe	
myrrh	equal parts
Roman earth	
glaucium	
red and white sandalwood	
litharge	1/2 part of each
coriander water	
fat from a ram's tail on a chard leaf	

Grind equal parts of buckthorn, aloe, and myrrh together with 1/2 part of Roman earth, glaucium, two sandalwoods, and litharge into a flour. Pound and knead into dough in coriander water. Apply on the opening of the vein, and cover with a light cloth. Cover the opening of the vein itself with fat from a ram's tail on a chard leaf.

Dressing V: Another dissolving dressing (§ 13:9)

egg yolk, roasted
rose oil

Take the egg yolk of a roasted egg and mix with rose oil according to the need. Knead the ingredients into a dough and cover the spot with it. Cover with a light cloth.

Dressing VI: A more dissolving dressing (§ 13:10)

chicken fat	
rose oil	5 *miṯqāls*
white wax	3 *miṯqāls*
tragacanth	
litharge	
ceruse	equal parts

Melt five *miṯqāls* of chicken fat and rose oil in three *miṯqāls* of white wax on fire. Remove from the fire, and add tragacanth, litharge, and ceruse. Use according to the need.

•••

This section presents some prescriptions for drugs that are mentioned, yet not described, in Ms. Escorial. In general, for an abundance of prescriptions for treating a great number of medical conditions with drugs, ointments, ligatures, cataplasms etc., see Kahl, *The Dispensatory of Ibn al-Tilmīḏ*, and *al-Kindī, Aqrābāḏīn*.

Fruit syrups: Several drinks prepared with different fruits are featured in Ms. Escorial. According to Fellmann, these syrups, or potions (in Arabic *šarāb*, pl. *ašriba*), are prepared of fruit and other juices, boiled with more sugar in relation to fruit, until a thick consistency is achieved.[14] For example, a citron syrup by *Ibn al-Tilmīḏ* is prepared of sour citrons and superb sugar. The juice of the sour citrons is pressed after the seeds are removed. Into each *raṭl* of sour citron juice one adds one *mann* of superb sugar. It should be left until the sugar melts without boiling, and then boiled on low fire. At the end, the syrup is removed from the fire, the scum removed, and the syrup is left to gain consistency.[15]

Rose syrup
by Ibn al-Tilmīḏ[16] (§ 10:3 & 11:6)

red roses	1 part
water	10 parts
pure sugar	similar amount of the remaining water

Cook one part of red roses in ten parts of water until one part of the water is gone. Press the roses and keep immersing them depending on the strength of the purgative effect you wish to achieve—stronger if one tenth of the water is left, weaker if half of it remains. Take the water in which the roses have been immersed and melt into it a similar amount of pure sugar. Cook until the mixture reaches the consistency of oxymel. Serve it by using four *ūqiyyas* of the

14 Fellmann, *Das Aqrābāḏīn al-Qalānisī*, p. 269.
15 Kahl, *The Dispensatory of Ibn al-Tilmīḏ*, p. 240.
16 Adapted from Kahl, *The Dispensatory of Ibn al-Tilmīḏ*, p. 237.

product with thirty *dirhams* of ice. The ice makes the purgative effect stronger, and yellow bile and other fine humours are purged.

Rose syrup
by Qusṭā ibn Lūqā[17] (§ 10:3 & 11:6)

dry Damascene rose	6 *ūqiyyas*
rain water (or fresh water)	20 *raṭls*
sugar water*	1/2 *raṭl* per each *raṭl*
(*alt. skimmed honey)	

Pour rain water or fresh water on the Damascene rose. Put into a long-necked bottle, close firmly. Boil profusely, remove from the fire, bury in straw for a day and a night. The following day, filter the extract, throw away the rose, pour half a *raṭl* of sugar water or skimmed honey over each *raṭl* of the extract. Boil until it reaches the consistency of julep. Take before and after meals, God willing.

Oxymel
by Ibn al-Tilmīḏ[18] (§ 10:3, 10:6, 11:4, 11:6, 11:12)

water
wine vinegar
sugar
egg white

For each *mann* of sugar, take eight *ūqiyyas* of wine vinegar and 1/4 *raṭl* of fresh water. Beat the white of two eggs into the water, mix, and boil. Skim off the scum repeatedly until the mixture is clear and ready to be stored. Alternatively, you may let the sugar dissolve naturally, without cooking on fire.

Qūqāyā pill
by Ibn al-Tilmīḏ[19] (§ 11:3)

aloe
mastic
absinthe sap or leaves

17 Adapted from Qusṭā ibn Lūqā, *Numbness*, 210, p. 74.
18 Adapted from Kahl, *The Dispensatory of Ibn al-Tilmīḏ*, p. 237.
19 Adapted from Kahl, *The Dispensatory of Ibn al-Tilmīḏ*, pp. 197–198.

scammony	
colocynth pulp	equal parts of each
celery water	

Take equal parts of aloe, mastic, absinthe, scammony, and colocynth pulp. Mix with celery water. Make pills by using 1.5–2 *dirhams* of the mixture. According to Ibn al-Tilmīḏ, a dose comprising two *dirhams*, with the amount of 4 *dāniqs* of both scammony and colocynth pulp, is very strong. He says that a dose of 0.5 *dirham* would result in a weak remedy, while a dose of one *dirham* is optimal.

Julep
by Ibn Sīnā[20] (§ 2:5, 10:3, 10:9, 11:5, 11:6)

water	1/2 cup
sugar	2 pounds
rose water	1/4 cup

Simmer 2 pounds of sugar with 1/2 cup water. Before removing the pot from the fire, add 1/4 cup rose water. The syrup may be diluted with water, or chilled with ice. Honey may be used instead of sugar.

Bitter hiera
by Ibn al-Tilmīḏ[21] (§ 3:8)

white turpeth	10 *dirhams*
yellow myrobalan	
chebulic myrobalan	
anise	5 *dirhams*
Indian salt	2 *dirhams*
scammony (grilled in quinces)	2.5 *dirhams*
Nabataean celery water	

Pound and knead all the ingredients with Nabataean celery water. A potion comprises 2.5 *dirhams* of the mixture.

20 Adapted from Ibn Sīnā's prescription in Nasrallah, *Annals of the Caliphs' Kitchens*, p. 552.
21 Adapted from Kahl, *The Dispensatory of Ibn al-Tilmīḏ*, p. 195.

Bitter hiera
by Sābūr ibn Sahl[22] (§ 3:8)

Greek mastic	
saffron	
Indian spikenard	
balm seeds	
asarabacca	
cassia	
cinnamon	1 *dirham* of each
Socotra aloe	15 *dirhams*
(balm twigs)	1 *dirham*

Pound and strain the ingredients, then store the mixture. Some physicians add the balm twigs. When a potion is needed, use 2 *dirhams* of the mixture, taken with honey.

Stomachic pill
by Ibn al-Tilmīḏ[23] (§ 3:8)

balm seeds	
balm twigs	
cassia	
Indian spikenard	
asarabacca	
cinnamon	
citronella root	
saffron	
mastic	
rootstock of sweet flag	
absinthe sap	
'rolled' birthwort	
Indian salt	1 *dirham* of each
Socotra aloe	15 *dirhams*
scammony	

22 Adapted from Kahl, *Sābūr ibn Sahl; The Small Dispensatory*, p. 72.
23 Adapted from Kahl, *The Dispensatory of Ibn al-Tilmīḏ*, pp. 196–197.

agaric	
colocynth pulp	4 *dirhams* of each
celery water	

Pound and strain the ingredients, then knead them with celery water. Form into small pills. A suitable portion comprises 2 *dirhams*, and is taken with hot water.

Drugs to stanch nosebleed
There are abundant varieties of drugs to stanch nosebleed (§ 7:9). Two examples below.

Snuff to stanch nosebleed by Ibn al-Tilmīḏ[24]

burnt papyrus	
gum Senegal	
alum	
Egyptian opium	
date *rāmik*	
camphor	5 *dirhams* of each
vitriol	
pomegranate flowers	
black bryony	
oak gall *rāmik*	
burnt mussel shells	
burnt oak galls (slaked with wine vinegar)	
plantain	10 *dirhams* of each
salsify sap	
dragon's blood	
burnt wormwood	7 *dirhams* of each
dry burnt coriander	8 *dirhams*

Pound and knead the ingredients with plantain water, and form into pastilles. When needed, use two *dāniqs* with plantain water.

24 Adapted from Kahl, *The Dispensatory of Ibn al-Tilmīḏ*, pp. 302–303.

A drug for nosebleed by al-Kindī[25]

wild ginger	
hematite	2 parts of each
sempervivum	
ben nut	powdered
myrrh	
wine vinegar (or vinegar only)	
cobweb	
Chinese ink or fragrant aloeswood	

Mix wild ginger and hematite with finely powdered sempervivum and ben nut. Add some myrrh and wine vinegar, alternatively wine vinegar only. Add cobweb into the mixture. The inside of the nose is rubbed with Chinese ink or fragrant aloeswood. [The mixture is then put inside the nose.]

Enema
by Qusṭā ibn Lūqā[26] (§ 3:8)

"One takes:

salix water	
purslane water	
waybread water	
knot-grass water	of each, a quarter of a *raṭl*
water of unhulled rice	half a *raṭl*

This is brought together, mixed with two *dirhams* of Armenian earth and the yolk of a fried egg, and used as treatment."

25 Adapted from al-Kindī, *Aqrābāḏīn*, p. 216.
26 Adapted from Qusṭā ibn Lūqā, *Al-adwiya al-mushila*, p. 94.

11 Index of Some Medical Terms

This index is for central technical terminology. Specific terms for drugs are presented in the index of *materia medica*. This index follows the Latin alphabet.

Arabic transliterated	Arabic	English
āfa	آفة	ailment
al-aḫdaʿān	الأخدعان	occipital arteries; the lateral parts of the neck
aḥšāʾ	أحشاء	viscera
aǧfār	أجفار	eyelids
al-akḥal	الأكحل	median cubital vein
amʿāʾ	أمعاء	intestines, guts
ašfār	أشفار	palpebral margin
awǧāʿ al-mafāṣil	أوجاع المفاصل	arthritis
ʿāda	عادة	custom, habit
ʿaḍal	عضل	muscle
ʿaḍw	عضو	body part; organ
ʿaraq	عرق	sweat
ʿašāwa	عشاوة	nyctalopia
ʿaṣab	عصب	nerve
bāb	باب	porta
bāb al-kabid	باب الكبد	portal vein
badan	بدن	body
bāh	باه	sexual desire
balġam	بلغم	phlegm
al-bāsilīq	الباسليق	basilic vein, vena basilica
bāsūr, bawāsīr	باسور ج. بواسير	haemorrhoid, haemorrhoids
baṯr, buṯūr	بثر ج. بثور	pustule
bawwāb	بواب	pylorus
bawl	بول	urine
balādat al-ḏihn	بلادة الذهن	want of intellect
buḥḥat al-ṣawt	بحة الصوت	hoarseness of voice
buḫār	بخار	vapour

(cont.)

Arabic transliterated	Arabic	English
dāʾ al-fīl	داء الفيل	elephantiasis
dam	دم	blood
damawī	دموي	sanguine
damʿa	دمعة	rhyas
dalīl	دليل	indication
al-dawālī	الدوالي	varicose veins
dawāʾ	دواء	drug
dimāġ	دماغ	brain
dummal	دمل	boil
duwwār	دوار	vertigo
ḏabūliyya	ذبولية	marasmus
ḏāt al-ǧanb	ذات الجنب	pleurisy
ḏirāʿ	ذراع	forearm
ḍarba	ضربة	blow
ḍarabān	ضربان	throbbing pain
ḍuʿf	ضعف	weakness
faṣd	فصد	phlebotomy
fam al-maʿida	فم المعدة	orifice of the stomach
fatq	فتق	rupture
fawadān	فودان	agitation
fiʿl	فعل	activity; effect
futūʾ	فتوء	protrusion
ǧabha	جبهة	forehead
ǧaḏb	جذب	drawing
ǧild	جلد	skin
ǧimāʿ	جماع	coitus, sexual intercourse
ǧuḏām	جذام	leprosy
ġašy	غشي	unconsciousness
ġaṯayān	غثيان	nausea
ġaṭīṭ	غطيط	snoring
ġiḏāʾ	غذاء	nutriment

(cont.)

Arabic transliterated	Arabic	English
ġišāʾ	غشاء	membrane
ġudda	غدّة	gland
haḍm	هضم	digestion
halāk	هلاك	death, annihilation
huzāl	هزال	emaciation
al-ḥārr al-ġarīzī	الحار الغريزي	innate heat
ḥabl al-ḏirāʿ	حبل الذراع	vena cephalica pollicis
ḥadbat al-kabid	حدبة الكبد	convex side of the liver
ḥarāra	حرارة	heat
ḥayḍ	حيض	menstruation, menses
ḥazāz	حزاز	dandruff
ḥiǧāb	حجاب	diaphragm
ḥiǧāma	حجامة	cupping
ḥikka	حكة	itching
ḥummā	حمى	fever
ḥumra	حمرة	redness
ḫadar	خدر	numbness
ḫāṣṣiyya	خاصّية	peculiar virtue
ḫawānīq	خوانيق	diphtheria; choking
ḫayfa	خيفة	fear
ḫilṭ, aḫlāṭ	خلط ج. أخلاط	humour, pl. humours
al-ibṭī	الإبطي	axillary vein
ifsād	إفساد	spoilage
iḫrāǧ	إخراج	extraction
iḫtilāf al-dam	أختلاف الدم	bloody diarrhoea
iḥtibās al-ḥayḍ	احتباس الحيض	amenorrhea
iḥtilām	احتلام	nocturnal emission
iḥtirāq al-dam	احتراق الدم	combustion of blood
iḥtiqān al-dam	احتقان الدم	congestion of blood
iltihāb	التهاب	inflammation
iʿtiqāl	اعتقال	detention
imāla	إمالة	deflection

(*cont.*)

Arabic transliterated	Arabic	English
imtilāʾ	امتلاء	plethos, overfilling
imtilāʾ bi-ḥasb al-awʿiya	امتلاء بحسب الأوعية	plethos due to vessels; overfilling relating to vessels
imtilāʾ bi-ḥasb al-quwwa	امتلاء بحسب القوة	dynamic plethos; overfilling affecting the strength
infiǧār al-dam	انفجار الدم	phleborrhagia
intišār	انتشار	*Liderweiterung*
ishāl	إسهال	diarrhoea
istifrāġ	أستفراغ	evacuation
istirḫaʾ	استرخاء	feebleness
ʿilāǧ	علاج	treatment
ʿilla	علّة	illness
ʿirq	عرق	vein, vessel
ʿirq al-ǧabha	عرق الجبهة	frontal vein
ʿirq ḍārib	عرق ضارب	pulsatile vein
ʿirq ġayr ḍārib	عرق غير ضارب	non-pulsatile vein
ʿirq al-nasā	عرق النسا	sciatic vein; sciatica; vena saphena externa
kaʿb	كعب	ankle
kabid	كبد	liver
kadar al-ḥawāss	كدر الحواس	cloudiness of sensations
kāhil	كاهل	interscapular region
kalaf	كلف	freckles
kammiyya	كمية	quantity
kasal	كسل	laziness
kaṯrat al-dam	كثرة الدم	surplus of blood
kayfiyya	كيفية	method
labba	لبة	jugular fossa
lahā	لهاة	uvula
liṯa	لثة	gums
luzūm	لزوم	adhesion
maʾbiḍ al-rukba	مأبض الركبة	popliteal fossa
mādda	مادة	matter, substance

(*cont.*)

Arabic transliterated	Arabic	English
mafṣil	مفصل	joint
maġṣ	مغص	gripes
maʿida	معدة	stomach
mālinḫūniyyā	مالنخونيا	melancholy
manfaʿa	منفعة	benefit
manḫar	منخر	nostril
maqʿada	مقعدة	anus
maʾq	مأق	canthus
maraḍ	مرض	illness, disease
maṯāna	مثانة	bladder
mawḍiʿ	موضع	site, spot
mirfaq	مرفق	elbow
mirra	مرّة	bile
miʿṣam	معصم	wrist
mizāǧ	مزاج	disposition
nabḍ	نبض	pulse
nafṯ al-dam	نفث الدم	haemoptysis
al-naḫīla	النخيلة	callous hardenings of the face
naḫs	نخس	pricking pain
nāsūr, nawāsīr	ناسور ج. نواسير	polyp
natn	نتن	bad smell
nawba	نوبة	paroxysm, crisis
nazf	نزف	haemorrhage
nazla	نزلة	catarrh
niqris	نقرس	gout
nuqra	نقرة	the hollow of the neck
nuzūl al-māʾ	نزول الماء	defluxion; cataract
qayʾ	قيء	vomiting
qalb	قلب	heart
qarḥ, qurūḥ	قرح ج. قروح	ulcer
qawlanǧ	قولنج	colic
al-qīfāl	القيفال	cephalic vein
qulāʿ	قلاع	aphthae
quwwa	قوة	strength; faculty

(*cont.*)

Arabic transliterated	Arabic	English
rabw	ربو	asthma
raḥim	رحم	uterus
ramad	رمد	ophthalmia
ra's	رأس	head
ri'a	رئة	lungs
rīḥ al-sabal	ريح السبل	wind of pannus
ruʿāf	رعاف	epistaxis; nosebleed
sabab	سبب	cause
saʿfa	سعفة	cradle cap
sahar	سهر	insomnia
sakta	سكتة	apoplexy
saqṭa	سقطة	fall
sawrat al-dam	سورة الدم	surplus of blood
silliyya	سلية	phthisis
suʿāl	سعال	cough
sulāq	سلاق	ptilosis
šabakat al-dimāġ	شبكة الدماغ	arachnoid mater
šaqīqa	شقيقة	migraine
šarsūf, šarāsīf	شرسوف ج. شراسيف	false rib, pl. false ribs
šarṭ	شرط	scarification
šawṣa	شوصة	pleuritis
šayḫūḫa	شيخوخة	old age
širsām	شرسام	phrenitis
širyān	شريان	artery
šuqāq	شقاق	fissures
al-ṣāfin	الصافن	saphenous vein
ṣadr	صدر	chest
ṣarʿ	صرع	epilepsy
ṣinf	صنف	sort, species, kind
ṣimāḫ	صماخ	auditory meatus
ṣudāʿ	صداع	headache
ṣulb	صلب	spinal column

(*cont.*)

Arabic transliterated	Arabic	English
tabṯīr	تبثير	vesication
tadbīr	تدبير	regimen
taḥlīl	تحليل	dissolution
tamaddud	تمدد	expansion, tension
tamaṭṭin	تمط	stretching
tarquwa	ترقوة	clavicle
tasāwin	تساوٍ	balance
taṯāʾub	تثاؤب	yawning
taṯniya	تثنية	epaphairesis
ṯarb	ثرب	omentum
ṯiqal	ثقل	heaviness
ṭabʿ	طبع	natural disposition
ṭabīʿa	طبيعة	nature, natural disposition
ṭabaqa	طبقة	tunic
ṭamṯ	طمث	menstruation, menses
ṭiḥāl	طحال	spleen
al-unṯayān	الأنثيان	testicles
al-usaylim	الأسيلم	vena salvatella
wadağān	ودجان	jugular veins
wağaʿ	وجع	pain
wağaʿ al-ʿayn	وجع العين	ophthalmalgia
wağh	وجه	face; kind
waram, awrām	ورم ج. أورام	swelling, pl. swellings
wirk	ورك	hip
zand	زند	antebrachium
ziyāda	زيادة	excess
zukām	زكام	rheum

PART 2

Ma'amar baHaqqaza le'al-Rāzī

מאמר בהקזה לאלראזי

0:1 מאמר בהקזה לאלראזי מאשר הכריחני נכבד א׳ ומעולה ואוהב החכמה מכבד אנשי המזמה במעלה רמה ושאל ממני לחבר לו כלל קצר בענין ההקזה ותועלותיה והדרכים הראויים אליה ענינה ומעשיה ופעלותיה. 91r

0:2 וחברתי אליו המגלה הזאת מה שזכרתי מה צריך עליה כל מי אשר לא יסתפק בלעדיה.

0:3 וקבצתי במאמר זה כל הצריך והראוי בהקזה.

0:4 והקדמתי כל זה בלב טוב ובנפש חפצה והלכתי בחבורי אל דרך אשר לא השיגהו מי שקדמני בו.

0:5 ואשאל מהאל יתברך[a] להדריכני בדרך ישרה ולהצילני מהשגגה ולזכני בנפש ברה וטהורה.

שערי המאמר

0:6 וחלקתי המאמר הזה אל י״ד שערים.

0:7 השער הא׳ בתועלת הדם אל האדם ותולדתו ואיך ענינו עד שיהיה מזון ומתי נשלם.

0:8 הב׳ יזכור בו הענינים הצריכים לראות ולהשגיח בהם מי שיצטרך אל ההקזה.

0:9 הג׳ בסבות המחייבות ההקזה.

0:10 הד׳ בכמות מה שיוציא מן הדם.

0:11 הה׳ בגידי ההקזה.

0:12 הו׳ באיכות הקזת הגידים ומה שיגיע הטעות בהם והשמירה ממנו.

0:13 הז׳ במשיכת הליחות.

a יתברך: ית׳

Al-Rāzī's Treatise on Phlebotomy

0:1 Al-Rāzī's treatise on phlebotomy, as I was compelled [to compose] by an honoured, eminent person who loves science and respects intelligent and high-ranking individuals, who asked me to compose a concise summary, dedicated to him, concerning phlebotomy and its benefits, appropriate methods, matter, deeds, and effects. 91r

0:2 I composed this treatise for him based on what I remembered and what those who are not satisfied without it need.

0:3 I have gathered everything that is necessary and appropriate regarding phlebotomy in this treatise.

0:4 I preceded all this with a good heart and a willing soul, and while composing it I pursued a path unattained by my predecessors.

0:5 I ask God—may He be blessed!—to guide me on a righteous path and to save me from error, and to grant me a pure and untainted soul.

Chapters of the Treatise

0:6 I have divided this treatise into fourteen chapters.

0:7 The first chapter on the benefit of blood for a human being, its origins, and how it is until it becomes nutriment, and when it is completed.

0:8 The second [chapter] on the circumstances that someone in need of phlebotomy needs to observe and consider.

0:9 The third [chapter] on the causes that require phlebotomy.

0:10 The fourth [chapter] on the quantity of blood that should be extracted.

0:11 The fifth [chapter] on the phlebotomised veins.

0:12 The sixth [chapter] on the method of venesection, and the mistake deriving from it, and how to avoid it.

0:13 The seventh [chapter] on drawing matters.

0:14 הח׳ בזמנים הטובים להוציא הדם והשמירה מיציאתו.

0:15 הט׳ בחזרת ההקזה השנית.

0:16 הי׳ במזון מי שהוקז[a] ושתיתו.

0:17 הי״א במזונות המכבים חמימות הדם.

0:18 הי״ב בתועלת הקזת הגידים רפואתה אל החוליים תהיה ההקזה להם.

0:19 הי״ג ברפואת השגגה הנופלת בהקזה.

0:20 הי״ד בכוסות המציצה עם שריטה ובלתי שריטה הנקרא אלחג׳אמה.[b]

השער הא׳

1:1 השער הא׳ בתועלת הדם באברים ותולדתו ואיך ישוב אל האברים עד שיהיה מזון אמתי נשלם.

1:2 אמר אבובכר: בעבור היות הדם יותר ישר משאר הליחות אשר באדם ובו החמימות הטבעית[c] אשר הוא קיום החיות והוא כמו העצים אל האש והוא ישמין ויבריאהו וישמחהו ויסיר האנחות וימנעהו ממנו החלי היבש הנקרא אלסליאה[d] או אלדבוליא[e] ויבריא הכבד אשר בבריאותו יהיה בריאות הגוף כמו שאמר גלינוס: כי נחיה בטוב חיינו בבריאות כבדנו.

1:3 וכבר הגיד גלינוס על ארסיסטרטוס[f] כי הוא היה מונע וחס וחומל על הדם והיה עושה במקומה המניעה מן האכילה או מעוטה. וזה היה אפשר עליו אם לא יקרהו פתאם רבוי הדם רק מה שלא ישאר עם החולה רבויו ואם ימעט מזונו.

a מי שהוקז: מי שהקיז

b الحجامة

c החמימות הטבעית: החמימות הטבעי

d السلية

e الذبولية

f ארסיסטרטוס: ארס׳

0:14 The eighth [chapter] on the appropriate times to extract blood, and when to guard against extracting it.

0:15 The ninth [chapter] on additional removal of blood.

0:16 The tenth [chapter] on the food and drink of the phlebotomised person.

0:17 The eleventh [chapter] on the foods that extinguish the heat of blood.

0:18 The twelfth [chapter] on the benefit of venesection and treatment of illnesses for which phlebotomy is conducted.

0:19 The thirteenth [chapter] on the treating the error that may befall during phlebotomy.

0:20 The fourteenth [chapter] on cupping with and without scarification, called *al-ḥiǧāma*.

The First Chapter

1:1 The first chapter on the benefit of blood in the parts,[1] its origin, and the manner it circulates into the parts until it becomes proper and complete nutriment.

1:2 Abū Bakr said: blood is the most balanced of the humours in man, containing the innate heat that is the foundation of life, as wood for fire, that fattens the man and makes him healthy, brings him happiness, obliterates sighs, protects him from the dry illness called *al-silliyya* [i.e., phthisis] or *al-ḏubūliyya* [i.e., marasmus], and heals the liver, in the health of which the body is healthy, as Galen said: "For we shall live our lives in goodness through the health of our liver."

1:3 Galen has spoken about Erasistratus,[2] who used to avoid [phlebotomy] and have pity and mercy on blood, and that he, in its stead, used to abstain from the intake of food or consume it in small quantities. This would be possible for him if a sudden increase in blood did not occur, provided that the patient is not left with an excess [quantity of blood], and if his intake of food is reduced.

---

1 Ms. Escorial: "in man."

2 See commentary.

1:4 והדם גם כן[a] הוא המזון האמתי אשר זכרו אבוקראט במאמרו כי המזון יהיה על ג׳ פנים: האמתי והנכון שיקרא מזון והוא מה שידמה אל הנזון וימשכו אותו האברים מהגידים אשר יצא אליהם בדמיון העשן והוא יהיה במקום מה שנתך תמיד מהם.

1:5 והב׳ דומה אל המזון והוא הדם המתהוה בגידים בעבור כי זה הדם יפל בו מקרה החסרון בסבת פתיחת הגידים מאיזה מקום שיהיה מהגוף או זולת זה מנפילה או הכאה וימעט הדם הזה מהגוף ולא יזון ממנו.

1:6 והג׳ מה שנזון בו במה שעבר והוא המאכל המתהוה באצטומכא אשר הסבה[b] בו שיהיה חמר המזון האמתי רק אם יקרה בו מקרה מקיא או משלשול או שישוב אל גבול מה שידמהו אל המזון ואחר יקרה בו המקרה אשר זכרנו ולא יזון ממנו גם כן.[c]

1:7 ואם אמר אומר: ואיך ישוב הדם וילך אל האברים על דרך[d] העשן להזנתם תשובתו כי האצטומכא מונחת כמו קדרה עצומה וסביבה הבערת אש רבות בימין הוא הכבד ובשמאל הוא הטחול ולמעלה ממנו המסך | הנקרא אלחג׳אב[e] והחלב המכסה את הקרב. ועל אלה 91v
האברים כלם אל האדם בלבד וזה לחולשת עכולו ורכות[f] עורו והעדר שערו בהקשתו וערכו אל שאר בעלי חיים.[g]

1:8 וכאשר תרגיש האצטומכא בצרכה אל המזון עם העצבים הבאים אליה מהמוח או במציצת הגידים שתחת האצטומכא והכבד ולקיחתם המאכל הם נדבקין ומקיפים עליה ונסתם השער אשר תחתיה הנקרא אלבואב.[h]

1:9 ובקצת בעלי חיים[i] הושם במקום אלבואב[j] דמיון הבשר †התרוה† הנקרא אלגבה[k] להוסיף הדבקות. ולא יוסיף כן[l] עד שישלים העכול וישוב המאכל בדמיון המיץ ואז ידחה הרע ממנו ויתך השאר וישנו אותו הגידים אל הדם שנוי קרוב משנויו בכבד בעבור כי טבעם קרוב

a גם כן: ג״כ
b הסבה: הסנה
c גם כן: ג״כ
d על דרך: ע״ד
e الحجاب
f ורכות: וירקות
g בעלי חיים: ב״ח
h البواب
i בעלי חיים: ב״ח
j البواب
k الغدة
l Ms. Escorial: فلا يزال كذلك

1:4 Blood is also the real nutriment that Hippocrates mentioned in his treatise, stating that there are three kinds of nutriment: the real and proper, called nutriment, which resembles what is nourished. The parts attract it from the veins where it flows like vapour, and it replaces what is constantly dissolved from them.

1:5 The second [kind] is that which resembles nutriment [i.e., quasi-nutriment], and it is the blood in the veins. If affected by an ailment due to the opening of veins anywhere in the body, or alternatively due to a fall or a blow, this blood is reduced in the body, and the body cannot be nourished from it.

1:6 The third [kind] is destined nutriment, which is the food in the stomach destined to be a matter of proper nutriment, unless it is afflicted by vomiting or diarrhoea, or that it reaches the degree of what resembles nutriment [i.e., quasi-nutriment], being afterwards afflicted by what we mentioned, in which case it does not provide nutriment either.

1:7 If someone asks, 'how does blood flow and reach the parts as vapour, thus nourishing them?' the answer is that the stomach is placed like an enormous cauldron, surrounded by many burning fires: on the right side the liver, on the left side the spleen, above it a veil | called *al-ḥiǧāb* [i.e., diaphragm], and the 91v
omentum. Only a human being has all these parts, and that is due to his weak digestion, delicate skin, and lack of hair in comparison to the other animals.

1:8 Whenever the stomach feels the need for nutriment, [this happens] through the nerves that reach it from the brain or by the suction of the veins below the stomach and the liver. To take nutriment, they get firmly attached and surround it, and the pylorus below it, called *al-bawwāb*, gets closed.

1:9 In some animals, a meat-like †*htrwh*†[3] called *al-gabba*[4] [i.e., a gland] is placed in the pylorus, to increase its adhesion. It does not increase[5] until the digestion is completed, and the food begins to resemble juice. At that time, it expels what is bad, and the rest is dissolved. The veins transform it into blood in a manner that resembles its transformation in the liver, since their nature is close to the nature of the liver. [Its expulsion to the liver takes place via one

3 See commentary.
4 In Arabic *al-ġudda*.
5 Ms. Escorial: "it remains that way."

מטבע הכבד וצורתו גיד רק שלא תקיף הדם כמוהו ויצמחו משרשה ענפי גידים מתחלקים בעצם הכבד חלקים דקים נתבשל בהם הדם ונבחר מהלחות. ולולי מה שנתערב עם הדם אשר בגידים הדבוקים במעים באצטומכא ובכבד מהלחות המימיי כשיגיע הדם אל אלו המקומות היו צרים וסתומים ממנו לעביו[a] ולא יזונו ממנו כלל.

1:10 ויצמח מגבנינות הכבד גיד עצום ממנו יצמחו כל הגידים הבלתי[b] דופקים כמו שזכרו המנתחים. ושרש אלו הגידים נחלק בכבד אל חלקים דקים בתחלת השער ומתחברים עם החלקים הנחלקים אל המעבר הנקרא השער לקחת ממנו הדם הנקי מרב המרירות ומהלחות המימיי עם הכלים המונחים בזה.

1:11 ואחר יקחו הדם קצתם בקצתם לדבקותם כמו שאמר[c] אבוקרט בספר המזון שלו כי האדם גוף א׳ משותף מגידים רבים וכאשר יתחלק ויהיו ענפים רבים מתפשטים ומגיעים עד קצות הגוף ידבק כל אחד מאלו[d] אל עצם יחלק מזונו. רצונו בזה כי נדבקו אל העצמות גידים דקים בעבור כי הם קשים האריגה הקרים הצריכים אל מזון מועט. והלב ואם הוא קשה צריך אל גידים גדולים לרוב התכתו והמוח ואם הוא רך הוא צריך אל מזון מועט במעוט חמימותו. וכן שאר האברים על זה ההקש בעצמו. ישתבח יתברך הבורא כל זה והמנהיג עולמו.

1:12 ואחר כך[e] יצא זה הדם באלה הגידים אל האברים אשר זכרנו. אין לו מקום יציאה מהם[f] אחר השלמת בשולו וחלוקו רק על דרך[g] העשן או המשוש כמו הדבר המתחמם או מתיבש או מתלחלח או מתקרר מסבת משושו או קירובו אליו. הוצרך להיות הגידים מתפשטים בכל הגוף כי הם מביאים המזון אליו.

1:13 והיה האדם מתוכו דבוק עם גידים וזה כי אם ידקר הגוף עם מחט יצא הדם ממקום הדקירה על הרוב והדם לא יצא כי אם מהגיד. מה יורה כי בכל מקום אשר ידקר ויצא הדם ממנו הגיד דבוק אליו.

---

a + ~~לעברו~~

b Added in tiny script above the line.

c כמו שאמר: כש׳

d כל אחד מאלו: כא״מ

e ואחר כך: ואחכ׳

f ואין לו מקום יציאה מהם: ואין להם מקום יציאה ממנו

g על דרך: עד׳

path that is called *porta*][6] and its shape is like the shape of a vein, except that it does not contain blood as a vein does. Branches of veins, distributed as thin parts, sprout from its origin in the body of the liver, in which the blood is cocted and separated from the two biles. Had it not been for the watery fluid that mixes with the blood in the veins attached to the intestines, the stomach, and the liver, when the blood arrives at these places, they would be too narrow and blocked due to its thickness, so that they would not be nourished from it at all.

1:10 A large vein [i.e., *vena cava*] grows from the convex side of the liver, from which all the non-pulsatile veins grow, as the surgeons have mentioned. The root of these veins is divided into capillary parts in the liver, at the base of the *porta*, and they connect to the divided parts in the passage called *porta*, taking from it the blood that is cleansed from the major portion of the two biles and the watery fluid through the instruments assigned for it.

1:11 Thereafter, they take blood from each other, as Hippocrates said in his book, *Nutriment*, that a human being has one body with many communicating veins, and when being divided, many branches spread and reach the extremities of the body, each attached to a bone,[7] distributing its nutriment. His intention with this is that thin veins are attached to the bones,[8] that are of solid texture, and cold, and consequently require a little nutriment. But the heart, even if it is solid, needs large veins since it dissolves a lot. And the brain, being tender, needs a little nutriment due to its low temperature. And the same holds good for the rest of the parts. Blessed and praised is the Creator of all this, who governs his World!

1:12 Then, this blood flows through these veins into the mentioned parts. There is no other way for it to exit them after the completion of its concoction and division than through vapour or by contact, just as something heating, drying, moistening, or cooling, because of its contact or closeness to it. The veins must be dispersed in the whole body, because they provide it with nutriment.

1:13 Veins pervade the inside of a human being, and that is [evident] if the body is punctured with a needle, as in most cases blood flows from the site of the puncture, and blood only flows from a vein. What indicates this is that every site that you puncture and blood flows out from it, is attached to a vein.

---

6 [...] lacking in Ms. Parma.

7 Ms. Escorial: 'part.'

8 Ms. Escorial: 'parts.'

השער הב׳

2:1 השער הב׳ בענינים אשר יצטרך לראות ולהשגיח בהם מי שצריך אל הקזה.

2:2 הא׳ הכח הב׳ האומנות הג׳ המנהג הד׳ המזג הה׳ הזמן הו׳ העת הז׳ המקום הח׳ מה שיאכל וישתה הט׳ בערך אל הליחות אשר בגוף ואם הם שוות או מתחלפות.

2:3 אמנם הכות הוא קיום האדם ועמוד ענינו והוא כמו הצידה אל האורח אשר לא תפסק הליכתו כפי שעור צידתו. וכן הכח כאשר[a] יקצר לא תשיג החולה אל תכלית מחלתו ואין להקדים ההקזה והמשלשל רק עם קיומו ועמידתו כי הרופא המשכיל בעת הצרך אפשר שיתיר אל החולה במזון הרע כאשר יאוה אותו או יערכהו עם הטוב |[b] בעת תקותו בשמירת כחו 92r
ויאכל בעל הקדחת בזמן ההקפה ובעת חזק רעתו בעבור שלא יפל כחו על כי המזון בזמן ההקפה[c] יוסיף מחלתו. וכבר העיד בזה אבוקרט באמירתו: ויומנע המזון בזמן ההקפה.

2:4 וכן כאשר יתאמת אל הרופא כי חלי החולה ארוך ויושן יתירנו אל המזון אחר אשר יעברו עליו יב׳ ימים ולילות. ואם הוא מוסיף על מחלתו הרבה מפחדו שיפל[d] כחו קודם תכלית מחלתו וירידתו ויהיה סבה אל מיתתו. וצריך שיומנע החולה מן המזון לגמרי כאשר יתאמת אליו כי הכח משלים ומספיק בזה. וכבר באר זה אבוקרט באמירתו כי החלי המגיע אל הדקות הרבה צריך שיתנהג בהנהגה הדקה הרבה ורצונו בזה הנחת המאכל לגמרי.

2:5 וכאשר ידע כי הכח לא יספיק אל זה ישתה החולה ג׳לב.[e] ואם ידע כי הכח לא יעמידנו זה יקח מי בשול השעורים או לביבות הפת רחוצים עם סכרי ודומיהם.

---

a כאשר: אשר

b הטוב + Ms.

c ההקפה: התרופ׳

d שיפל: שלא יפל

e جلاب

The Second Chapter

2:1 The second chapter on the circumstances that whoever is resolute about phlebotomy needs to consider and notice.

2:2 The first is the strength, the second the occupation, the third the custom, the fourth the disposition, the fifth the time, the sixth the season, the seventh the geographical location, the eighth what is eaten and drunk, and the ninth the relation of the humours in the body, whether they are equal or unbalanced.[9]

2:3 As to the strength, it is the essence of a human being, the foundation of his condition, as the provisions for a traveller that does not cease his journey unless by his provisions. When the strength reduces, the patient does not reach the end of his illness. One should not proceed to phlebotomy nor purgation unless [allowed by] his state and condition. At the necessary moment, a skilled physician may permit the patient [some] bad food if he has appetite for it, or prescribe him some good [food], | hoping to preserve his strength. During the 92r
paroxysm [of fever] and its peak, the fevered should eat so that his strength would not diminish, although nutriment at the time of the paroxysm intensifies his illness. Hippocrates testified this as he said: "Nutriment should be prohibited at the time of the paroxysm."

2:4 And thus, when the physician is certain that the patient's illness is long and chronic, he may allow the patient to consume food after twelve days and nights have passed.[10] Even if this may lead to increased fear that the patient's strength would diminish before the end and decline of his illness, being the cause of his death, he must be restrained from food completely. [He may only do so] when it is certain that the strength is complete and suffices this. Hippocrates already explained this by saying that "a very acute illness needs to be managed by a very restricted regimen"[11] by which he means complete abandonment of food.

2:5 Whenever he [the physician] knows that the strength is not sufficient for it [i.e., the complete abandonment of food], the patient should drink julep. If he knows that the strength does not get him to his feet, he should take barley broth or bread pith washed with sugar, and the like.

9 This chapter in Ms. Parma is incomplete: not all these topics are covered.
10 Ms. Escorial: "the patient may be fed with coarse food for a period of fourteen days."
11 See commentary.

2:6 אמנם השנים כי הנערים אשר לא הגיעו אל שנות הבחורים והם י״ד שנים לא נצטרך להקיז דם וזה כי הם צריכים אל ההבערה והוא המזון הרב וכן נתך מהם מזון רב לח ובהם קצת חולשת האיברים העצביים. וכן הזקנים וגבולם מבן ס׳ שנה ומעלה לא יקיזו לעולם. ותועיל ההקזה במה שבין אלו השנים. ולמעלה לא יסבלו ההקזה והמשלשל על הרוב למעוט דמם וחולשת עכולם. וכבר זכר גלינוס כי הוא הקיז זקן בן ע׳ שנה וזה יקרה מעט.

2:7 וכבר היה במצרים איש א׳ מעבדי המלך והיו ימיו יותר מע׳ שנה והקזתיו פעם א׳ בכל כ״ה ימים וקרוב מהם בכל הזמנים. ואפשר שיקרה לחולה שיצטרך אל ההקזה והזמן חד בסבת החום והקור אז משתנה אותו מזה וצויתי להשקותו מהמשקים המכבים הדם כמשקה הבסר ומשקה אלריבס ומשקה אלענאב[a] והמאכלים הנקראים אלחצרמיא[b] אלרמאניאה[c] ואלסמקיא[d] ואלעדסיא.[e] ולא הועיל כל זה ונצטער הרבה בענין ונשבר גופו עד שנדמה אליו כאילו פורחת נפשו והוא נחנק עד אשר נחוסר כל זה עם ההקזה ונתחזק. והיה האיש ההוא עב הגוף אדום המראה טוב הבנין והוצאתי אליו בין ב׳ פעמים כמו ג׳ ליטרים.

2:8 ואין ליציאת הדם גבול מיוחד ברב או במעט. וכבר זכר גלינוס כי הוא הקיז אנשים והוציא מהם כמו ו׳ ליטרים ומצאו בזה תועלת ואחרים הוציא מהם ליטר והזיק להם. וזכר קוסטא בשם עבד אללה אלראזי כי הוא הקיז חולה בה׳ חדשים תכופים י״ו הקזות והוציא ממנו דם ברב ההקזות ת״ת זוז במשקל.

a العناب
b الحصرمية
c الرمانية
d السماقية
e العدسية

2:6 As to the age, the boys that have not reached the age of adolescents, that is fourteen years, should not be phlebotomised. That is because they need burning, which is the large amount of nutriment, and thus, a lot of moist nutriment is diffused from them, and their neural parts are a bit weak. The same holds good for old people from sixty years and above, they should never be phlebotomised. Phlebotomy is beneficial for what is between these ages. [Who are] above [that age] do generally not tolerate phlebotomy nor purgation due to their low blood quantity and weak digestion. Galen mentioned that he phlebotomised an old, seventy-year-old man,[12] yet this does not happen often.

2:7 There was a man in Egypt,[13] one of the servants of the king, who was over seventy years old. I used to phlebotomise him once every twenty-five days or close to it during all seasons. Sometimes it happened that the patient required phlebotomy, but the season was severely hot or cold, causing his appetite to differ.[14] Thus, I commanded him to drink the syrups that extinguish the [combustion of] blood, such as verjuice, rhubarb syrup,[15] jujube syrup, and the dishes called *al-ḥiṣrimiyya, al-rummāniyya, al-summāqiyya*, and *al-ʿadasiyya*.[16] If all this did not help, he was very disappointed regarding the matter, and got into a precarious state, so much that it seemed that whilst suffocating his soul would depart from him. [This lasted] until all that was alleviated by phlebotomy, and he gained strength. That man had a fleshy, well-built body with red complexion, and I extracted from him around three litres [of blood] in two sessions.

2:8 There is no determined limit regarding how much and how little blood should be extracted. Galen mentioned that he phlebotomised people and extracted from them around six litres, and they benefitted from that, while from others he extracted one litre, which harmed them. Moreover, Qusṭā[17] reported that ʿAbdallāh al-Rāzī said that he phlebotomised a patient during five consecutive months sixteen times, and in many sessions, he extracted from him 800 *zuz*[18] of blood in weight.

---

12 Ms. Escorial reads "old men at the age of seventy years" in plural.
13 Ms. Escorial: *Madīnat Miṣr*, i.e., al-Fusṭāṭ.
14 Ms. Escorial: "I would postpone it for that sake."
15 Ms. Escorial: "syrup of [two types of] pomegranates."
16 Ms. Escorial lists also *sikbāǧ*.
17 Qusṭā Ibn Lūqā.
18 Ms. Escorial: *dirham*.

2:9 ואמנם האומנות מי שיהיה רופא ברב העמל והמשגל והתנועה והיגיעה והאנחות והתעורה ורוב המחשבות בחכמות הדקות צריך שימעט הדם וההפך בהפך.

2:10 ואמנם המנהג כבר אמרו החכמים כי הוא טבע וצריך שלא יקדים על ההקזה מי שלא הוקז[a] מימיו וכבר עברו משנות חייו זמנים אשר הוצרכה ההקזה אז[b] לא יקיז רק אחר ההשגחה והעיון.

2:11 אמנם המזג הגופים אשר יסבלו יותר ההקזה הם החמים והלחים העבים השמנים בעלי בשר אשר יתערב במראיהם האדמימות רחבי הגידים הנראים עבי השער. ויהיה גבולי ההקזה כפי הרחוק האלה והקורבא. לפעמים גופים עבים ושמנים מעטי הדם וגופים רזים רבי הדם.

2:12 וכבר הגיד גלינוס בספר אפידימיא[c] בשם כי אשה א׳ נעצר אליה הוסת ח׳ חדשים והיתה בתכלית הרזון והקיזה ושב גופה אל איתנו וענינו הראשון. והיו הרופאים מונעים אותה מזה הרבה וכל שכן[d] בהיות תאותה אל המאכל מתחלף. והוציא אליה[e] מהדם כמו ג׳ ליטרים בג׳
ימים: ביום הא׳ ליטר וחצי ובב׳ ליטר ובג׳ חצי ליטר ומיד נתרפאה. | ומלבד עצירת הוסת היו 92v
הגידים מלאי דם ובעת ההקזה יצא הדם שחור כזפת נגר וחייבהו זה להרבות יציאתו.

2:13 ואמנם הזמן מבחר הזמנים אל ההקזה הוא תקופת ניסן הנקרא אלרביע.[f] וזכר גלינוס כי רבים במדינת רומא היו מקיזים בתקופה הזאת מבלי הצרך אל ההקזה למנהג והיו מרויחים בזאת ההנהגה כי כאשר היתה נופלת בהם השגגה לא היתה מזקת להם הרבה ברעתה. ואנשים הרבה בשאר המדינות הגדולות היו נוהגים על זה המנהג. ואחריו בחשיבות הוא תקופת טבת הנקראת אלשתא[g] ואחריו הקיץ ואחריו וחרף. ואמנם העת הנמצא כבר זכרתי אותו למעלה בזה הספר במקום ההקזה כמו שזכרו חנין בן אסחק.

---

a הוקז: הקיז

b אז: או

c אפידימיא: אפידימי׳

d וכל שכן: וכש׳

e אליה: אליו

f الربيع

g الشتاء

2:9 As to the profession, whoever is a hard-working physician, has a lot of sexual intercourse, exercises a lot, with a lot of exertion, sighs [i.e. worries], insomnia, and bears many thoughts in exacting sciences needs to reduce the [evacuation of] blood, and vice versa.

2:10 As to the custom, the wise men[19] have said that it is [an acquired] nature. Therefore, one ought not to rush into phlebotomising those who have not yet undergone this procedure, even if they have reached an age when phlebotomy would have been necessary. They should be phlebotomised only after careful consideration and deliberation.

2:11 As to the disposition, the most tolerant bodies for phlebotomy are those that are hot, moist, wide, fat, with flesh combined with reddish complexion, with wide visible veins and with dense hair. The limits of bloodletting are according to what is far from or near to these. Sometimes thick and fat bodies have a small quantity of blood, and thin bodies have a large quantity of blood.

2:12 Galen spoke in his book called *Epidemics* about a woman whose menstruation stopped for eight months, and she was very emaciated, so he phlebotomised her and her body returned to its former strength and condition. The [other] physicians were strongly preventing her from doing so, especially since her appetite was different [from the usual]. He removed from her blood around three litres in three days: on the first day one and a half litres, on the second day a litre, and on the third day half a litre, and she got cured immediately. | In addition to the amenorrhea, the veins were full of blood, and at 92v
the time of the phlebotomy the blood flowed out black like liquid tar, which forced him [Galen] to increase its extraction [i.e., to extract more than he initially intended].

2:13 As to the season, the most suitable of the seasons for phlebotomy is the season of Nisan, that is called *al-rabīʿ* [i.e., spring]. Galen mentioned that many people in Rome used to phlebotomise during this season without any need for phlebotomy for the sake of tradition, and gained from that the regimen, for if an error befell, it did not cause any severe harm. People in many of the other big countries used to follow the same custom. After it in importance is the season of Tevet, called *al-šitāʾ* [i.e., winter], and after it the summer, and after it the autumn. As to the current time, I already mentioned it above in this treatise [while discussing] phlebotomy, as it was mentioned by Ḥunayn ibn Isḥāq.

[*lacuna*][20]

---

19 I.e., the Ancients.

20 See 2:17–2:19 in the edition of Ms. Escorial.

השער הג׳

3:1 השער הג׳ בסבות המחייבות ההקזה.

3:2 מהסבות לזה הוא המלוי ונחלק לב׳ חלקים. הא׳ מהם כפי החללים והם הגידים והוא שיהיו הגידים והשרינים מלאי דם ורוחות ושאר הליחות הן בערכן ושעורן אשר היו קודם תוספת הדם בהיות הגוף בריא. וישיג אל הגוף[a] מזה הדפוקה[b] וכאלו הגידים נמתחים ויהיו הפנים עם זה אדומים כאלו מטיפים הדם ורוב[c] השינה והתפשטות האיברים ורוחות הפה הנקראות אלתמטא[d] ואלתתאב[e] וכובד הראש וגדל הדופק ועבי השתן ואדמימותו וכובד הרגשת[f] האיברים ורפיון הדעת ומתיקות הפה ונגעיו ויציאת הדם מצדדין[g] והצמחים הנקראים אלדממאל[h] הנפתחים מהרה. ואם יתחבר עם זה שיהיה משוש הגוף חם נוטה אל הרכות כאלו יצא מן המרחץ[i] מהמים החמים הנקראים אלמוחמתא[j] והשנים שנות הבחרות והגידים רחבים והמזון הנקדם יחייב זה יהיו האותות יותר אמתנים.[k]

3:3 ואפשר להוסיף בזה החלומות כמו שזכר אבוקרט בספרו אפידימיא[l] וזכרו רופאש בספרו וזה כי מי שראה בחלומו חבורות ודם נגר ומראים אדומים מודה על הצרך ביציאת הדם. וזה הדרך אל שאר הליחות כי מי שיראה השלג והמטר יורה על רוב הלחה.[m]

3:4 ואמנם המלוי כפי הכוח והוא אשר יוסיפו בו הליחות בשעור אשר לא יספיק הטבע לשמרו ולהנהיגו. וישיג אל הגוף מזה הכובד והעצלה והרפיון מקשי התנועה ומעוט התאוה אל האכילה וחולשת הכח להוציא מה שבגוף מהליחות עד שהטבע לא יוכל להתבשל מה שיהיה בגידים להשיבו מזון. ונשאר על ענינו מעצלת הטבע עליו לשנותו.

---

a ~~הזק׳~~ + Deleted

b הדפוקה: והדפוקה

c ורוב + .Ms

d التمطي

e التثاؤب

f הרגשת: הרעשת

g Could also be read as מצדדיו

h الدمل ج. الدماميل

i מן המרחץ: מהם מרחץ

j [*sic*]

k אמתנים: אמתיים

l אפידימיא: אפידימי׳

m הלחה: הלכוה

The Third Chapter

3:1 The third chapter on the causes that make phlebotomy necessary.

3:2 [One] of those causes is overfilling, which is divided into two parts. The first of them is relating to vessels, i.e., the veins. It occurs when the veins and the arteries are filled with blood and *pneuma*, and the other humours are in their respective proportion and extent as they were before the increase of blood when the body was still healthy. This is followed by spoilage of the body, as if the veins are being ruptured, accompanied by a reddened face as if dripping blood, excessive sleep, stretching of the body parts, winds of the mouth called *al-tamaṭṭā* [i.e., stretching][21] and *al-taṯā'ub* [i.e., yawning], heaviness of head, magnitude of pulse, thick and red urine, heaviness of the parts,[22] want of intellect, sweetness of mouth pustules in it, bleeding from its sides, and boils, called *al-dummal*[23] that burst out quickly. If this is combined with the sensation that the body is hot to touch, leaning towards tenderness, as if he [i.e., the patient] got out of a bathhouse, from the hot waters called †*al-mwḥmt'*†,[24] and he is in the age of adolescence, the veins are wide, and the preceding food requires it, then the indications are stronger.[25]

3:3 Perhaps it comes with the addition of the dreams, as Hippocrates mentioned in his book *Epidemics*, and [as] Rufus mentioned in his book, that dreaming of bruises, flowing blood, and red colours indicates the need for extraction of blood. This is the manner to [draw prognostic conclusions from] the other humours, since dreaming of snow and rain indicates a large quantity of phlegm.

3:4 As to the overfilling affecting the strength, it occurs when the humours increase to the extent that Nature is insufficient to protect and process it. This results in heaviness of the body, laziness, difficulty of movement, lack of appetite, and weakened ability for the body to expel humours, until Nature cannot digest what is in the veins, thus returning the food to it. It remains that way since Nature is unable to transform it.

---

21 See commentary.

22 Ms. Escorial: *kadar al-ḥawāss*, 'troubled sensations.'

23 Ms. Escorial: *al-damāmīl*, in plural.

24 See commentary.

25 Ms. Escorial: *aqwā*, 'stronger.' See commentary.

3:5 ואם יהיו אלה האותות בהרגשת[a] המלוי כפי החללים כבר חלקו ביניהם בשתן ובדפק וזולתם ממה שזכרנו כי הדפק אל המלוי כפי הכח קטן והשתן עם נאות והמראה בלתי אדום ועל הרוב הוא מוליד חליים קודם שלמות האותות.

3:6 וכל אלה המלויים יחייבו חליים וצריכים הרקה. אמנם המלוי הראשון והוא אשר כפי החללים יצטרך אל ההקזה בלבד ואל מעוט המזון. ואמנם המלוי הב׳ והוא אשר כפי הכח יצטרך אל ההקזה ואל ההרקה וצריך השגחה ועיון ולקחת האותות אשר ימצאו אל החולה ורפואתם ממקומותם המיוחדים אליהם וזה כי אפשר שיהיו בגופותם ליחות נאות ואם יקיזו אותם אשר כזה ענינם יקרה להם רפיון וחולשה וקרירות המזג ויהיו מזומנים אל החליים הקרים עד שאי אפשר[b] להם לשוב אל ענינם הראשון. והשגגה עצומה הרבה וכל שכן[c] בהיות זה בזמן הקיץ והאצטומכא והכבד שלו קרים והמזג רך.

3:7 ויועיל למי שיהיה בזאת התכונה משיחים עם השמנים הישרים ולהתמיד הסמים החותכים הליחות העבות ומעוט המזון ודקותו ומאכלים מעטי המזון. ואפשר להוציא להם מהדם מעט ויעשה זה בפעמים הרבה.

3:8 ומי שיקרה לו רוק הדם ונתרפא צריך שיקדים להקיז בתחלת תקופת ניסן |[d] ואם לא יהיה 93r
בגופו מעט מלוי או יפחד פן יבקע או שישבר גיד בחזהו. וכן אל מי שיפחד עליו מחלי הכפייה או חלי אלסכתה[e] או פתיחת גידי פי הטבעת או המורסות המתהוות בראות[f] או מורסת הצלעות הנקראת שוצא[g] והחניקות וכאבי הפרקים והקדחות הדבקות הדמיות.

3:9 ובכלל כל החליים הבאים ונופלים מסבת הדם או שאר הליחות צריך להקדים אליהם ההקזה והמשלשל כפי הצרך בתקופת ניסן. ואם לא יהיו אותות הרבוי נראים ונופלים למה שיתחדש אחרי זה[h] וזה כי הוא יבא אל הקיץ ויבקשו[i] הליחות מקום רחב יותר. ואפשר לעשות

a בהרגשת: בהרעשת
b עד שאי אפשר :עד שא״א
c וכל שכן: וכש׳
d ניסן + .Ms
e السكتة
f בראות: בריאו
g الشوصة
h אחרי זה: אח״ז
i ~~ממנו~~ +.Deleted in the Ms

3:5 Even if these indications occur, you may feel overfilling relating to vessels. The two may be differentiated by urine, pulse, and the other factors we have mentioned, since the pulse in overfilling affecting the strength is weak, the urine is somewhat raw and its colour is not red. In most cases, it is generating illnesses before the symptoms are developed.

3:6 Both of these [two kinds of] overfillings impose illnesses and require evacuation. As to the first [kind of] overfilling, that is the one relating to vessels, it requires only phlebotomy and reduction of food. As to the second [type of] overfilling, that is the one affecting the strength, it requires phlebotomy and evacuation. It [also] requires hesitation and consideration regarding the patient's symptoms and their treatment in their specific sites. This is because their bodies may contain raw humours, and whenever someone in this condition is phlebotomised, they become weak, their disposition becomes cold, and they become susceptible to cold illnesses so that they cannot return to their former condition. And the mistake[26] is very great, especially if it is summer, his stomach and liver are cold, and his disposition is tender.

3:7 Those characterised by this condition benefit from massages with moderate oils, continuous use of drugs that cut coarse humours, reduction of food and making it finer, and taking scarcely nourishing foods. One may extract a small quantity of their blood, and this may be done in several sessions.

3:8 For those who have suffered from haemoptysis and have healed from it, one may proceed to phlebotomy in the beginning of the period called | Nisan [i.e. 93r
springtime], even if there is not [even] a slight [indication of] overfilling in his body, since [otherwise] one would be afraid of a vein splitting or bursting in his chest. This also applies to those who are afraid of epilepsy, apoplexy, burst veins in the anus, swellings in the lungs, or swelling of the ribs called *šawṣa* [i.e., pleuritis], as well as diphtheria, arthritis, and continuous [and] sanguine fevers.

3:9 In general, all illnesses that arise and befall because of [a surplus of] blood or the other humours must be tackled by phlebotomy and purgation as needed during Nisan [i.e., in the springtime], even if no indications of a surplus are apparent or occur. This is done [in anticipation] of what may follow, for as the summer approaches, the humours demand a wider space. It is possible to evac-

26 Ms. Escorial: 'danger.'

להם הרקה גם כן[a] עם ההקזה ואם לא יהיה הגוף מלא מא׳ המלויים בעת התחלת המורסה חמה או בסבת הכאה ונפילה או צער חזק או חולשת האבר כי אם יהיה בו כאב או חולשה ימשוך על זה דם אם יהיה הליחה נמשכה לזה כמו שימשכו כוסות המציצה הדם.

השער הד׳

4:1 השער הד׳ בכמות שיצא מן הדם.

4:2 אמנם אמתה שעור הדם ושאר הליחות בגוף ושעור מה שצריך להוציא להם בעת הצרך[b] וכמות שעור המשלשל אשר בו ההרקה בערכו ובהקשתו אל הליחות זה יקשה הרבה כמו שזכרנו כי רק ההרקה עם הקזה היא יותר בטוחה מהשלשול הרבה בעבור כי יוכל אדם להפסיקה כשירצה. ואמנם המשלשל כאשר הוא בבטן לא יוכל לחסם ממנו ולא מפעלתו.

4:3 וכאשר יהיה הדם הרבה בגוף ונתחמם ונרתח ונתחדשה ממנו קדחת יעשה הרקתו פתאם בעת ירידת הקפת הקדחת וקודם שיהיה נגר אל האברים המעולים בעבור כי זאת הקדחת ואם היא דבקה יהיה לה על הרוב התחלה התוספת ותכלית וירידה. וצריך להוציא מהדם עד שיתעלף בעבור כי הדם הרע כאשר נשאר בגוף הפסיד זולתו. ופעמים הרבה תמהר ותתחיל הזיעה אחר העטוף ויזיע מעט או ישלשל הטבע ויסור החלי מהרה. ואין ליציאת הדם גבול ידוע ברב או במעט.

4:4 והראוי והנכון להשתדל ולהשגיח בו בעת ההקזה לעיין ולראות הדפק מהצד המתחלף כל עת התמדת הגרת הדם בעבור כי כאשר יקרהו העלוף שלא יקרהו המות. וכאשר יראה הדפק משתנה ומתחלף בגדלו או בהשואתו ויתיין הכח עם חולשא או שנחלש ונחסר רוע מראה הדם צריך להפסיקו מיד. ופעמים הרבה לא ישתנה העצם והמראה מהדם.

---

a גם כן: ג״כ

b והשגחה + .Ms

uate them by means of phlebotomy even if the body is not afflicted by either type of overfilling, at the onset of a warm swelling caused either by a blow or a fall or severe sorrow,[27] or weakness of a part—since when a part aches or weakens, it attracts blood if the humour is drawn to this area, just as the cupping vessels draw blood.

The Fourth Chapter

4:1 The fourth chapter on the quantity of blood that should be extracted.

4:2 Really knowing the quantity of blood and other humours in the body, the quantity of what needs to be extracted from them when necessary, and the quantity of the purgative drug in its proportion and relation to the humours, is very difficult, as we have mentioned. However, evacuation by phlebotomy is much more secure than purgation, because one can end it whenever desired. As to the purgative drug, once it has reached the stomach, one cannot undo it nor its effect.

4:3 When there is a lot of blood in the body, and it gets hot and boils, generating a fever, one should proceed to evacuating all at once at the time of the decay of the paroxysm of fever before it flows into the vital parts, because this fever, even if it is a continuous fever, will in most cases have a beginning, increase, culmination, and decline. One needs to extract blood until [the patient] faints because when bad blood remains in the body, it corrupts the rest. In many cases, sweating begins quickly after unconsciousness, and he sweats a little,[28] or the Nature gets purged, and the illness terminates quickly. There is no known limit regarding how much or how little blood should be extracted.

4:4 At the time of phlebotomy, it is preferable and correct to be careful and consider, and to observe and monitor the pulse from the opposite side throughout the continuous flow of blood, so that if fainting occurs, death does not follow. When one sees the strength and regularity of the pulse differ and change, in addition to weakening or diminished force, and the colour of the blood is bad, it is necessary to stop it immediately. Many times, the consistency and the colour of blood do not change.

27 Ms. Escorial: 'severe pain.'

28 Ms. Escorial: "the body becomes cold immediately after unconsciousness, and moist."

4:5 ומי שיהיה בו מורסא קרוב למקום ההקזה כמו השוצ׳א[a] וזולתה הטוב והנכון לו יותר מכל דבר להוציא מהדם עד שישתנה בו מראה ועצם כי הדם באלו החליים[b] אם הוא בענין טבעו נא או אדום אם יהיה במורסא בסבת הרתיחה הדם יוצא אדום והאדום השחור צריך להרחיק העטוף בעת ההקזה הרחקה רבה רק מה שצריך אליו בהכרת.

4:6 וכאשר תהיה ההקזה ברבוי הדם צריך להגיע ההקזה עד העלוף. ואם תהיה ההקזה לשריפת הדם אז צריך להגיע עד שישתנה מראהו.

השער הה׳

5:1 השער הה׳ בגידי ההקזה.

5:2 הגידים המוקזים הם ב׳ מינים: מהם דופקים והם השרינים וצמיחתם וגדולם מהלב ומהם בלתי דופקים והם הורידים וצמיחתם וגדולם מהכבד. ואנחנו נבא לזכרם כלם בשמותם ומקומותם ותועלתם על הסדר ונתחיל בראש.

5:3 והם ד׳ גידים אחורי האזנים בראש | בכל צד ב׳ גידים א׳ מימין וא׳ משמאל ומתנגדים 93v
ובאים בקצה האזן העליון. וכאשר נדבקו אל הראש יהיה הגידים למעלה מן האזן בשעור מעט. ותועיל הקזתם מנגעים וחבורות הראש ואלסעפא[c] הלחה והיבשה ומהצרעות.

5:4 וג׳ גידים והם שרינים בחיצון כל אזן ב׳ מהם נסתרים וא׳ נראה. ותועיל הקזתם מחלי הנגעים הדקים הנקרא אלסעפא[d] ולכאב העינים. וזכר אבוקרט בספרו האוירים כי מי שנכרת לו אלו הגידים איננו מוליד ואמר זה במאמר מוחלט.

5:5 וב׳ גידים באחורי הראש סמוכים אל נקרת הראש והוא נקב הערף הנקרא אלנקרא.[e] ותועיל הקזתם מהעשן העולה ומהתחלת המים היורדים בעינים וחלי אלאנתשאר.[f]

a الشوصة

b Ms. + a deleted, smudged word.

c السعفة

d السعفة

e אלנקרא: אלסקרא، النقرة

f الانتشار

4:5 Whoever has a swelling near the phlebotomised site, such as *šawṣa* [i.e., pleuritis] and the like, the best and most appropriate treatment is to extract blood until its colour and consistency change. For in these patients, if the blood is naturally raw or red, and if it is in the swelling due to boiling, it will come out red or dark red. One must avoid unconsciousness during phlebotomy as much as possible, only reaching that point when necessary.

4:6 When you phlebotomise for the surplus of blood, phlebotomy should last until unconsciousness. If you phlebotomise for the combustion of blood, you should reach the point where its colour changes.

The Fifth Chapter

5:1 The fifth chapter on the phlebotomised veins.

5:2 There are two kinds of phlebotomised veins: the pulsatile, i.e., the arteries, that originate and grow from the heart, and the non-pulsatile, i.e., the veins, that originate and grow from the liver. We will mention them all by their names, sites, and benefit consecutively, and we will begin in the head.

5:3 There are four veins behind the ears in the head, | two veins on both sides, 93v
one on the right, one on the left. They run parallelly and reach the upper tip of the ear. As these connect to the head, the veins are slightly above the ear. Phlebotomising them is beneficial for pustules and ulcers in the head, wet and dry *al-saʿfa* [i.e., cradle cap], and leprosy.

5:4 Three veins that are arteries in the exterior of each ear, two of which are concealed, and one visible. Phlebotomising them is beneficial for the illness of fine pustules called *al-saʿfa* [i.e., cradle cap] and for ophthalmalgia. Hippocrates mentioned in his book, *Airs*, that whoever had these veins cut will not procreate, and he said it as an absolute statement.[29]

5:5 Two veins in the back of the head, near the occiput, [also called] the hollow of the neck, [in Arabic] *al-nuqra*. Phlebotomising them is beneficial for the rising fumes, watery discharge from the eyes, and for the illness called *al-intišār*.

29 See commentary.

5:6 וב׳ גידים באים אל המצח מאמצע הראש יתחלקו שם לב׳ חלקים ואפשר שיהיו יותר. ויהיה הא׳ בימין והאחר בשמאל. וצריך להקיזם לעולם כאשר יהיו מלאים. ותועיל הקזתם מכאב העינים הקדום והישן והכובד המתהוה באחורי הראש.

5:7 וב׳ גידים נפתלים בצדעים והם שרינים. ותועיל הקזתם לכאב הראש התמידי וכאב חצי הראש הנקרא אלשקיקא[a] ולחלי העינים הנקרא אלאנתשאר[b] ולכאב העין אשר יפחד ממנו על המות. ותהיה הקזתם בדקירה או בכריתה.

5:8 והכלל צריך להקיז דם מהגידים הדופקים מה שידע כי הוית החלי מליחה חמה וחדה ודקה עוקצת הקרומים הדקים וירגיש הכאב כאלו הוא מרכז והכאב ההוא עוקץ ומתפשט סביב המרכז.

5:9 וב׳ גידים בקצות העורקים הנקראים אלמאקין.[c] ותועיל הקזתם משארית חלי העינים הנקרא אלרמאד[d] והדמעות וחולשת הראות הנקרא אלעשוא.[e]

5:10 וגיד א׳ בקצה החוטם ותועיל הקזתו מהכתמים הנקראים אלכלוף[f] ומשנוי המראה והחמימות[g] והנגעים והחבורות אשר בחוטם והשפה והעצר הדם בהם והמורסות הקשות הנקראות אלנואסיר[h] והבקוע המתחדש בהם.

5:11 וב׳ גידים בפנימי הלשון ותועיל הקזתם מנפיחת הלשון ומהחניקות אשר מסבת הדם.

5:12 וב׳ גידים בתוך הזקן לפנים ואם יגבה הלשון יראה הא׳ אל הימין והאחר אל השמאל. ותועיל הקזתם ממורסת העצל אשר בושט.

---

a الشقيقة
b الانتشار
c المأقيين
d الرمد
e العشاوة
f الكلف
g الحزاز Ms. Escorial
h אלנואסיר: אלבואסיר

5:6 Two veins[30] reach the forehead from the middle of the head, dividing there into two parts, possibly more. One is on the right and the other on the left. One should always phlebotomise them when they are full. Phlebotomising them is beneficial for long-lasting, chronic ophthalmalgia, and for the heaviness that occurs in the back of the head.

5:7 Two curved veins in the temples, and they are arteries. Phlebotomising them is beneficial for chronic headache, pain affecting one side of the head called *al-šaqīqa* [i.e., migraine], for the eye illness called *al-intišār*, as well as for ophthalmalgia that makes one afraid of dying. Phlebotomising them is done by puncturing or by cutting.

5:8 In general, the pulsatile veins should be phlebotomised if it is known that the illness is caused by a hot, sharp, fine, pricking humour in the membranes, and the pain feels as if it is concentrated, and that pain is pricking and spreading around the centre.

5:9 Two veins by the edges of the veins that are called *al-ma'qayn* [i.e., *canthus internus*]. Phlebotomising them is beneficial for remains of the eye illness called *al-ramad* [i.e., ophthalmia], tears [i.e., rhyas], and the visual impairment called *al-ʿašāwa* [i.e., nyctalopia].

5:10 One vein in the tip of the nose. Phlebotomising it is beneficial for the stains that are called *al-kaluf* [i.e., freckles],[31] discoloration, dandruff,[32] pustules and ulcers in the nose and the lips, congestion of blood in them, and the hard swellings called *al-nawāsīr* [i.e. polyps][33] and fissures in them.

5:11 Two veins inside the tongue: phlebotomising them is beneficial for swelling of the tongue and for diphtheria caused by blood.

5:12 Two veins inside the inner part of the chin. If the tongue is lifted, one can be seen on the right and the other on the left. Phlebotomising them is beneficial for the swelling of the muscle in the oesophagus.

---

30 Ms. Escorial: 'a vein.'

31 In Arabic *al-kalaf*.

32 Ms. Escorial: *ḥazāz*, 'dandruff,' apparently read and understood as *ḥarāra*, 'heat' by the copyist of Ms. Parma.

33 See commentary.

5:13 וב׳ גידים הנקראים אללודג׳ין[a] ומקומם בצואר ותועיל הקזתם לנמיכות הקול הנקראת בחוחא אלצות[b] ולכאב הריאה ולקשי הנשימה הנקרא אלרבו[c] ולחלי הצרעת.[d]

5:14 וב׳ גידים בב׳ הזרועות ונקראים אלבטאן[e] וימצא כל א׳ מהם בין פרק הזרוע הנקרא אלמרפק[f] ובין בית השחי הנקרא אלאבטא[g] מהצד הפנימי. ותועיל הקזתם מהגרת הדם אל הלב ולכאב הריאה והחזה והשוצ׳א.[h]

5:15 וו׳ גידים באמות הזרוע בכל אמות הזרוע מהם ג׳ גידים. הא׳ נקרא אלקיפאלי[i] והוא שם יוני. ותועיל הקזתו מהחליים אשר למעלה מהמקום הנקרא אללבא[j] והראש והפנים בפרק שלהם.

5:16 והב׳ הנקרא אלבסליק[k] והוא שם משותף מן הראשות ומקומו מן הצד הפנימי ותועיל הקזתו מן החליים אשר למטה מהמקום הנקרא אללבה[l] כי לשם תכליתו ואחר הוא הולך ויורד אל הרגלים.

5:17 והג׳ הוא הנקרא אלאכחל[m] והוא ענף מהבסליק[n] וענף מהקיפאל[o] יתחברו במקום א׳ באמצע שניהם. ותועיל הקזתו מהחלי הכול הגוף כלו בעבור כי הוא מחובר משניהם.

5:18 וכאשר יהיה החלי בראש צריך להקיז הקיפאל[p] כי הוא מיוחד אליו רק אם ירצה למשוך הליחות. וידוע כי בין הקזת הגיד המיוחד אל החלי ובין הגיד אשר איננו מיוחד הפרש גדול.[q]

---

a الودجان
b אלבחוחא אלצות: אלבחוסא אלצות، بحة الصوت
c الربو
d חלי הצרעת: חלי הצער
e الإبطان
f المرفق
g الإبطي
h الشوصة
i القيفال
j اللبة
k الباسليق
l اللبة
m الأكحل
n الباسليق
o القيفال
p القيفال
q גדול וב׳ added below the line.

5:13 Two veins called *al-wadağayn* [i.e., the jugular veins], located in the neck. Phlebotomising them is beneficial for the raspy voice called *al-buḥūḥa al-ṣawt* [i.e., hoarseness of voice],[34] for lung pain, difficulty of breathing called *al-rabw* [i.e., asthma], as well as for leprosy.

5:14 Two veins in the two upper arms that are called *al-*[*i*]*bṭān* [i.e., the axillary veins], each located between the joint of the upper arm, called *al-mirfaq* [i.e., elbow], and the armpit, called *al-ibṭa*, on the inner side. Phlebotomising them is beneficial for blood flowing into the heart, for pain in lungs and chest, and for pleuritis.

5:15 Six veins in the forearms, three in each forearm. One is called *al-qīfāl* [i.e., the cephalic vein], which is a Greek name. Phlebotomising it is beneficial for the illnesses that occur above the site called *al-labba* [i.e., jugular fossa], the head, and the face in their part.[35]

5:16 The second is called *al-bāsilīq* [i.e., the basilic vein], which is a name derived[36] from the [Greek word for] leadership,[37] located on the inner side. Phlebotomising it is beneficial for the illnesses below the site called *al-labba* [i.e., jugular fossa], because its utmost scope is there, and afterwards it continues going down towards the feet.

5:17 The third is called *al-akḥal* [i.e., the median cubital vein], which is a branch of the basilic vein and a branch of the cephalic vein which unite at one spot in the middle of the two. Phlebotomising it is beneficial for illnesses in the whole body, since it is composed of the two.

5:18 Whenever the illness is in the head, one needs to phlebotomise the cephalic vein, because it is specifically intended for it, unless one wants to draw matters. It is known that there is a great difference between phlebotomising a vein specifically intended for [treatment of] an illness and a vein that is not specifically intended.

---

34 In Arabic *buḥḥat al-ṣawt*.

35 Ms. Escorial: *liʾannahu murtaq ilayhā*, "because it ascends to them."

36 Ms. Parma reads 'common name,' see commentary.

37 Arabic *riʾāsa*, Greek *basilikós*.

5:19 וב׳ גידים בחיצוני המקומות הנקראים אלמעצמין[a] והם האמות בזרוע ונקראים יתרי 94r
הזרוע והם מגיד אלבסליק[b] ויעמדו בהקזה במקומו.

5:20 וענף א׳ הולך בין האצבע הנקרא אלבנסר[c] והאצבע האמצעי. ותועיל הקזתו מכאבי הכבד והלב והטחול והריאה.

5:21 וענף א׳ הולך בין האצבע הנקרא אלבנצר[d] ובין אלכנצר[e] ונקרא אלאסילם.[f] ותועיל הקזתו מכאב החזה והכבד והטחול והריאה.

5:22 וב׳ גידים נמצאים במקום הנקרא מאבץ אלרכבתאן[g] והם עבים ומלאים מהגידים אשר בשוקים. ותועיל הקזתם מנפיחת השוקים ומחלי פתול הגידים הנקרא אלדואלי[h] ולהוריד דם הוסת.

5:23 וב׳ גידים הנקראים וידועים כגיד הנשה[i] ונמצאים בחיצוני העקבים אשר בצד החיצוני ותועיל הקזתם מהכאב החזק אשר יתחדש מתחת הירך וחיצוני השוק עד אחרית הרגל. ואפשר שלא יגיע הכאב עד הרגל.

5:24 וב׳ גידים הנקראים אלצפאן[j] ונמצאים על העקבים מהצד הפנימי. ותועיל הקזתם מהנגעים וחכוך הביצים ולהוריד דם הוסת.

5:25 ואפשר שימצאו גידים נקראים אלערק אלמדיני[k] ותולדתם מסבת המאכלים והמשקים ורפואתם יוצא מכונת הספר.

a المعصمين
b الباسليق
c البنصر
d البنصر
e الخنصر
f الأسيلم
g مأبض الركبتين
h الدوالي
i عرق النسا
j אלצפאן: אלצפאפן، الصافنان
k العرق المدني

5:19 Two veins on the outer sides of the sites called *al-miʿṣamayn* [i.e., the wrists], which is the forearms in the arm, called 'extensions of the forearm' [i.e., *vena cephalica pollicis*]. They come from the basilic vein and serve in phlebotomy instead of it. 94r

5:20 One branch runs between the finger called *al-binṣir* [i.e., ring finger], and the middle finger. Phlebotomising it is beneficial for pain in the liver, heart, spleen, and lungs.

5:21 Another branch runs between the finger called *al-binṣir* [i.e., ring finger] and *al-ḫinṣir* [i.e., little finger], and it is called *al-usaylim* [i.e., *vena salvatella*]. Phlebotomising it is beneficial for pain in the chest, liver, spleen, and lungs.

5:22 Two veins located at the site called *ma'biḍ al-rukbatān* [i.e., *popliteal fossa*], that are thicker and fuller than [the other] veins in the legs. Phlebotomising them is beneficial for the swelling of the legs, the illness of twisting veins called *al-dawālī,* [i.e., varicose veins], and to make the menstruation flow.

5:23 Two veins that are called and known as *gid ha-naše* [i.e., the sciatic veins], located on the outer side of the ankles, on the outside. Phlebotomising them is beneficial for the strong pain that occurs below the thigh and the external part of the leg until the tip of the foot. Perhaps the pain does not reach the foot.

5:24 Two veins that are called *al-ṣafān* [i.e., saphenous veins],[38] located on the inner side of the ankles. Phlebotomising them is beneficial for pustules, itching testicles, and to make the menstruation flow.

5:25 One may find veins that are called *al-ʿirq al-madīnī* [i.e., Guinea worm],[39] that are generated from foods and drinks—their treatment is outside the intention of this book.

38 In Arabic *ṣāfin,* dual *ṣāfinān.*

39 In Arabic *al-ʿirq al-madanī.*

השער הו׳

6:1 השער הו׳ באיכות הקזת הגידים ומה שישיג בהם מהטעות והמשגה להשמר ממנו.

6:2 בעבור היות גידי ההקזה דופקים ובלתי דופקים כמו שזכרנו ויש בהקזת הגידים הדופקים סכנה בסבת עבי עורם וקשי הפסק דמם וסתומם. והם מורכבים מב׳ מחיצות רק כי הגיד אשר ישקה הריאה הוא לבדו מורכב במחיצה א׳ והמחיצה הפנימית מהם עביה ה׳ פעמים כעבי המחיצה החיצונה.

6:3 ונתחיל תחלה גיד אלקיפאל.[a] אלקיפאל[b] צריך להקיזו ממקום העצל כנגד הבשר הרך ולא יהיה מקום ההקזה צר.

6:4 ויהיה בעת שריפת הדם מקומה רחב לעבי הליחה ובעת משיכת[c] הליחה יהיה מקומה צר להאריך המשיכה ובעת רבוי הדם בינוני בעבור כי אם היה רחב פוחד מהגרת הדם בכוח חזק ותתחדש[d] במקום ההקזה נפיחה. וכאשר תעכב ותמנע הגרת הדם ממקום ההקזה אז ימשח עליו עם עכירות שמרי השמן והוא יותר טוב לזה מהזך ממנו.

6:5 אלאכחל[e] צריך להשגיח ולעיין בהקזתו כי אם היה העצב[f] ממנו אל הימין או אל השמאל יקיז אותו עם חדות ברזל ההקזה הנקרא אלשפרה אלמבצע[g] אל הפך צד העצב. ואם יהיה בין ב׳ העצבים יקיזהו בארך.[h]

6:6 אלבסליקי[i] צריך להשגיח ולעיין השרין אשר תחתיו וצריך שתהיה הקזתו עם ברזל רך קצר החדות בעבור כי הוא גיד[j] עצבי כי אם יצא הדם אדום אז דע כי הוא מהשרין.

---

a القيفال
b القيفال
c משיכת: משיך
d ותתחדש: ותתחזק
e الأكحل
f העצב: העצל
g شفرة المبضع
h בארך in the margin.
i الباسليق
j גיד: גידי

The Sixth Chapter

6:1 The sixth chapter on the method of venesection and the mistake deriving from it, and how to avoid it.

6:2 Since the veins used in phlebotomy are pulsatile and non-pulsatile, as we have mentioned, there is a danger in phlebotomising the pulsatile veins, because their skin is thick and stanching the blood and blocking them is difficult. They are composed of two tunics, apart from the vein that nourishes[40] the lungs, that alone is composed of one tunic, and the thickness of the inner tunic of them is five times the thickness of the outer tunic.

[*lacuna*][41]

6:3 We begin with *al-qīfāl* [i.e., the cephalic vein]. The cephalic vein should be phlebotomised from the site of the muscle opposite the soft flesh. The site of phlebotomy should not be narrow.

6:4 During a combustion of blood, a wide vein should be phlebotomised due to the coarseness of the matter; and when drawing matter, a narrow vein, to lengthen the drawing. During a surplus of blood, a medium-size vein should be phlebotomised, since if a wide vein was cut, one would be afraid of an intense blood flow, causing a swelling at the phlebotomised spot. When blood flow is hindered and prevented from the phlebotomised site, one should anoint it with the sediment of oil, which is better for it than pure oil.

6:5 *Al-akḥal* [i.e., the median cubital vein] needs to be examined carefully when phlebotomised, because if the nerve is to the right or to the left, one phlebotomises it with the blade of the phlebotomising iron called *al-šafra al-mibḍaʿ* [i.e., scalpel],[42] on the opposite side of the nerve. And, if it is between two nerves, one phlebotomises it lengthwise.

6:6 *Al-bāsilīq* [i.e., the basilic vein], one must examine and observe the artery below it, and one should phlebotomise it with a fine, short-bladed scalpel, since it is a nerval vein. Should the blood flow out red, then you know that it is from the artery.[43]

40 Lit. irrigates.

41 See 6:2–6:8 in the edition of Ms. Escorial.

42 In Arabic *šafrat al-mibḍaʿ*.

43 See commentary.

6:7 הנקרא חבל אלדרע[a] והוא מיתר הזרוע והוא סר ממקומו הרבה וצריך להקיזו עם ברזל ההקזה רך ובו חדות הנקראת שפרה.[b] וצריך שתהיה השקיעה עם הברזל כפי שעור קשי העור. וידוע כי העור השחור לעולם יותר קשה והלבן יותר רך.

6:8 אלאסלים[c] צריך שישים הכף במים חמים עד שתעלה עליו נפיחה ויקשור המקום הנקרא אלמעצם[d] היטב עם מצנפת ואחר יקיז וישיב הכף במים חמים בעבור שלא יקפא הדם.

6:9 ערק אלניסא[e] הוא נסתר ומכוסה והוא גיד הנשה וצריך אם לא יכירנו להכניס החולה במרחץ או לשום הרגל במים חמים וישגיח וישקיף עליו עד שיראהו.

94v 6:10 ואם לא יראהו יקיז במקומו קצת מהענפים אשר על גב הרגל | והטוב והראוי יותר מהם הוא הגיד הנמצא בין האצבעות הקטנות אלכנצר[f] ואלבנצר.[g]

6:11 וידוע כי במקום הנקרא מכאן אלרכבא[h] ב׳ גידים, הא׳ מהם גיד הנשה והאחר אלצפאן.[i] אלצפאן[j] זה הגיד אם יקיז אותו או על העקב או בקצת ענפיו אשר זכרנו יהיה יותר טוב מהקזת השרש הרבה מאד. וכן כל מה שתהיה הרחקת ההקזה יותר ממקום החלי והחליים הישנים יהיה יותר טוב מהקזת השרש הרבה.

השער הז׳

7:1 השער הז׳ במשיכת הליחות.

7:2 בעבור היות הליחות בהתחלת החליים אשר מסבת הדם נגרות בעת תכליתם עומדות ונעצרות יתחייב להחליף ולשנות כפי זה מקומות ההקזה.

---

a حبل الذراع חבל אלדרע: זבל אלדרע
b شفرة
c الأسيلم
d المعصم
e عرق النسا
f الخنصر
g البنصر
h مأبض الركبة
i الصافن
j الصافن

6:7 [Then a vein] that is called *ḥabl al-ḏirāʿ* [i.e., *vena cephalica pollicis*],[44] the cord of the forearm. It deviates from its site a lot. One should phlebotomise it with a fine phlebotomy iron that has a blade, called *šafra* [i.e., scalpel]. The depth of the [incision with the] scalpel must be according to the hardness of the skin. It is known that black skin is always harder, and white [skin] softer.

6:8 *Al-usaylim* [i.e., *vena salvatella*]: one needs to put the palm of the hand into hot water until it swells, tighten the site called *al-miʿṣam* [i.e., wrist] well with a bandage, and then phlebotomise it, and return the palm of the hand back into the hot water to prevent the blood from coagulating.

6:9 *ʿIrq al-nasā* [i.e., the sciatic vein] is concealed and covered; it is the sciatic vein [*gid ha-naše*]. If it is not visible, the patient should be put in a bathhouse, or the leg put into hot water, and [the site] carefully observed until one sees it.

6:10 If it does not become visible, one phlebotomises instead of it some of its branches on the external part of the foot. | The best and the most appropriate 94v
thing to do is [to phlebotomise] the vein between the small toes *al-ḫinṣir* [i.e., pinkie toe] and *al-binṣir* [i.e., ring toe].

6:11 It is known that there are two veins in the site called *makān al-rukba* [i.e., *popliteal fossa*], one of them the sciatic vein, and the other *al-ṣafān* [i.e., the saphenous vein].[45] It is preferable to phlebotomise the saphenous vein at the heel or through any of its previously noted branches, rather than at its origin. And thus, the further away phlebotomy is conducted from the affected site, including chronic illnesses, is a lot better than phlebotomising the origin.

[*lacuna*][46]

The Seventh Chapter

7:1 The seventh chapter on drawing matters.[47]

7:2 Since the matters at the first stage of sanguine illnesses are flowing, and at the end still and stagnant, the phlebotomised sites must vary according to that.

---

44 In Arabic *ḥabl al-ḏirāʿ*; Ms. Parma reads *z-b-l al-ḏirāʿ*.

45 In Arabic *al-ṣāfin*.

46 See 6:21–6:22 in the edition of Ms. Escorial.

47 See commentary.

7:3 משל לזה כי מי שיקרהו חלי מורסת הצלעות הנקרא אלשוצא[a] מסבת הדם בצד הימין צריך להשתדל לרפאתו בתחלת החלי ולעיין ולראות כי אם יהיה הדם בגוף הרבה יקיז החולה מהיד השמאלי וישים חזרת ההקזה שנית הנקראת אלתתניא[b] מהיד הימני. ועל זה הדרך בהיות הדם בין הרבוי והמעוט כי אם יהיה הדם בגוף מועט ישים ההקזה בצד החלי עצמו. וזה הענין יוצא מהמחשבה וההקש. ואם עברו על החולה ד׳ ימים ויותר יעשה ההקזה בכל הענינים בצד החלי עצמו וזה בעבור כי הליחות ישובו רובם אל צד החלי עצמו. וכבר הרבו בחייותינו ונסיונותינו בזה על חליים רבים.

השער הח׳

8:1 השער הח׳ בזמנים הטובים להוציא הדם בהם והשמירה ממנו.

8:2 הטוב והראוי יותר בזמנים לזה הוא תקופת ניסן הנקראת אלרביע[c] כמו שזכרנו ומהזמן הזה היום השוה בחום ובקור ומהיום השעה הב׳ והג׳ מהשעות הישרות. ויתחלף זה כפי קרירות המזג וחמימותו.

8:3 כי אם הוא חם המזג או שימהר אליו העלוף צריך להתחיל בהקזתו בשעה ראשונה מן היום. ומי שהוא קר המזג צריך לאחר ההקזה עד שיפוח היום ויתחמם מעט.

8:4 ואנחנו עתידים לזכור מתי יתחייב לקחת המזון קודם ההקזה במקומו.

a الشوصة
b التثنية
c الربيع

7:3 An example of that is that whoever suffers from a sanguine swelling in the ribs called *al-šawṣa* [i.e., pleuritis] on the right side, one must strive to cure it at the onset of the illness, and observe and monitor: if there is a lot of blood in the body, one phlebotomises the patient from the left hand, and does the second, additional removal of blood, called *al-taṯniya* [i.e., epaphairesis], from the right hand. According to this, depending on the quantity of blood—between surplus and scarcity—, since if there is a little blood in the body, one phlebotomises from the affected side itself. This is beyond rational thinking and analogy. If the patient has been ill for four days or more, one conducts the phlebotomy in all cases from the defected side itself, and that is because most of the humours will return to the defected site itself. We have experienced this several times in our experiments on many patients.

[*lacuna*][48]

The Eighth Chapter

8:1 The eighth chapter on the appropriate times to extract blood, and when to guard against extracting it.

8:2 The best and the most appropriate time for this is the season of Nisan called *al-rabīʿ* [i.e., the spring], as we have mentioned, and during this time a day that is moderate in heat and cold, and on such a day the second and the third hours of the equinoctial hours. This may vary depending on whether the natural disposition is cold or hot.

8:3 If the patient is of hot disposition, or faints quickly,[49] one should get started with his phlebotomy at the first hour of the day. For whoever is of cold disposition, one should postpone the phlebotomy until the day breaks and becomes slightly warmer.

8:4 We will mention when he must take some food before being phlebotomised in its proper place.[50]

48 See 7:4–7:9 in the edition of Ms. Escorial.

49 Ms. Escorial: "or quickly becomes hungry."

50 I.e., chapter 10.

8:5 ואם הקיז צריך שלא יקשור על המקום בחזקה כי זה יביא עליו המורסא ולא ירבה אחריה הדאגה והאבל. וימנע מהמשגל רק בעת התשוקה החזקה כי הוא יתרון הזרע המקובץ ויציאתו יותר טובה מהנחתו הרבה. וצריך שישמר מהמאכלים הרעים קודם ההקזה ואחריה כב׳ ימים. וישמר מההקזה כל אשר התמידו בו החליים הקרים או שהוא חלוש העצבים או הרבה דאגה או התעורה או הרבה המשגל או הרבה זמנו בהליכה או שקרב זמנו מהשלשול או הקיא או מי שנתחמם או נתקרר גופו יותר מהנהוג או בעל הקדחת או השכור או המלא מהמזון או הרעב או מי שהפסיד עכולו או מי שיש לו באצטומכא ליחות נאות.

8:6 זה כלל כל מה שישבר הכח ומתיכו או ישנה אותו. רק אם יקרהו פתאם ויפלו בו חליים עצומים מאשר כפי נמצאים כמו חלי אלסכתא[a] והחניקה ודפיקת הלב או בטול הגוף העצום הנקרא אלסכתה אלעטמא[b] כי אז באלה החליים ודומיהם צריך להקיז החולה מהם באיזה עת שיקרה ביום או בלילה.

8:7 וכאשר יחשוב על החולה להקיזו והוא חלוש ורזה או נשבר הגוף או עם חלי ישן ויצטרך להקזה ולהוציא הדם. צריך לפתוח הגיד ואם יראה הדם שחור מעט וקצף יוצא ממנו מה שיחשוב להוציאו. ואם הוא או ירוק או כמראה רמון צריך לסתום מיד בעבור כי יש ביציאתו סכנה.[c]

8:8 ולא נמנע[d] | מהקזת החולה אשר נמשך חליו ימים. וכבר הקיז אבוקרט חולא א׳ ביום הח׳ 95r
לחליו ואמר [גלינוס[e]]: ולא ימנע מההקזה ביום הכ׳ מהחלי על דרך משל[f] עם בריאות הכח ושלמות העכול.

a السكتة
b السقطة العظيمة
c סכנה below the line, in the margin.
d נמנע + ולא נמנע below the line, in the margin, Ms.
e وجالينوس يقول :Ms. Escorial
f על דרך משל: עדמ׳

8:5 If phlebotomised, one should not tighten the ligature very tight, because that causes a swelling. Neither should it be followed by a lot of worries and sadness.[51] One should also abstain from sexual intercourse, except during strong desire, for the accumulation of semen is beneficial, and releasing it is better than its prolonged retention. One should also be cautious with bad foods approximately two days before and after phlebotomy. Whoever constantly suffers from cold illnesses should be cautious with phlebotomy. The same applies to whoever has weak nerves, a lot of worries, insomnia, a lot of sexual intercourse, or who has been walking a lot,[52] or recently has been purged or vomited, whose body has become hotter or colder than customary, who is fevered,[53] drunk, full of food, hungry, whose digestion is corrupted, or who has raw humours in his stomach.[54]

8:6 As a general rule, [one should be cautious in the case of] everything that exhausts the strength and dissolves or alters it. Only in case severe illnesses—such as the illness of *al-sakta* [i.e., apoplexy], choking, heart palpitations, or the severe collapse of the body called *al-sakta al-ʿaẓīma*[55]—or similar ones suddenly develop and befall, the patient needs to be phlebotomised no matter what time it happens, day or night.

8:7 When one considers phlebotomising a patient who is weak and emaciated, severely exhausted, or suffers from a chronic illness, he surely needs phlebotomy and extraction of blood. [In such a case] a vein must be opened, and if the blood is slightly black and foamy, one extracts whatever one intended to extract. If it is either green or dark red,[56] one needs to tie it off immediately, because there is a danger in its extraction.

8:8 One should not avoid | phlebotomising a patient whose illness has lasted 95r
for several days. Hippocrates phlebotomised a patient on the eighth day of his illness. And [Galen] said: "One should not avoid phlebotomy on the twentieth day of the illness, for instance, if the strength is sound and the digestion completed."[57]

51 Ms. Escorial: "do not apply many cloths on it."
52 Ms. Escorial: "who has recently travelled or been phlebotomised, or who is very tired, who suffers from constipation …"
53 Ms. Escorial: "who suffers from indigestion."
54 Ms. Escorial: "in his body."
55 In Arabic *al-saqṭa al-ʿaẓīma*.
56 Lit. "colour of a pomegranate."
57 Ms. Parma does not mention the quote as Galen's words, which is clearly expressed in Ms. Escorial. See commentary.

השער הט׳

9:1 השער הט׳ בחזרת ההקזה הנקראת אלתתניה.[a]

9:2 מי שיהיה כונתו אל ההקזה בשמירת בריאותו צריך להוציא מהדם בשעה אשר זכרנו ויחזיר אותה שנית אחר השעה[b] הד׳ מהשעות הישרות מזמן ההקזה ועל הרוב עד תחלת השעה הו׳. וימהר אותה אל החזק ויאחר אותה אל החלש וכל שכן[c] למי שיקרה עליה העטוף. כי זה צריך להוציא הדם בין פעמים הרבה אחר שיקח מהמזון בין ההקזה ובין החזרה.

9:3 וכאשר ירצה להקיז שנית יספיק להתיר המקום ההוא ולקשור למעלה ממנו ולקבץ הכף הרבה. ואם לא יצא הדם יפתל ויטה הזרוע מעט. ואם נעדרת יציאתו ימשוך הדם עם מריחה אל צד פתיחת הגיד. ואם לא יצא הדם או שנקפא בפי הגיד ואז אפשר שתתחדש מזה מורסא ונפיחה. וכאשר תתחדש הנפיחה במקום ההקזה אין צרך להשתדל להחזירה שנית רק אחר ב׳ ימים או ג׳.

9:4 והחזרה[d] הוא דבר גדול כאשר הטבע לא יסבול ביציאת הדם פתאם ואם הוא יפחד על החזרה.

9:5 וכאשר יפחד על סתום הגיד בעת החזרה שנית או בסבת עבי הדם או לסבת דקות וצרות ההקזה אז צריך שישים מלח שחוק מעורב עם שמן ורדים וישים על ההקזה ויצנוף עליה. ואם יהיה עור ההקזה דק ישים בו שמן ורדים בלבד שלא יעשה בו חבורה.

a التثنية
b השעה: בשעה
c וכל שכן: וכש׳
d והחזרה: וההקזה

The Ninth Chapter

9:1 The ninth chapter on the additional removal of blood called *al-taṯniya* [i.e., epaphairesis].

9:2 Whoever is phlebotomised with the intention of preserving his health, his blood should be extracted at the hour that we have mentioned, and an additional removal of blood should be conducted after the fourth equinoctial hour after the time of phlebotomy, and no later than at onset of the sixth hour. This should be conducted earlier for the strong, and later for the weak, especially for those who lose consciousness. For these, the blood needs to be extracted in several sessions after taking some food between phlebotomy and epaphairesis.

9:3 When one wants to conduct epaphairesis, it is enough to untie that spot, tighten above it [a band], and to hold the palm of the hand a firmly. If no blood flows out, one twists and tilts the arm a little. In case its extraction is [still] absent, one should draw the blood with anointment towards the opening of the vein. If blood [still] does not flow out, or what comes out is coagulated at the opening of the vein, it may provoke a swelling and an inflammation. When a swelling occurs at the phlebotomised spot, one should not conduct it an additional time [on the same day], but after two or three days.

9:4 Epaphairesis[58] is a significant matter when Nature does not tolerate the extraction of [a lot of] blood in one session, [and can be done] even if one is afraid of an additional removal of blood.

9:5 When one is afraid of an obstruction of the vein at the time of epaphairesis, either because of coarse blood, or because the phlebotomy is fine and narrow,[59] it is necessary to apply ground salt mixed with rose oil on the phlebotomised [spot] and to bind it. If the phlebotomised skin is fine, one applies only rose oil on it, so that it does not become ulcerated.

---

58 See commentary.

59 Ms. Escorial: "or because the pulse is thin."

9:6 ואין כל הגידים סובלים ההקזה שנית בעבור כי יש מהם גידים לא ימשכו הדם. וכאשר יהיה רך צריך שיחזק הקשירה עליו בחזרה ויצנוף מצנפת באמתו וזרועו ויתמידהו בשינה בעבור שלא יגר הדם ממנו ויבא לידי סכנה.

השער הי׳

10:1 השער הי׳ במזון מי שהוקז[a] ושתיתו.

10:2 צריך שיהיה הבית אשר הקיז בו ישר האויר עליון התקרה פתוח אל הצפון שטוח עם סמי הריח הטובים והורדים ומיני הפירות והמגדים.

10:3 ושישתה אחר ההקזה מיד הסכנג׳ביז[b] והג׳לב[c] ומשקה הורדים כפי חזק הכח והביצים הרכים. ויאכל החזרת ואלהנדבא[d] עם חמץ. ויאכל בשר הגדיים או הטלאים או תרנגולים[e] עם חמץ ויהיה המאכל ביום ההקזה ומחרתו בינוני. ומהפירות הרמונים והחבושים אחר המזון.

10:4 ואשר יחלש כחו בעת ההקזה או שיקרה עליו העלוף זה צריך שיאכל קודם ההקזה מרק התרנגולים[f] והמאכלים הנקראים אלחצרמיא[g] ואלרומניאה[h] או לבות לחם במיץ רמונים חמוצים וישתה משקה הורדים. ויוציא הדם בין פעמים כמו שזכרנו ויאכל בין כל פעם ופעם. וישתה ממשקה הדבש והמיבא[i] כי אלה יעמדו במקום היין כמו שנזכור אחר זה.

10:5 וידוע כי סבות העלוף רבות ורפואתו מתחלפת ופעלתו א׳ והוא התכת הכח החיוני ומנוחת הלב. ואם ירצה לקרא אל העלוף נפילת הכח בחדות ובמהירות וכבר אמרו אנשים כי העלוף יקרה לסבות דוחקות המוח ומונעות אותו מלשלח החוש אל הלב וישיג הלב מזה

a הוקז: הקיז
b السكنجبين
c الجلاب
d الهندباء
e תרנגולים: תרנוגלים
f התרנגולים: התרנוגלים
g الحصرمية
h الرمانية
i الميبة

9:6 Not all veins tolerate epaphairesis, because there are veins that do not draw blood.[60] When it is delicate,[61] one needs to strengthen the tightening on it during epaphairesis and apply a ligament in his [the patient's] forearm and his upper arm, and his sleep should be overseen so that the blood would not dribble out from it, exposing him to danger.

The Tenth Chapter

10:1 The tenth chapter on the food and drink of the phlebotomised [patient].

10:2 The house in which one phlebotomises should have moderate air, a high ceiling, be open towards the north, decorated with fragrant herbs, roses, and a variety of fruit and pleasant things.[62]

10:3 Immediately after phlebotomy, one should drink oxymel, julep, and rose syrup according to strength,[63] and [consume] soft-cooked eggs. He should also eat lettuce and *al-hindibāʾ* [i.e., endive] with vinegar. He should also eat goat meat, mutton, or soured pullets, and the food on the day of phlebotomy, as well as the day after, should be moderate.[64] Of the fruit, [one may eat] pomegranate and quince after the meal.

10:4 Whoever gets weak or unconscious during phlebotomy should eat pullet soup and the dishes called *al-ḥiṣrimiyya* and *al-rummāniyya* or breadcrumbs in sour pomegranate juice before being phlebotomised, and drink rose syrup. His blood should be extracted in [several] sessions, as we have mentioned, and he should eat between each session. He should also drink melicratum and *mayba*, because these substitute wine, as we will mention later.

10:5 It is known that there are several causes to losing consciousness, and its treatment varies, yet its cause is one, which is the dissolution of the animal faculty, the seat of which is the heart. If one wants to define unconsciousness as a sudden and rapid decay of strength, some people have said that unconsciousness occurs due to pressuring causes on the brain that prevent it from sending sensory signals to the heart, from which the heart obtains unconsciousness. As

60 Ms. Escorial: "there are veins that do not react positively to that."
61 In Ms. Escorial this is the way to treat a drunk person (*wa-man kāna sakīran*), which is not mentioned in Ms. Parma.
62 Ms. Escorial: "a variety of fruit spread out in it."
63 Ms. Escorial: "according to appetite".
64 See commentary.

העלוף. ובעבור כי כונתנו בזה הספר אמנם הוא העלוף המתחדש בעת ההקזה ובסבתה נאמר
95v כי אשר תהיה בו הרוח החיונית בכבד דקה תצא ממנו הרבה | עם יציאת הדם המעט ויתחדש
לזה העלוף אל הלב בסבת השתוף אשר ביניהם. ואמנם מי שתהיה בו הרוח החיונית בכבד
עבה לא תצא ממנה עם יציאת הרבה מהדם כי אם מעט ולא יתחדש העלוף.

10:6 והדרך ברפואתו כי הוא כאשר ימצאנו עמו האסטניסות צריך לעשות הקיא עם נוצה ושתית המים הפושרים עם הסכנג׳בין[a] כי הוא יורה על לחה נגרת אל האצטומכא. וצריך להזות עליו ועל פניו מי הורדים ומים קרים ולעורר אותו ולקראו וימרח פי האצטומכא וידיו ונחיריו.

10:7 ואם לא שבה רוחו עליו בזה צריך שיריח אלמסך[b] ואלגליא.[c] וכאשר יהיה העלוף בלי אסטניסות יורה על רע וצריך למהר תחלה להשקותו מי הבשר ומי הדבש והמיבא[d] ולבקע לפניו תרנגולים[e] צלויים ויריח אלמוסך[f] ויזו על פניו המים ולזמר לפניו עם הקולות העליונים והנגונים.

10:8 וכאשר יקרהו נפילת הכח מרב יצאת הדם או לדקות הלב אז צריך למהר תחלה בזאת ההנהגה מלבד הקולות והנגונים.

10:9 תכונת מי הדבש: יוקח מן[g] הדבש הנקי המסונן ליטר ויערב אותו בקדרה חדשה עם ה׳ ליטרים מים ויבשל באש ויסונן וכשישוב קרוב לתכונת הג׳לב[h] יקח פלפל ארוך ודרציני[i] סנבל[j] מסתק[k] קרנפל[l] מכל אחד[m] זוז ישחקם וישים אותם בצמר בגד פשתן וישימהו בקדרה ויבשל היטב עד שישוב בתכונת המשקים ויקח ממנו בעת הצרך.

---

a السكنجبين
b المسك
c الغالية
d الميبة
e תרנגולים: תרנוגלי׳
f المسك
g מן: מי
h الجلاب
i دارصيني
j سنبل الطيب
k مصطكى
l قرنفل
m מכל אחד: מא׳

our intention in this book, indeed, is unconsciousness that occurs during phlebotomy and its cause, we say that for someone in whose liver the vital pneuma is fine, a lot of it will get extracted | with a little blood, causing unconsciousness 95v
to the heart due to the connection between the two. As to a person in whose liver the vital pneuma is coarse, only a little of it will be extracted with the blood, and unconsciousness will not occur.

10:6 The manner of treating a patient to whom nausea occurs with it is to induce vomiting by using a feather, and to make him drink lukewarm water with oxymel, because this indicates that a humour has flowed into the stomach. One also needs to sprinkle rose water and cold water on him and on his face, wake him up and shout at him, and massage the orifice of his stomach, his hands[65] and his nostrils.

10:7 If this does not help him regain consciousness,[66] one should make him smell musk and *al-ġāliya*.[67] When no nausea occurs with unconsciousness, it is a bad indication, and one needs to hurry. First, make him drink meat broth, melicratum, and *mayba*, grilled pullets should be chopped in front of his face, make him smell musk and sprinkle water on his face, and play loud sounds and musical instruments.

10:8 When the abundance of the blood extracted or the delicateness of the heart causes the patient a decay of strength, one needs to quickly begin this regimen without the [loud] sounds and musical instruments.

10:9 The prescription of melicratum: one takes clean, filtered honey, one litre, and mixes it in a new pot with five litres of water. It is cooked on fire and skimmed, and as it gets close to the consistency of julep, one takes long pepper,[68] cinnamon, Indian nard, mastic, cloves, one *zuz*[69] of each, grinds them well, and puts them in a linen cloth, and inserts it all in a cooking pot to be cooked well until it reaches the consistency of syrups. One consumes it when necessary.

---

65 Ms. Escorial: "his body."

66 Lit. "if his soul does not return to him."

67 A men's perfume with several variations, the basic components of which are must, ambergris, and balsam oil.

68 Ms. Escorial: + ginger.

69 Equals *dirham* in Ms. Escorial.

10:10 ויתמיד משקה המיבא[a] וכבר נכתב בספר אלמנצורי[b] שלנו.

השער הי״א

11:1 השער הי״א בסמים[c] ובמזונות הטובים לכבות הדם.

11:2 בעבור כי יש מן האנשים מי שהוא חלוש ההרכבה או שלא נהג בהקזה צריך שנזכור מהמזונות והסמים מה שיעמדו במקום ההקזה. ומהמשקים הידועים לזה הם משקה חמוץ האתרוגים ומשקה הרמונים ומשקה אלענאב[d] ומשקה אלסכנג׳בין[e] החזק החמוץ הנעשה עם שרשים ועם הנדבא[f] לבדו או משקה הרמונים ומי בישול התמר הינדי ומשקה האגסים.

11:3 ומהמזונות מי בשול השעורים הנעשה עם אלענאב[g] ולבות לחם עם סכרי או עם מיץ רמונים. ומהתבשילים התבשילים הנקראים עדסיא[h] או הצרמיה[i] וסומקיא[j] ורומניה[k] ודלעיה[l] ורג׳ליה[m] ומי בשול הירקות וההנדבא[n] וחזרת.[o] ומהדגים הקטנים בני יומן המבושלים עם מעט חמץ. ומהפירות הרמונים והחבושים ואלכמתרה[p] והתפוחים והקשואים וקתא[q] ופקוס וימעט המזון.

11:4 [...] ומהתבשילים אלתפחיא ואלאספינך[r] וסויק השעורים[s] ודומים.

---

a المیبة
b الكتاب المنصوري
c בסמים: בסיוני״
d العناب
e السكنجبين
f هندباء
g العناب
h العدسية
i الحصرمية
j السماقية
k الرمانية
l قرع In Ms. Escorial
m رجلة In Ms. Escorial
n الهندباء
o וחזרת: ודחזרת
p الكمثرى
q القثاء
r الإسفاناخ
s سويق الشعير

10:10 He should also continue with the administration of *mayba*, as already written in our *al-Kitāb al-Manṣūrī*.[70]

The Eleventh Chapter

11:1 The eleventh chapter on the drugs and foods that are good to extinguish [the combustion of] blood.

11:2 As there are people whose constitution is weak, or who are not accustomed to phlebotomy, it is necessary for us to mention some of the foods and drugs that substitute phlebotomy. Among the syrups known for that: sour citron syrup, pomegranate syrup, jujube syrup, and very sour oxymel prepared with roots [of endive] and with endive alone,[71] or pomegranate syrup, boiled tamarind juice, and plum syrup.

11:3 Among the foods: barley broth made with jujube, and breadcrumbs with sugar or with pomegranate juice; among the dishes: the dishes that are called *ʿadasiyya, ḥiṣrimiyya, summāqiyya, rummāniyya, dullāʿiyya*, and *riǧliyya*,[72] vegetable broth,[73] endive, and lettuce; of the fish the fresh, small ones cooked in some vinegar;[74] of the fruit: pomegranate, quince, pear, apple, gourd, squirting cucumber, and melon;[75] and food should be decreased.

11:4 […] And of dishes *al-tuffāḥiyya*,[76] *al-isfīnāḫ* [i.e., spinach],[77] and barley gruel and the like.[78]

---

70 *Al-Kitāb al-Manṣūrī*, also written by al-Rāzī.

71 Ms. Escorial: "very sour oxymel, alternatively with the addition of endive roots and its seeds."

72 Ms. Escorial: "gourd and purslane." See commentary.

73 Vegetable broth is not mentioned in Ms. Escorial.

74 Ms. Escorial: "Of fresh fish the small ones prepared as *sikbāǧ*".

75 Ms. Escorial: melon, i.e., *dullāʿ*, also described *as al-biṭṭīḫ al-madanī* and *al-biṭṭīḫ al-dalasī*.

76 *Al-tapuḥiyya*, understood as *al-tuffāḥiyya*, a dish made with apples. Not mentioned in Ms. Escorial.

77 Spinach, in Arabic *al-isfānāḫ*, is mentioned as a plant or an ingredient, not as a dish in Ms. Escorial.

78 This short passage seems to be the only thing left from what in Ms. Escorial describes the diet and regimen of a patient whose disposition needs to be cooled down.

11:5 תכונת מטבד[a] לשלשל הטבע ויומנע מרתיחת הדם: יקח תמר הנדי ב׳ אוקיא אגס[b] ענאב[c] סבסתן[d] מכל אחד[e] ורדים בנפסג[f] עדשים ברבריש[g] מכל אחד[h] רביע אוקיא כזבורי[i] יבש ב׳ זוזים עלי הנדבא[j] חצי אוקיא. יבושל הכל במים עד שיתעבו. ואחר יקח מהמים המסוננים חצי ליטר ויסחוט וימרס בהם אוקיא לב כיאר שנבר[k] מנוקה מהגרעינים ואחר יחמם מעט וישתה. ואם לא נתחמם הטבע ישוב לקחת מהם ג׳ ימים רצופים.

11:6 תכונת אקראץ[l] לכבות רתיחת הדם ולחזק האצטומכא ולפתוח סתום הכבד: ורדים
96r אדומים י׳ זוזים זרע רג׳לא[m] וזרע הנדבא[n] |[o] ברבריס[p] צמג ערבי[q] כתירא[r] מכל אחד[s] זוז וחצי
סנדל[t] לבן טבשיר[u] מכל אחד[v] זוז וחצי. ואם יהיה בו חמימות יוסיף בו רביע זוז כאפור[w] ישחקם
וינפם וילוש אותם במיץ ענבי[x] אלתעלב[y] מרותח ומסונן ויעשה מהם אקרץ[z] כל אחד[aa] זוז וחצי.
ויקח מהם בכל יום קרצה[bb] עם אוקיא סכנג׳בין.[cc]

---

a مطبوخ
b إجاص
c عناب
d سبستان
e מכל אחד: מא׳
f بنفسج
g برباريس
h מכל אחד: מא׳
i كزبرة
j هندباء
k خيارشنبر
l أقراص
m رجلة
n هندباء
o הנדבא + Ms
p برباريس
q صمغ عربي
r كثيراء
s מכל אחד: מא׳
t صندل
u طباشير
v מכל אחד: מא׳
w كافور
x ענבי: ענבים
y عنب الثعلب
z أقراص
aa כל אחד: כא׳
bb قرصة
cc سكنجبين

11:5 The prescription of a decoction that loosens the bowels[79] and prevents the combustion of blood:[80] one takes tamarind, two *ūqiyyas*, plum, jujube, sebesten, [ten grains][81] of each; roses, violet, lentils, barberry, of each a quarter *ūqiyya*;[82] dry coriander seeds, two *zuz*;[83] endive leaves,[84] half an *ūqiyya*.[85] All that is boiled in water until it thickens. Thereafter, one takes filtered water, half a litre,[86] and squeezes and soaks in it one *ūqiyya* of the pith of cassia fistula that is cleansed from seeds. Thereafter one heats it a little[87] and drinks it. Should the natural constitution not get warmer,[88] one should take this for three consecutive days.

[*lacuna*][89]

11:6 Prescription of pastilles that extinguish the combustion of blood, strengthen the stomach, and open [the obstructions of] the liver: red roses, ten *zuz*; purslane seeds and endive seeds, | barberry, gum Arabic, gum traga- 96r
canth, one *zuz* and a half of each;[90] white sandalwood, bamboo chalk, one *zuz* and a half of each.[91] If it is very hot, one adds in it a quarter *zuz* of camphor. [Thereafter the ingredients are] pulverised, sieved, and kneaded in boiled, filtered nightshade pulp, and formed into pastilles of approximately one *zuz* and a half each.[92] One takes a pastille every day with one *ūqiyya* of oxymel.[93]

79 Lit. purges the natural constitution.
80 Ms. Escorial: "surplus of blood."
81 The amount of the mentioned ingredients is not mentioned in Ms. Parma; Ms. Escorial reads "ten grains."
82 Ms. Escorial adds endive seeds and purslane seeds, three *dirhams* of each.
83 In Ms. Escorial the measure is *dirham*.
84 Ms. Escorial adds nightshade leaves.
85 In Ms. Escorial "one part of each."
86 Litre corresponds to *raṭl* in Ms. Escorial.
87 Ms. Escorial: "it is filtered for a second time."
88 Ms. Escorial: "If it loosens the bowels, [then that is fine], but if not …"
89 See 11:8–11:11 in the edition of Ms. Escorial.
90 Ms. Escorial: "two *dirhams* of each."
91 Ms. Escorial adds three *dirhams* of peeled liquorice root, one *dirham* of Chinese rhubarb, and half a *dirham* of saffron.
92 Ms. Escorial: "one *dirham*."
93 For an additional prescription of pastilles, see 11:13 in the edition of Ms. Escorial.

השער הי״ב

12:1 השער הי״ב בתועלת הקזת הגידים.

12:2 הקזת הקיפאל[a] יועיל מההכאה והנפילה המתחדשות בראש ומכובד הגוף ומכאב הראש ומגלגולו בעת התנועה ומסבוב הראש הנקרא אלדואר[b] אשר עם אדמימות הפנים ומלוי הגידים וממורסת המוח החמה הנקראת אלשרסאם[c] ומחלי אלסכתה[d] אשר עם אדמימות הפנים ומכובד התנועה הנקרא אלכדר[e] עם אדמימות המראה ומהזלות הראש הנקראות זכאם[f] ואלנזלה[g] אשר עם אדמימות הפנים ומחלי העינים הנקרא אלרמד[h] אשר עם אדמימות העינים ומחליים המתחדשים בהם הנקראים אלסבל[i] ואלסלאק[j] ואלאנתשאר[k] בעפעפים עם אדמימות וכובד הראש והמצח ומדם הנחירים וכאב השנים אשר עם נפיחת הלסתות ומחלי נגעי הפה הנקרא אלקלע[l] אשר עם אדמימות וחמימות הפה ומנפילת הלהאה אשר עם חזק האדמימות והחמימות ומנפיחת הלשון עם אדמימות וחמימות והחניקות אשר עם אדמימות הפנים והעינים ומתוח הגוף.

12:3 אלבסליק[m] יועיל ממורסת הצלעות והשוצ׳א[n] וביניהם הפרש גדול כמו שזכרנו ואם יהיה הכאב נוטה אל צד המתנים הנקרא אלשראסיף[o] יהיה המשלשל תחלה ואחריו ההקזה.

12:4 ויועיל לקשי הנשימה הנקרא אלרבו[p] עם אדמימות הפנים ומדפיקת הלב עם חמימות החזה וגדל הדפק ומנפיחת האצטומכא עם חמימות נראה ונפיחת הכבד עם חזק הצמא וקדחת דבקה ומחלי מלנכוניא[q] אשר עם שנוי מראה והפסד העכול וקיא חמוץ ורוחות

---

a القيفال (three dots above the word, repeated in the margin).
b الدوار
c الشرسام
d السكتة
e الخدر
f الزكام
g النزلة
h الرمد
i ريح السبل Ms. Escorial
j السلاق
k الانتشار
l القلاع
m الباسليق
n الشوصة
o الشراسيف
p الربو
q مالنخونيا

The Twelfth Chapter

12:1 The twelfth chapter on the benefit of phlebotomy.[94]

12:2 Phlebotomising the cephalic vein is beneficial for a blow and a fall that occur to the head; for the heaviness of the body and the head;[95] headache and dizziness while moving; vertigo called *al-duwwār* combined with redness of face; overfilling of veins; for the hot swelling of the [arachnoid mater of the] brain that is called *al-širsām* [i.e., phrenitis]; and for the illness of *al-sakta* [i.e., apoplexy] combined with redness of face; for the heaviness of movement called *al-ḫadar* [i.e., numbness] combined with redness of complexion; for the secretions of the head called *zukām* [i.e., rheum] and *al-nazla* [i.e., catarrh] combined with redness of face; for the eye illness called *al-ramad* [i.e., ophthalmia] combined with redness of the eyes, and for the illnesses that occur in them, called *al-sabal* [i.e., wind of pannus], *al-sulāq* [i.e., ptilosis]; *al-intišār* of the eyelashes combined with redness and heaviness of the head and the forehead; for epistaxis and toothache combined with swelling of the gums; for pustules of the mouth called *al-qulāʿ* [i.e., aphthae] combined with redness and heat of the mouth; for prolapse of the uvula that is severely red and hot; swelling of the tongue combined with redness and heat; and for diphtheria combined with redness of the face and the eyes and expansion of the body.

12:3 [Phlebotomising] the basilic vein is beneficial for the swelling of the ribs [i.e., pleurisy] and *al-šawṣa* [i.e., pleuritis], and there is a big difference between the two, as we have mentioned. If the pain is leaning towards *al-šarāsīf* [i.e., the false ribs], one should employ purgation in the first place, and thereafter phlebotomy.[96]

12:4 It is [also] beneficial for the respiratory difficulty called *al-rabw* [i.e., asthma] combined with redness of face; palpitation combined with heat in the chest and strong pulse; the visibly hot swelling of the stomach; the swelling of the liver combined with strong thirst and continuous[97] fever; melancholy that occurs with the change of complexion, decay of digestion, sour vomiting and chronic winds in the waist[98]—one has to phlebotomise it from the left side and

94 Ms. Parma omits mentioning the benefits of phlebotomising the frontal vein.
95 Ms. Escorial: "headache combined with heaviness of the body and the head."
96 Comparison between these two, extant in Ms. Escorial, is missing in Ms. Parma.
97 Ms. Escorial: "unavoidable fever."
98 Ms. Escorial: "chronic winds towards the false ribs."

תמידיות במתנים וצריך להקיזו בצד שמאל ולראות ולעיין אם יהיה הדם שחור יוציאהו ואם לא יפסיקהו ומכאב הטחול עם נפיחה וחמימות ומחלי המים הרעים הבשריים אשר סבתו מעצירת דם הטחורים ודם הוסת או מסבה אחרת מהמלוי ומכאב המעים הנקרא אלמגץ[a] הבא פתאם ומשלשול הדם מחלי אלסחג׳[b] עם בריאות הכח ומהשלשול מסבת השחורה הנגרת אל האצטומכא יהיה הקזתו מהצד השמאלי ומחלי אלקולנג׳[c] המתחדש מסבת נפיחת המים או הקיא ודפיקת הבטן ומנפיחת מורסת הכליות וישיגנו בהתחלה קדחות על בלתי סדר ומחולשת הכליות אשר עם כאב השדרה ומעוט המשגל ויהיה השתן כמו מי בשר או מי השתנת הדם והגרת הזרע הנקראת אלאחתילאם[d] ומרוב דם הוסת עם חזק הכח וממורסות קשות ברחם ובעת מלוי הגוף וממורסת הרחם המתחדשת מסבת עצירת הוסת או מקשי הלידה או מההכאה על הרחם ומכאבי הטחורים ובקוע פי הטבעת ונפיחת הביצים עם חמימות ומכאב השדרה עם חמימות ודפיקה ומכאב | הירך עם מעט חמימות ומכאב גיד הנשה[e] עם 96v
חמימות המשוש ועכירות המראה וזה החלי יעבו בו הלשון והרגל.

12:5 הקזת אלאכחל[f] אמנם תועלתו כמו שזכרנו שהוא כולל הגוף וצריך אם ירצה להקיזו בזה החלי לראות ולעיין אם הדם לא יתחיל להתעפש ימהר להוציאו כי הוא לא יבטח כאשר יתעפש שיצא ממנו וישאר בו ויפסיד הנשאר. והאות המורה על העפוש באוש השתן או באוש הזיעה ושהוא יפחד בעת הזאת שיהיה החלי בעליתו וחזוקו ותהיה יציאת הדם בעת ההיא הזק הרבה.

12:6 הקזת אלאסילם[g] יועיל לכאב הטחול ולקשי הנשימה אשר עמהם חמימות אחר הקזת הבסליק[h] ואל מלנקוניאה.[i]

a المغص
b Ms. Escorial reads: سحج الأمعاء
c القولنج
d الاحتلام
e Ms. Escorial: ومن داء الفيل
f الأكحل
g الأسيلم
h الباسليق
i مالنخونيا

monitor and observe whether the blood is black, in which case one extracts it, and if not, then one ends it[s extraction]—; and for pain in the spleen combined with swelling and heat; fleshy dropsy[99] caused by the obstruction of blood of the haemorrhoids, menstruation, or other causes of overfilling; for sudden intestine pain called *al-maġṣ* [i.e., gripes]; bloody diarrhoea; *al-saḥaǧ* [i.e., the abrasion of guts] with sound strength; for diarrhoea caused by a melancholic humour flowing into the stomach—it is phlebotomised from the left—; and for the illness *al-qawlanǧ* [i.e., colic] caused by a swelling [of the guts, followed by thirst of] water, or vomiting; and throbbing pain in the stomach [i.e., ileus];[100] for swelling [or] tumour in the kidneys that in the initial stage is followed by irregular fevers; for the kidney weakness combined with pain in the spinal column, reduced sexual desire, and urine that resembles meat broth, or bloody urine; for the spilling of semen called *al-iḥtilām* [i.e., nocturnal emission]; for heavy, strong menstrual bleeding; hard swellings [i.e., polyps] in the uterus during an overfilling of the body,[101] and for swellings in the uterus caused by amenorrhea, difficult birth, or a blow on the uterus; for pains of haemorrhoids; fissures in the anus; swelling of the testicles with heat; for spinal pain with heat and throbbing; and for | thigh pain with some heat; for sciatica pain 96v
that occurs with heat of touch, cloudiness of complexion—this is the illness in which the tongue[102] and the foot become thick [i.e., elephantiasis].

12:5 Phlebotomising the median cubital vein: as to its benefit, as we have mentioned, it comprises the [whole] body. If one wants to phlebotomise it in the case of this illness [i.e., sanguine fever],[103] one needs to monitor and observe: [even] if the blood has not begun to putrefy, one needs to quickly extract it, since when it decays, one cannot be certain that it is expelled, thus it remains in it and corrupts the rest. The symptom indicating the putrefaction is bad smell of urine or sweat, which, at that moment, make one afraid that the illness is escalating and getting severe. At that moment, extraction of blood is very harmful.

12:6 Phlebotomising the *vena salvatella* is beneficial for pain in the spleen and for respiratory difficulties, both combined with heat, after phlebotomising the basilic vein; as well as for melancholy.

---

99 Lit. "illness of bad, fleshy waters."

100 Important parts missing in Ms. Parma.

101 Ms. Escorial: "polyps in the uterus that bleed in cycles that are not menstrual cycles."

102 Ms. Escorial: *al-sāq*, 'leg.' See commentary.

103 This central part mentioning sanguine fever, extant in Ms. Escorial, is missing in Ms. Parma.

12:7 הקזת אלמבאץ[a] ואלצפאן[b] מועילים מעצירת דם הוסת קודם עתו בשני ימים מחבורות השוקים וחכוכם ומחכוך הביצים ומחלי פתול הגידים ומחלי הכפיה מסבת הדם ומחולי הקולנג׳[c] אחר הקזת הבסליק.[d]

12:8 הקזת גיד הנשה[e] עם חמימות ויועיל מכאב אשר בו אחר הקזת הבאסליק.[f]

השער הי״ג

13:1 השער הי״ג ברפואת השגגה הנופלת בהקזה.

13:2 כאשר יקרה בהקזת הבסליק[g] שיראה הדם אדום ויקפוץ וידלג אז ידע כי הוא מהשרין וצריך שיתרפא ברפואת גלינוס אשר נאמר עליה שהיא טובה הרבה להפסיק הדם.

13:3 תכונתו: יוקח צבר[h] כנדר[i] שיאן חלקים שוים ישחקם וינפם וילוש עם לובן ביצים ויעשה פתילה מצמר גפן על ראש המול והוא כלי ויבלול אותו עם הרפואה וישים אותו במקום ההקזה וישים עליו שער ארנבת הנקרא ובר אלארנב[j] בלול עם לובן ביצים[k] ויקשור עליו ויניחנו ויתיר אותו על הדרך הנזכר.

13:4 ואם נתחדשה בו קדחת או שנפחד מזה יזה עליו פעם אחר פעם עם מי ורודים ולא יתיר.

13:5 תכונה אחרת רבת ההתכה: יוקח[l] שומן תרנגולת ושמן ורדים מכל אחד ז׳ זוזים שעוה לבנה ד׳ זוזים יתיך הכל על האש ויניחנו לקרר מעט וישים עליו[m] כתירא[n] מרדסאג׳[o]

a المأبض
b الصافن
c القولنج
d الباسليق
e عرق النسا
f الباسليق
g الباسليق
h صبر
i كندر
j وبر الأرنب
k ויעשה פתילה מצמר גפן Deleted in the MS
l יוקח: יוקס
m עליו: עלי
n كثيراء
o مرداسنج

12:7 Phlebotomising the *popliteal fossa* and the saphenous vein is beneficial for amenorrhea two days before its time; itchy ulcers in the legs; itchy testicles; varicose veins; sanguine epilepsy; and for colic, after phlebotomising the basilic vein.

12:8 Phlebotomising the sciatic vein with heat is beneficial for the pain occurring in it after phlebotomising the basilic vein.

The Thirteenth Chapter

13:1 The thirteenth chapter on treating the mistake that occurs during phlebotomy.

13:2 Whenever it happens while phlebotomising the basilic vein that one sees the blood red, jumping and hopping, it is evident that it is from an artery, and it needs to be treated with Galen's remedy that is said to be excellent to cease blood flow.

13:3 Its prescription: one takes equal parts of aloe and premium quality frankincense,[104] and mixes, grinds, and kneads them with egg white. One makes a roll of cotton wool on the tip of a probe[105]—which is an instrument—, mixes it with the preparation, applies it on the site of the incision, and covers it with hare's fur, called *wabar al-arnab*, mixed with egg white. It is tightened on the spot, allowed to remain, and untied as previously mentioned.

13:4 If the patient develops a fever, or if one is afraid that it could happen, one sprinkles rose water time after time on it [i.e., the wound], and does not untie it.[106]

[*lacuna*][107]

13:5 Another prescription of a very much dissolving [preparation]: one takes chicken fat, rose oil, of both seven *zuz*,[108] white wax, four *zuz*.[109] All that is

104 Ms. Escorial: "one part of frankincense, and half a part of aloe."
105 *ṭrʾš hmwlṭ*, see commentary.
106 This is mentioned as a part of another prescription Ms. Escorial (13:4).
107 See 13:4–13:9 in the edition of Ms. Escorial.
108 Ms. Escorial: five *miṯqāls* each.
109 Ms. Escorial: three *miṯqāls*.

אספידאג׳[a] חלקים שוים עד שיתעבה וימשח ממנו בעת הצרך ולא יכנס במרחץ כל עת החמימות באבר.

השער הארבעה עשר

14:1 השער הארבעה עשר בתועלת כוסות המציצה עם שריטה ובלי שריטה הנקראות אלחג׳אמה.[b]

14:2 זאת ההרקה נחלקת לב׳ חלקים הא׳ עם שריטה והב׳ בלא שריטה והמקומות |[c] הנהוגים 97r
לעשות שריטה בהם הם נקרת הראש[d] והצדדים[e] הנקראים אלארדעין[f] ותחת הזקן ואלכהאל[g] ואלמעצמין[h] ועל השוקים.

14:3 ואלחג׳אמה[i] תקח הדם ותוציא מהגידים הדקים ויקל המלוי מהגוף. ואפשר שיקרה מעט עד פלא שיצא עמה דם הרבה וכל שכן[j] מהשוקים.

14:4 ואמנם תועלותיה כי הנעשית בנקרת הראש[k] תועיל מכובד הראש עם חמימות.

14:5 והנעשית במקום אלכדעאן[l] תקל כאב הראש והפנים והעינים ותועיל לכאב שרשי השנים אשר יצא מהם דם.

14:6 ואשר תחת הזקן תועיל מאלקלע[m] האדום והגרת דם הלסתות.

14:7 ואמנם אלקאהל[n] תועיל מדפיקת הלב עם חמימות.

---

a إسفيداج
b الحجامة
c והמקומות + .Ms
d النقرة
e והצדדים: והצדעים
f الأخدعان
g الكاهل
h المعصمان
i الحجامة
j וכל שכן: וכש׳
k النقرة
l الأخدعان
m القلاع
n الكاهل

melted on fire, then removed to cool down a little, and then one adds gum tragacanth, litharge, and ceruse, equal parts until it thickens. It is used when necessary. The patient should not bathe as long as the part is hot.

The Fourteenth Chapter

14:1 The fourteenth chapter on the benefit of cupping with and without scarification, called *al-ḥiǧāma*.

14:2 This [manner of] evacuation is divided into two parts, the first with scarification and the second without scarification. The | sites that are usually used 97r
for scarification are the hollow of the neck, the lateral parts of the neck[110] called *al-aḫdaʿayn*,[111] below the chin, *al-kahāl* [i.e., the interscapular region],[112] *al-miʿṣamayn* [i.e., the wrists], and the legs.

14:3 Cupping takes blood from thin veins, extracts [it], and eases the overfilling in the body. Occasionally, although utmost rarely, it may happen that a large quantity of blood is extracted, especially in the legs.

14:4 As to its benefits, when applied on the hollow of the neck, it is beneficial for the heaviness of the head combined with heat.

14:5 When applied on the lateral parts of the neck, it eases the pain occurring in the head, the face, and the eyes, and is beneficial for the pain in the roots of the teeth with which bleeding occurs.

14:6 [Cupping] what is below the chin is beneficial for the red *al-qulāʾ* [i.e., aphthae] and for bleeding gums.

14:7 As to *al-kāhil* [i.e., the interscapular region], [cupping] it is beneficial for palpitation accompanied with heat.

---

110 See commentary.

111 In Arabic *al-aḫdaʿān* in nominative.

112 In Arabic *al-kāhil*.

14:8 והנעשית במקום הנקרא אלמעצמין[a] תועיל מהנגעים אשר בזרועות.

14:9 ואשר בשוקים תועיל מאלסכתה[b] והכפיה אשר הם מהדם או מפתילי הגידים הנקראים אלדואלי[c] עם חמימות ומחלי אלסלאק[d] הישן ומכאב המקוה והכליות והרחם והמורסות החמות הנקראות אלדמאמיל[e] ומהנגעים אשר בירכים ומעצירת הוסת. ואשר תהיה מהנשים בעלת בשר עם מראה לבן תועיל אליה זאת האלהג׳מא[f] הרבה באלה המקומות יותר מכל דבר ומההקזה ותעשה אותם קודם עת הוסת בג׳ ימים.

14:10 ואמנם כוסות המציצה מבלי שריטה הנקראות אלחג׳מא[g] תועיל למשוך מה שצריך למשוך מהליחות ולהביא הדם אל המקום הצריך והיא נעשית בב׳ ענינים עם מציצה ועם אש והיא יותר נדבקת ומושכת הרבה.

14:11 ותועלתה כי אם תהיה נתלית על הראש או תחת המתנים או הצדדים אחר ההקזה היא פוסקת דם הנחירים ואם תעשה בערף או תחת הגרון למי שיקרה לו החניקות בעבור מאכל או סם.

14:12 ותועיל הרבה למשוך הליחה הנגרת על העינים אם תתלה אותה על הראש ואם תתלה אותה על השדים פוסקת הגרת דם והסת.

14:13 ותועיל מהכאב ואם תהיה סבתו מהעשן ואם תהיה סבתו מהליחה ישוב אחר ג׳ או ד׳ ימים.

14:14 ותועיל לבעלי חלי המלנכוניא[h] אם היא נתלית תחת המתנים הנקראים אלשראסיף[i] מצד השמאל ועל הבטן ואם היא נתלית על הטחול תהיה פוסקת השלשול אשר מסבת השחורה ותגברת[j] הטחורים בפי הטבעת.

---

a المعصمين
b السكتة
c الدوالي
d السلاق
e الدماميل
f الحجامة
g الحجامة
h مالنخونيا
i الشراسيف
j [*sic*]

14:8 Applied at the site that is called *al-miʿṣamayn* [i.e., the wrists] is beneficial for pustules in the forearms.

14:9 [Cupping] the legs is beneficial for sanguine *al-sakta* [i.e., apoplexy] and sanguine epilepsy; or[113] for the twisted veins called *al-dawālī* [i.e., varicose veins] combined with heat; chronic ptilosis; pain in the bladder, the kidneys, and the uterus; the warm swellings called boils and pustules in the thigs; and for amenorrhea. For women who are fleshy and have a white complexion, cupping these sites is much more beneficial compared to other procedures and phlebotomy. This should be done three days before the time of her menstruation.

14:10 As to cupping without scarification, called *al-ḥiǧāma* [*bi-lā šarṭ*], it helps to draw the humours that need to be drawn, and to transport the blood to the necessary site. It is done in two manners: either with suction or with fire, which adheres and draws better.

14:11 Its benefit is that if applied on the head, below the false ribs or on the flanks after phlebotomy, it stanches epistaxis. If applied on the back of the head or below the throat, [it is beneficial] for whoever suffers from choking because of food or drugs.

14:12 It is very beneficial for drawing humours that flow towards the eyes if applied on the head, and when applied on the breasts, you stanch the flow of menstrual blood.

14:13 It is also beneficial for pain caused by vapour. If it is caused by a humour, [the pain] should return after three or four days.

14:14. It is also beneficial for the melancholic if suspended below *al-šarāsīf* [i.e., costal cartilages of the false ribs] on the left side and on the stomach. If applied on the spleen, it ceases melancholic diarrhoea, and defeats haemorrhoids in the anus.

---

113 And?

14:15 אמר אבו בכר: הפסקנו מאמרנו זה בזה המקום אשר באנו עד תכלית מה שיעדנו בו. והיה דעתנו לחבר אל מאמרנו זה מאמר אחר בכויה וראינו בזה קצת אריכות והיציאה מכונת המאמר בהקזה וכל שכן[a] כשכבר זכרנו זה בספרנו במלאכת הידים.

14:16 תם ונשלם שבח לאל בורא עולם.[b]

a וכל שכן: וכש׳

b תושלבע

14:15 Abū Bakr said: we have completed this treatise, reaching the limit of what we intended to cover. Our intention was to attach another treatise on cauterisation into this treatise of ours, but we considered it a bit lengthy and deviating from the purpose of the treatise on phlebotomy, especially as we already have mentioned it in our book *Be-malʾaḵat ha-yadayim*.[114]

14:16 Finished and Complete, Praise be to God, Creator of the Universe.

114 See commentary.

Commentary

This commentary discusses some key concepts within the medical framework and specific cases related to Ms. Parma. Given the overlap in the subject matter, many parts of the commentaries of Ms. Escorial and Ms. Parma contain the same information. For additional information, see the commentary of part 1.

1:1 **Nutriment:** For Galen's theory on how food becomes nutriment, see e.g., Galen, *On the Usefulness of the Parts of the Body*, and Galen, *On the Properties of Foodstuffs*.

1:2 **Humours:** The principle of the humours explained by Hippocrates: "The body of man has in itself blood, phlegm, yellow bile and black bile; these make up the nature of his body, and through these he feels pain or enjoys health."[1]

Innate heat: Innate heat in Galen's system: "There are two kinds of heat; the ordinary variety, which burns things up, and the *innate heat* of living creatures, which makes the body grow instead of consuming it, and also has the power of generation. The innate heat is often equated with nature in Galen's works; it is the life of the body, which dies when it is extinguished. Since it is distributed to every part with the arterial blood, it is often also equated with blood. The innate heat, as its name suggests, is not acquired from outside; it comes to the embryo through the semen, which contains the hot principle, and resides in the arterial blood of the left ventricle when the heart is formed."[2]

1:3 **Erasistratus:** Ms. Parma reads ארס׳ which could be interpreted both as Erasistratus and Aristotle. Ms. Escorial reads Aristotle, but most probably Erasistratus, notorious for rejecting bloodletting and preferring fasting, is meant. See e.g., *Galen's Book on Venesection against Erasistratus*, and *On Venesection against the Erasistrateans at Rome* in Brain, *Galen on Bloodletting*.[3]

1 Hippocrates, *Nat. Hom*, IV (LCL 150: 10–11).

2 Brain, *Galen on Bloodletting*, p. 8.

3 Both works, *Galeni de Venae Sectione adversus Erasistratum Liber* (pp. 15–37), and *Galeni de Venae Sectione Adversus Erasistrateos Romae Degentes* (pp. 38–66) extant in Brain, *Galen on Bloodletting*.

1:4 **Hippocrates … three kinds of nutriment**: “Nutriment is what nourishes, what can nourish, and what will nourish.”[4] Galen’s views on this topic, based on Hippocrates’ statement above are discussed in Galen, *Nat. Fac., I. XI*: “For to that which is already being assimilated he gave the name of *nutriment*; to the similar material which is being presented or becoming adherent, the name of *quasi-nutriment*; and to everything else—that is, contained in the stomach and veins—the name of *destined nutriment*.”[5]

1:9 **A meat-like …**: The word featuring in Ms. Parma is unintelligible and reads התרוה. The term likely comes from the root רוה and refers to being moist, hence ‘a moist tissue,’ i.e., a gland, might be a satisfactory interpretation.

Had it not been for the watery fluid that mixes with the blood: Galen: “For the chyle resulting from the food could not be taken up successfully from the stomach into the veins and could not pass easily through the many fine veins in the liver unless some thinner, watery fluid were mixed with it as a vehicle. In fact, this is the reason why water is useful to the animal; for although no part can be nourished by water, nutriment could not be distributed from the stomach if it were not conducted in this way by moisture of some sort.”[6]

1:10 **A large vein:** i.e., *vena cava*. Galen: “Another vessel, a vein, which is called hollow because of its size [the vena cava], passes from the convexity of the liver upward and downward and resembles a sort of double trunk; for some parts of our body are higher than the liver and some are lower.”[7]

1:11 … **as Hippocrates said**: Perhaps Hippocrates in *Places In Man*: “All vessels communicate and flow into one another.”[8] See also commentary for 1:10 in the edition of Ms. Escorial.

2:1 **The circumstances**: All these topics are not covered in Ms. Parma. For the lacking content, i.e., the geographical location, what should be eaten and drunk, and the relation of the humours in the body, see § 2:17–2:19 in the edition of Ms. Escorial. These correspond to what Galen and Qusṭā ibn Lūqā have

4 Hippocrates, *Nutriment*, 8 (LCL 147: 328–329).
5 Galen, *Nat. Fac., I.* XI (LCL 71: 42–43).
6 Galen, *UP*, Fourth Book, 1, p. 207.
7 Galen, *UP*, II, 378, p. 682.
8 Hippocrates, *Places In Man*, 3 (LCL 482: 26–27).

written on the topic.[9] However, the topic of age, lacking in this introductory passage in Ms. Parma, is covered.

2:2 **Disposition**: in Greek *diathesis*, a term that Galen uses for any stable condition of body, whether it be normal or abnormal.[10]

2:3 **Hippocrates testified that as he said**: Cf. Hippocrates in *Regimen III*: "And if through lack of forethought there is an attack of fever, nothing should be given for three days except water. If the fever go down in that time, well and good; if it does not, treat the patient with barley water, and on the fourth or the seventh day he will sweat and be quit of the trouble."[11]

2:4 **Twelve days and nights**: Ms. Escorial reads "the patient may be fed with coarse food for a period of fourteen days" which corresponds to Hippocrates: "Acute diseases come to a crisis in fourteen days."[12]

"a very acute illness needs to be managed by a very restricted regimen": Ms. Parma reads: החלי המגיע אל הדקות הרבה צריך שיתנהג בהנהגה הדקה הרבה which corresponds to Ms. Escorial: *al-maraḍ al-bāliġ fī l-laṭāfa ğiddan yanbaġī an yudabbar bi-l-tadbīr al-bāliġ fī l-laṭāfa ğiddan*. As discussed in the commentary of Ms. Escorial, it is likely that the copyist mistakenly duplicated the words *al-bāliġ fī l-laṭāfa ğiddan*. The intended reference may be to an acute (*ḥādd*) illness. Compare with Hippocrates: "Where the disease is very acute, immediately, not only is the pain extreme, but also it is essential to employ a regimen of extreme strictness."[13] The Arabic term for 'very restricted regimen' is attested as *al-tadbīr mā huwa fī l-ġāya min al-laṭāfa*,[14] whereas *tadbīr laṭīf* is simply 'a light diet.'[15] Light foods, Ar. *aṭʿima laṭīfa*, are foods that are low in density and generate thin blood. These foods include wheat starch, shelled grains and seeds, pullets, bird wings, small fish with tender flesh, and gourd.[16]

9 Galen, *Cur. Rat. Ven. Sect.*, p. 67; Qusṭā ibn Lūqā, *Kitāb fī l-Faṣd*, pp. 330–331.
10 Brain, *Galen on Bloodletting*, p. 178.
11 Hippocrates, *Regimen III*, LXXII (LCL 150, pp. 390–393).
12 Hippocrates, *Aphorisms*, XXIII (LCL 150: 112–113).
13 Hippocrates, *Aphorisms*, I.VII (LCL 150: 102–103).
14 Translated from Galen by Ḥunayn ibn Isḥāq in Galen, *Opt. Med. Ex.*, pp. 80–81.
15 Translated from Galen by Ḥunayn ibn Isḥāq in Galen, *Opt. Med. Ex.*, pp. 66–67.
16 Nasrallah, *Annals of the Caliphs' Kitchens*, p. 732.

Regimen: Cf. Powell in Galen, *Alim. Fac.*: "The way to this state of excellence, many believed, was through *diaita*, which we usually translate as regimen, and which meant much more than the word diet that is derived from it, embracing as it did virtually everything to do with the lifestyle of the individual. According to Celsus it was one of three forms of therapy available to the physician (although therapy was only a part of its purpose)—the others being surgery and pharmacology. The concerns of regimen were with the whole of an individual's activities, covering such things as how often and when one should bathe; the nature of one's work and leisure; sexual activity; and, of course, the food one ate and its preparation. This was a holistic approach to personal health two millennia before the word was coined and the concept popularized in the twentieth century."[17]

2:5 **Barley broth**: Cf. Nasrallah, *Annals of the Caliphs' Kitchens*: "recommended as a healthy and nourishing food for the sick".[18]

2:6 **As to the age …**: Cf. Galen: "Those who have large veins, who are moderately slender and neither fair nor soft-fleshed, you will evacuate freely. Those of the opposite type, however, must be sparingly evacuated, since they have little blood and flesh that transpires well. For the same reason you will not phlebotomise children up to the age of fourteen."[19]

The same holds good for old people …: "Some sixty-year-olds can no longer bear phlebotomy, while some people of seventy still can. But obviously you will remove less from these, even if they appear to be in the same condition as a body in the prime of life."[20]

An old, seventy-year-old man: Cf. Galen: "You have learned to trust the strong, regular pulse as an infallible sign of strength of the faculties; this applies even more strongly to the large pulse. Thus you will phlebotomise even the seventy-year-olds, if the kind of pulse I have mentioned is present, whenever their condition demands it."[21]

2:7 **Egypt**: See commentary for § 2:7 in the commentary for Ms. Escorial.

---

17 Galen, *Alim. Fac.*, pp. 4–5.
18 Nasrallah, *Annals of the Caliphs' Kitchens*, p. 610.
19 Galen, *Cur. Rat. Ven. Sect.*, p. 87.
20 Brain, *Galen on Bloodletting*, p. 131.
21 Galen *Cur. Rat. Ven. Sect.*, p. 87.

2:8 **There is no determined limit**: Corresponds to Galen: "we cannot lay down in black and white a fixed amount to be removed in each of the conditions mentioned."[22]

2:12 **Galen …**: Cf. Galen's commentary of Hippocrates' *Epidemics*, book 6: "Galen reports [the case] of a woman whose menstruation was retained for eight months and who was extremely emaciated. When he saw that the blood was flowing copiously in her vessels but that it had a livid color, he bled her and extracted on the first day a quantity of one and a half *raṭl* of dark blood resembling liquid tar. On the second day he extracted one *raṭl* and on the third day eight ounces. And he said that she was cured and her body returned to its [normal] condition in a short time."[23]

2:13 **I already … Ḥunayn ibn Isḥāq**: Perhaps referring to another script that is extant in the same volume, Ms. Parma 2283, *Ingenio Sanitatis*, that is a compendium of Galen's *De prudenti metodo medendi*, written by Ḥunayn ibn Isḥāq. This work is extant in Ms. Parma 2283, folios 97ᵛ–100ᵛ, right after the treatise on phlebotomy. The treatise deals with phlebotomy and evacuation by vomiting and drugs. However, a clear reference to what the author is referring to regarding the "current season" has not been found, but this part may be related. See 98ᵛ with my translation:

> בזמן הקיץ עם החום רב ובזמן הסתו עם הקור רב אין צריך להריק ולא להקיז. אבל בזמני׳ הבינוניים שיהי׳ הפרק ממוזג. אבל ישמור שלא יבא הזמן מעורבב כמו עם חום רב או קרירות או רוחיות על ההקזה ועל ההרקה או על המרחץ או על המשגל כי ענין כזה ישחית מהרה המזג. ואם ימטיר או יהיה הזמן לח לא ימנע מהקיז ולהריק כל זמן שלא יעשה קרירות.

> In the summer with great heat and in the winter with great cold, purging or phlebotomy is not needed. But in moderate times when the season is balanced, it should be ensured that the time is not mixed, such as with severe heat, coldness, or winds concerning bloodletting, purging, baths, or sexual intercourse, because such humours can quickly corrupt the temperament. If it rains or the season is moist, bloodletting and purging should not be avoided, as long as it does not cause coldness.[24]

---

22 Galen, *Cur. Rat. Ven. Sect.*, p. 89.

23 Maimonides, *Aphorisms 24*, 17, p. 79.

24 Ms. Parma, Biblioteca Palatina 2283, fol. 98ᵛ.

3:2 **Overfilling:** Cf. Galen: "Whenever the humors are increased to an equal degree to each other, [doctors] call this 'abundance' or 'plethora'. On the other hand, whenever the body is already full of yellow or black bile, or phlegm, or the serous humors, they call such a condition *kakochymia* and not plethora. Plethora is treated by the letting of blood, and by numerous baths, exercises and rubbings, as well as by discutient medications, and in addition by all fastings, which I covered comprehensively in the treatises on health. *Kakochymia*, however, is treated by the specific evacuation appropriate for each of the humors in excess."[25] Every excess is harmful, as stated by Hippocrates: "all excess is hostile to nature."[26]

Two parts: i.e., overfilling relating to vessels, and overfilling affecting the strength. In *Galen on Bloodletting*, Brain translates these as *plethos by filling* and *dynamic plethos*: "It has been shown in my book on plethos that plethos is of two kinds, both in origin and in terminology. One set of signs indicates dynamic plethos, another the variety due to dilatation of the vessels containing the humours, which some call plethos by filling."[27]

Pneuma: Galen identifies three types of pneuma: vital pneuma that is generated in the heart and the arteries, that is produced from the inhalation and vapourisation of the humours; psychic pneuma, that is generated from a further refinement of the vital pneuma in the retiform web through the carotid arteries, reaching the ventricles of the brain;[28] and natural pneuma, generated in the liver and distributed through the veins.[29]

Winds of the mouth: The copyist seems to have misunderstood something in this passage, as Ms. Parma reads ורוחות הפה הנקראות אלתמטא ואלתתאב, suggesting that both stretching and yawning are 'winds of mouth'—אלתמטא from the Arabic التمطي spelled التمطى in Ms. Escorial.

... from the hot waters called ...: The term featuring in Ms. Parma, אלמוחמתא, is an unidentified word that seemingly refers to a bathhouse. Ms. Escorial reads: *ka'annahu qad ḫarağa min al-ḥammām wa-huwa laḥim*. This might be either

25 Galen, *Meth. Med.* III, XIII, 891K (LCL 518: 344–345).
26 Hippocrates, *Aphorisms* II, LI (LCL 150: 120–121).
27 Galen, *Cur. Rat. Ven. Sect.*, p. 71.
28 Galen, *PHP* VII 3, pp. 444–445. For an explanation how this works, see Galen, *PHP* VII 3–4, pp. 442–453.
29 Galen, *UP*, p. 48.

the translations addition, or perhaps a corrupt term from another copy. Perhaps this error consists of the Arabic definite article *al*, the word for hot spring *ḥamma*, and possibly water, *mā'*, or simply the plural form of *ḥammām*.

… the indications are stronger: Ms. Parma seems to read יהיו האותות יותר אמתיים, "the indications are more real", chosen to be read as אמתנים to match Ms. Escorial, which reads *aqwā*, stronger. Gesenius gives the word אֶמְתָּנִי, from the Arabic root √mtn, متن, meaning 'strong, mighty.'[30]

Indication: Galen attests that the term 'indication' is "the discovery of the truth about the thing in question arising out of the nature of the thing and made through following out the clues given by what is clearly observable".[31]

3:3 **Dreams**: In *Epidemics I*, Hippocrates gives a story of Erasinus, who manifested a fever after supper, and suffered from delirium, distress, exacerbation, convulsions with sweating, discomfort, fear, and dreams. His urine was dark with round particles in it, and towards the end of the fifth day he died.[32] The symptoms resemble the indications of plethos described in this paragraph. Dreams indicating multitude of blood are not mentioned in *Dreams* or *Regimen IV* by Hippocrates. Ms. Escorial refers to Rufus' book *Medical Questions*, which does not contain this quoted part either. However, the passage is very similar to Galen in his commentary on Hippocrates' *Humours*: "Dreams belong to the things that regularly indicate the disposition of the body. If someone see fire in a dream, then this man suffers from yellow bile. If rain appears, then know that cold liquid is in overabundance. Likewise also if [someone see] snow, ice, or hail, this indicates cold phlegm; if he thinks that he is in a malodorous place, this indicates the putrefaction of the humours. If he sees the crests of cocks, or something flaming red, this indicates that blood is in overabundance. If he sees something dark-coloured or thinks that he is in a dark place, then this indicates breaths [i.e., flatulence.]."[33]

This is the manner …: Dreams are a strong prognostic sign. According to Mattern, Galen, following Hippocrates and other predecessors, identified various

30 Gesenius, *Gesenius' Hebrew and Chaldee Lexicon to the Old Testament Scriptures*, p. 63.
31 Galen, *Inst. Log.*, p. 42.
32 Hippocrates, *Epidemics I* (LCL 147: 207–209).
33 Galen's Commentary on Hippocrates' *Humours*, 2.2 [16.219.9–220.3 Kühn]. I am very grateful to Professor Peter Pormann for his generous help with identifying the quote in this passage.

origins of dreams, some of which may seem familiar to contemporary readers. He believed that dreams could indicate an imbalance of the humours. For instance, a wrestler with an excess of blood might dream of standing in a cistern of blood, while images of snow and rain could symbolise the cold and wet phlegm.[34] In the work quoted in Ms. Escorial, *Medical Questions*, Rufus of Ephesus provides many examples in which dream interpretation has been used in diagnostics of overfilling.[35]

3:6 **Raw humours**: "Crude or raw humour is material, derived from nutriment, that has not been properly cooked or concocted by the innate heat."[36]

3:7 **Scarcely nourishing foods**: Cf. Nasrallah, *Annals of the Caliphs' Kitchens*: Foods with poor nutrition include those low in density, excessively dry foods like salted meat, and those producing too much excretion such as trotters, tripe, intestines, tallow, ears, lungs, poultry, barley bread, bread with bran, and all vegetables. Astringent foods such as olives, pistachios, walnuts, and almonds also offer poor nourishment. Fish, gourd, pomegranate, mulberry, plums, and apricot are poor sources of nutrition due to their high moisture content and rapid nutrient dissolution.[37] This is in contrast with highly nourishing foods that are dense and nourishing when fully digested, even in small amounts. Travellers and convalescents who cannot eat a lot need such foods. Highly nourishing foods include beef, brain, heart, gizzards of all birds, fish with thick flesh, fine white flour, fava beans, chickpeas, beans, lentils, dates, acorn, chestnut, turnip, milk, and red sweet wine.[38]

3:9 **Springtime**: Cf. Galen: "And as for those who go down every year in summer with plethoric diseases, they too should be evacuated at the onset of spring."[39]

4:3 **This fever … a beginning, increase, culmination, and decline**: Corresponds to e.g., Maimonides who identifies four periods of illness: "The periods of a disease are four altogether: beginning, increase, culmination and decline."[40]

34 Mattern, *Prince of Medicine*, p. 174.
35 Rufus, *Quaestiones medicinales*, §§ 28–33 (pp. 74–77).
36 Galen, *Cur. Rat. Ven. Sect.*, p. 76, footnote 29.
37 Nasrallah, *Annals of the Caliphs' Kitchens*, p. 735.
38 Nasrallah, *Annals of the Caliphs' Kitchens*, p. 732.
39 Galen, *Cur. Rat. Ven. Sect.*, p. 88.
40 Maimonides, *Aphorisms 11*, 1, p. 20.

One needs to extract blood until [the patient] faints: Galen: "When, however, there is a plethos of seething blood, enkindling a very acute fever, there is need for copious evacuation. One must try to evacuate this blood to the point of fainting".[41]

Unconsciousness: Throughout the edition, Ms. Parma employs two interchangeable terms for 'unconsciousness': עטוף,[42] appearing in passages 4:3, 4:5, and 9:2; and a synonymous term, עלוף,[43] found in passages 4:4, 4:6, 8:3, 10:4, 10:5, and 10:7.

5:1 **Phlebotomised veins**: For what these veins may refer to, see the commentary section in Ms. Escorial.

5:4 **Hippocrates mentioned …**: Hippocrates talking about the Scythians: "They cure themselves in the following way. At the beginning of the disease they cut the vessel behind each ear. After the blood flows out, sleep comes over them from their weakness, and they go to bed. Later they wake up, some being cured and others not. Now, in my opinion, by this treatment their seed is destroyed; for by the side of the ear are vessels which, when someone cuts them, make the person cut sterile, and so I believe it is these vessels they are cutting."[44] While Ms. Escorial mentions that it was Galen who said that what Hippocrates has described is a convincing statement, Ms. Parma reads that Hippocrates said it as an absolute statement.

5:5 **The hollow of the neck, called *al-nuqra***: نقرة القفا *nuqrat al-qafā*, the hollow of the neck.[45]

Al-intišār: See commentary for § 5:5 in the edition of Ms. Escorial.

5:10 **Polyps**: Ms. Parma reads *al-bawāsīr*, haemorrhoids, as Ms. Escorial also does. However, in my edition, I have emended it to *nawāsīr*, polyps, while the term *bawāsīr* is used for haemorrhoids.

---

41 Galen, *Cur. Rat. Ven. Sect.*, p. 85.
42 Gesenius, *Gesenius' Hebrew and Chaldee Lexicon to the Old Testament Scriptures*, p. 621.
43 Gesenius, *Gesenius' Hebrew and Chaldee Lexicon to the Old Testament Scriptures*, p. 635.
44 Hippocrates, *Airs, Waters, Places*, Chapter 22. (LCL 147: 132–133).
45 Fonahn, *Arabic and Latin Anatomical Terminology: Chiefly from the Middle Ages*, p. 103.

5:13 **Leprosy**: Ms. Parma reads חלי הצער, not corresponding to 'leprosy' in Ms. Escorial. Therefore, emendation to the Hebrew term חלי הצרעת.[46]

5:16 ***Al-bāsilīq* … name derived:** While Ms. Parma reads שם משותף, 'a common name,' Ms. Escorial reads *wa-huwa muštaqq min al-riʾāsa*, 'derived from *riʾāsa*.'

5:23: ***Gid ha-naše***: The Hebrew term for the sciatic nerve, or tendon, that occurs also in Genesis 32:33.[47]

7:1 **Drawing matters:** This chapter in Ms. Parma is comprised to the minimum. See the edition of Ms. Escorial for several additional passages on drawing matters.

7:3 **… patients**: Another possible reading would be 'illnesses'; but see Ms. Escorial 7:7: "*qad imtaḥanā hāḏā fī ǧumla min al-marḍā,*" i.e., "we have examined this with a number of patients".

8:3 **Until the day breaks**: The phrase "עד שיפוח היום" is from Song of Songs, verse 2:17.[48]

8:5 **Sexual intercourse:** For more on al-Rāzī on sex, see e.g., *The Spiritual Physick of Rhazes*, pp. 83–84; and Pormann, 'Al-Rāzī (d. 925) on the Benefits of Sex: A Clinician Caught between Philosophy and Medicine,' in A. Vrolijk, & J.P. Hogendijk (Eds.), *O Ye Gentlemen: Arabic Studies on Science and Literary Culture, in Honour of Remke Kruk* (pp. 134–145), Brill.

8:6 **Severe illnesses, such as …**: Ms. Parma does not distinguish between the Arabic terms *sakta* and *saqṭa*: *al-sakta*, 'apoplexy,' and *al-saqṭa al-ʿaẓīma*, 'a severe collapse.'

Day or night: Corresponds to Galen: "you will not shrink from sometimes opening a vein even during the night."[49]

8:8 **Hippocrates phlebotomised a patient on the eighth day of his illness …**: Corresponds to Hippocrates in *Epidemics III*, in which he talks about a patient

46 Bos, *Novel Medical Hebrew Terminology Vol. 2*, p. 150.
47 Gesenius, *Gesenius' Hebrew and Chaldee Lexicon to the Old Testament Scriptures*, p. 570.
48 שיר השירים פסוק ב פרק יז.
49 Galen, *Cur. Rat. Ven. Sect.*, p. 86.

with acute fever: "Eighth day. I bled him in the elbow. There was an abundant, proper flow of blood: the pains were relieved, although the dry coughing persisted."[50]

[Galen] … twentieth day: Corresponds to Galen: "For on whatever day you observe the indications for phlebotomy in the patient, on that day you will apply the remedy, even if it is the twentieth day from the onset. And what are the indications? The disease severe; strength of the faculties; except in the stage of childhood, and when the ambient air is very hot. Since, in most diseases, the patient's strength will already have been diminished with the passage of time, the opportunity for phlebotomy is lost because of the number of days that have elapsed; this, however, is not a primary effect, but is due to the intervention of another factor, namely the antecedent dissolution of the faculties. Hence, if even on the second day after the onset the powers should appear to be dissolved, we shall refrain from phlebotomy."[51]

9:2 **Earlier for the strong, and later for the weak**: In Ms. Escorial, the concept clearly is that epaphairesis should be faster, *asraʿ*, for the strong and slower, *abṭaʾ*, for the weak. However, reading Ms. Parma suggests another possible interpretation, that epaphairesis should be conducted earlier for the strong, and later for the weak. The principles of epaphairesis confirmed by Galen: "As for the time for epaphairesis, in those patients in whom we decide simply to evacuate, this should take place on the same day; but for those who are revulsed, it is better that it should be done on two successive days. You should monitor the strength of the patient in all such cases, by feeling his pulse, since some patients are sensitive where strength is concerned, so that they cannot bear copious evacuation. In such cases, the patient should be allowed to recover on the first day, and epaphairesis should be performed on the second."[52]

9:4 **Epaphairesis is a significant matter …**: Judging by the context, emendation from הקזה to חזרה seems appropriate. The Hebrew version abbreviates the Arabic explanation of epaphairesis, omitting the description of how Nature distinguishes and expels corrupt blood through the wound. Ms. Escorial presents epaphairesis as a necessary adaptation when the body cannot tolerate the evacuation of a lot of blood in one session. If this was done, it might weaken Nature.

50 Hippocrates, *Epidemics* III, 8 (LCL 147: 268–269).
51 Galen, *Cur. Rat. Ven. Sect.*, p. 96.
52 Galen, *Cur. Rat. Ven. Sect.*, p. 97.

Ms. Parma refers to Nature in the masculine but seems to suggest that it is a patient who may be afraid of an additional removal of blood.

10:1 **The food and drink of the phlebotomised [patient]**: In general, Ms. Parma includes only a fragment of the various prescriptions presented in Ms. Escorial. For several prescriptions mentioned in Ms. Escorial, see chapter 10 and *index of prescriptions* in the edition of Ms. Escorial.

10:2 **Pleasant things**: Cf. Albucasis: "There should also be in the place where he is sitting such things as are customary for men to enjoy, such as various perfumes, aromatics, and music, and the like, as each one may."[53] In general, the atmosphere should be pleasant and relaxed—see chapter 95 in *Albucasis on Surgery and Instruments*.[54]

10:3 **Soured pullets**: It is not clear whether the recommendation is to eat goat meat, mutton, or soured pullets, the vinegar referring only to pullets, or if all these should be pickled, i.e., pickled goat meat, mutton, and pullets. The same is unclear in Ms. Escorial: *laḥm ǧady aw ḫarūf aw farārīǧ muḥammaḍāt.*

The food on the day of phlebotomy and the day after should be moderate: Whereas Ms. Parma reads ומחרתו, 'the day after,' Ms. Escorial reads *wa-ġayruhu*, understood as 'in general.'

10:4 ***Al-ḥiṣrimiyya* and *al-rummāniyya***: Both these dishes are sour. Sour stews were typically deemed suitable for individuals with hot temperaments, while those with cold temperaments should consume white, simple dishes to counterbalance their cold properties.[55] Of these dishes, *ḥiṣrimiyya* is a stew that is soured with juice of unripe grapes;[56] and *rummāniyya* a stew made of pomegranate and chicken.[57]

Syrup: Ms. Parma reads משקה for the Arabic *šarāb*, that could be translated as a drink. However, according to the Arabic pharmacological tradition, this should be called syrup, i.e., a potion prepared of fruit, sugar, and honey, with a

53 Albucasis, *Albucasis on Surgery and Instruments*, p. 642.
54 Albucasis, *Albucasis on Surgery and Instruments*, p. 642.
55 Nasrallah, *Annals of the Caliphs' Kitchens*, p. 607.
56 Nasrallah, *Annals of the Caliphs' Kitchens*, p. 607.
57 Nasrallah, *Annals of the Caliphs' Kitchens*, p. 614.

thick consistency that contains more sugar in relation to fruit.[58] According to Temkin, syrups were "an Arabic contribution to pharmacology."[59]

Rose syrup: A prescription by Ibn al-Tilmīḏ:[60]

red roses	1 part
water	10 parts
pure sugar	similar amount of the remaining water

Cook one part of red roses in ten parts of water until one part of the water is gone. Press the roses and keep immersing them depending on the strength of the purgative effect you wish to achieve—stronger if one tenth of the water is left, weaker if half of it remains. Take the water in which the roses have been immersed and melt into it a similar amount of pure sugar. Cook until the mixture reaches the consistency of oxymel. Serve it by using four *ūqiyyas* of the product with thirty *dirhams* of ice. The ice makes the purgative effect stronger, and yellow bile and other fine humours are purged.

10:5 **Animal faculty**: One of the three central faculties: the natural faculties which are the effects of nature, manifesting in conception, growth, and nourishment; the animal faculties which sustain life, evident in the systole and diastole of the heart and arteries; and the psychical faculties, responsible for reasoning, discernment, emotion, and voluntary movement.[61]

10:7 ***Al-ġāliya***: A men's perfume that comes in various types, the basic components of which are musk, ambergris, and balsam oil.[62] For its preparation, see Al-Kindī, Yaʿqūb b. Isḥāq (d. ca. 873), *Kitāb kīmiyā al-ʿiṭr wat-taṣʿīdāt = Buch über die Chemie des Parfüms und die Destillationen*, transl. by K. Garbers, Leipzig, 1948, pp. 56–57.

Meat broth: Cf. Nasrallah, *Annals of the Caliphs' Kitchens*: 'meat juice,' obtained by slicing the meat thinly and cooking it without adding any liquid until it

58 Fellmann, *Das Aqrābāḏīn al-Qalānisī*, no. 3. 87, p. 269.
59 Temkin, *Galenism*, p. 127.
60 Adapted from Kahl, *The Dispensatory of Ibn al-Tilmīḏ*, p. 237.
61 Ullmann, *Islamic Medicine*, p. 60.
62 Nasrallah, *Annals of the Caliphs' Kitchens*, p. 770.

'sweats' and releases all its moisture. This juice is then collected and provided to the sick as a nourishing food.[63]

10:9 **Prescription of melicratum**: Ms. Parma leaves out ginger as an ingredient. See the prescription in Ms. Escorial (10:9):

clear honey	1 *raṭl*
fresh water	5 *raṭls*
long pepper	
ginger	
cinnamon	
Indian nard	
mastic	
cloves	1 *dirham* each

Take one *raṭl* of honey and pour five *raṭls* of water on it in a new pot. Cook on low fire and skim. When it gets close to the consistency of julep, take one *dirham* of long pepper, ginger, cinnamon, Indian nard, mastic, and cloves, and grind them well. Then, compress them in a linen cloth and suspend the cloth in the pot and cook until the liquid reaches the consistency of julep. Let the cloth soak in the drink. Remove from the fire and let cool down.

New pot: Ms. Parma reads קדרה חדשה, 'a new pot,' corresponding to Ms. Escorial that reads *qidr ǧadīd* (قدر جديد). However, what possibly is meant is *qidr ḥadīd* (قدر حديد), an iron pot.

10:10 ***Mayba***: Ms. Escorial contains two prescriptions for *mayba* (10:10):

quince juice	20 *raṭls*
grape jelly	10 *raṭls*
skimmed honey	5 *raṭls*
ginger	
mastic	
black cardamom	
small cardamom	
cinnamon	
cloves	

63 Nasrallah, *Annals of the Caliphs' Kitchens*, p. 610.

saffron	20 *dirhams* each
musk	1/8 *dirham*

Take fresh, juicy, sour quinces, peel them, clean their inside and grind them in a stone mortar. Squeeze from their juice 20 *raṭls*. Add 10 *raṭl*s of grape jelly and infuse it with the residues of the quince in some quince juice. Filter. Put the juices in a pot, boil gently on embers, and skim until half of the liquid remains. Remove from the fire. Then filter it for three days, a few times every day, in a thick, twofold cloth. After three days, add five *raṭl*s of skimmed honey in the mixture. Then crush and grind 20 *dirhams* of ginger root, mastic, black cardamom, small cardamom, cinnamon, cloves, and saffron, and bind them tightly in a thin linen cloth. Suspend the cloth in the pot and cook it altogether for a second time on low fire. Soak the spices in the liquid time after time until the mixture reaches the consistency of syrup and becomes clear. Then add 1/8 *dirham* of ground musk. Put the syrup in a glass receptacle. Leave the cloth soaking in it for two weeks, after which you remove it. If you want, you can let the spices sink to the bottom of the glass receptacle.

Mayba II (§ 10:11)

quince juice	1 part
clear, skimmed honey*	1 part
(*alt. crystalline sugar)	
very sour vinegar	3/4 part

Cook one part of quince juice and one part of honey (or crystalline sugar for whoever is of hot disposition) gently on embers, skim it, keep boiling until it reaches the consistency of syrup. Whoever wants sourness may add vinegar.

Al-Manṣūrī: *Al-Kitāb al-Manṣūrī*, one of al-Rāzī's central contributions to medical literature. This treatise discusses topics such as anatomy, physiology, pathology, *materia medica*, general maintenance of health, diet, cosmetics, surgery, and toxicology.[64] As for the reference in the passage, perhaps the Hebrew translation by Shem Tov b. Isaac, extant in codex Parma 2283 (fol. 106^{v}) is meant.[65] However, the text on folio 106^{v} only briefly mentions drinking wine and what

64 Sezgin, *Geschichte des arabischen Schrifttums, Bd. 3*, p. 281.

65 Richler, *Hebrew Manuscripts in the Biblioteca Palatina in Parma: Catalogue*, p. 451.

is similar to that. Perhaps something else, such as another copy of *al-Kitāb al-Manṣūrī*, is intended.

11:2 **Sour citron syrup:** As an example, a citron syrup by *Ibn al-Tilmīḏ* is prepared of sour citrons and superb sugar. The juice of the sour citrons is pressed after the seeds are removed. Into each *raṭl* of sour citron juice one adds one *mann* of superb sugar. It should be left until the sugar melts without boiling, and then boiled on low fire. At the end, the syrup is removed from the fire, the scum removed, and the syrup is left to gain consistency.[66]

Pomegranate: Ms. Parma lists pomegranates both in the singular and plural form. In several instances, Ms. Escorial lists pomegranate in the dual form, referring to two types of pomegranates, i.e., sweet (*ḥulw*) and sour (*ḥāmiḍ*) pomegranates.[67]

Plum: The term אגאס usually refers to pear; however, in this case its counterpart in Ms. Escorial is plum, in Arabic *iǧǧāṣ*, while the term כמתרא, in Arabic *kummaṯrā*, is used for pear. See index of *materia medica*.

11:3 **Barley broth**: Ms. Escorial presents a simple prescription of barley broth (§ 11:10)

barley	2 parts
peeled lentils*	1 part
(*alt. plum or jujube)	

Cook the barley and the lentils [in water]—or if you want, you may use plum or jujube.

According to Ibn Māsawayh's prescription, barley broth is made by washing new or old barley with the husk, after which it is washed clean. It is soaked for a whole hour, drained, and covered with a thick cloth overnight. On the following day the barley is pounded in a mortar, cleaned from the husk, and put in a clean pot. Thereafter it is cooked with water, for each *kayl* of barley 14 *kayls* of water, simmering on low fire until it thickens. It is consumed with or without sugar.[68]

66 Adapted from Kahl, *The Dispensatory of Ibn al-Tilmīḏ*, p. 240.
67 Ibn al-Ǧazzār, *Zād al-Musāfir*, 1.10.4 no: 174 (p. 107).
68 Adapted from Nasrallah, *Annals of the Caliphs' Kitchens*, p. 448.

ʿAdasiyya* and *summāqiyya: *ʿAdasiyya* is a lentil dish with several varieties;[69] *summāqiyya* is a meat dish with strained juice of sumac,[70] i.e., Rhus coriaria L., and smokebush, Cotinus coggygria Scop.; Anacardiaceae.[71]

Dullāʿiyya* and *riğliyya: While Ms. Escorial seems to suggest gourd (*qarʿ*) and purslane (*riğla*) as vegetables to be eaten, in Ms. Parma, they seem to have been understood as dishes. The term in Ms. Parma, *dalʿiyya*, possibly related to the word דלעת, may perhaps be understood as *dullāʿiyya*. See also the entry below.

Melon: The term פקוס in Ms. Parma apparently replaces the Arabic *dullāʿ*. Ms. Parma lists והקשואים וקתא ופקוס, which in Nathan Ben Eliezer haMe'ati's Glossary all seem to refer to the same plant: קראתי קשואים או קשות מה שנקרא קתא בלשון ערבי והוא "פקוס קוקומרו ארוך".[72] Ms. Escorial reads "… quince, pear, apple, ⟨and cucumber, squirting cucumber, melon …⟩", *ḫiyār*, *qiṯṯā'*, *dullāʿ*. Hence, Ms. Parma possibly refers to *faqqūṣ*, a plant in the *Cucumis melo* family, that according to Lane denotes a melon before it has become ripe, alternatively cucumus sativus, i.e., common cucumber.[73]

11:4 This passage seems to be the only thing left from what in Ms. Escorial describes the regimen of a patient whose disposition needs to be cooled down. Ms. Escorial reads 'apple,' in Ms. Parma apparently understood as an apple dish, אלתפחיא, *al-tuffāḥiyya* (?). Spinach, in Ms. Escorial, is mentioned only as an ingredient, not as a dish.

11:5 **The prescription of a decoction**: This prescription in Ms. Parma deviates from Ms. Escorial. See Ms. Escorial (11:7):

[water]	
tamarind	2 *ūqiyyas*
plum	
jujube	
large sebesten	10 grains of each

69 Nasrallah, *Annals of the Caliphs Kitchens*, p. 293.
70 Nasrallah, *Annals of the Caliphs Kitchens*, p. 299.
71 Ibn Ğanāḥ II, no. 1003 (p. 1120).
72 Bos, *Novel Medical and General Hebrew Terminology from the 13th Century, Vol. 2*, p. 119.
73 Lane, *An Arabic-English Lexicon*, p. 2427.

dry, red rose	
blue violet leaves	
peeled lentils	
barberry	
endive seeds	
purslane seeds	3 *dirhams* each
dry coriander seeds	2 *dirhams*
endive leaves	
nightshade leaves	1 part of each
kernel of cassia fistula cane cleaned from its seed	1 *ūqiyya*

Take two *ūqiyyas* tamarind, 10 grains of plum, jujube and sebesten, three *dirhams* of dry, red rose, blue violet leaves, peeled lentils, barberry, endive seeds and purslane seeds, two *dirhams* of dry coriander seeds, and a part of endive and nightshade leaves. Boil on low fire until the water becomes red and thickens. Add half a *raṭl* of clear water and soak the kernel of the cane of cassia fistula in the decoction. Filter and consume.

Thereafter one heats it a little: Ms. Escorial reads "it is filtered a second time". Although Ms. Parma reads ויחמם מעט, a possible, alternative reading would thus be ויסנן שנית.

Should the natural constitution not get warmer: The prescription is for loosening the bowels and preventing the combustion of blood. This may have been misunderstood in Ms. Parma.

11:6 **Prescription of pastilles**: This prescription deviates slightly from the one presented in Ms. Escorial (11:12):

dry, red rose	10 *dirhams*
purslane seeds	
endive seeds	
barberry	
gum Arabic	
white tragacanth	2 *dirhams* of each
white sandalwood	
chalk	1.5 *dirham* of each
upper part of peeled liquorice root	3 *dirhams*
Chinese rhubarb	1 *dirham*

saffron	0.5 *dirham*
camphor (optional)	1/4 *dirham*

Pound the ingredients and knead them in boiled, filtered nightshade pulp. Form pastilles à one *dirham* of weight and let dry in the shade. Take one pastille with every meal with one *ūqiyya* of oxymel. If the patient has coarseness in the chest, consume the pastilles with sweeter syrups, such as cherry syrup or the syrup made of both types of pomegranates.

12:3 **Pleurisy and pleuritis**: In passages 3:8 and 7:3, Ms. Parma refers to pleuritis as *mursat ha-ṣelaʿot ha-niqret al-šawṣa*, 'swelling of the ribs called *al-šawṣa*,' while in 12:3 it differentiates between the two: *mursat ha-ṣelaʿot ve ha-šawṣa*, 'swelling of the ribs [i.e., pleurisy] and pleuritis.' The Arabic terms used in Ms. Escorial are *ḏāt al-ǧanb* for pleurisy,[74] and *al-šawṣa* for pleuritis.[75]

12:4 **Reduced sexual desire**: Ms. Escorial reads *qillat al-bāh*, understood as reduced sexual desire, followed later by *kaṯrat al-šahwa al-bāhiyya*, increased libido or abundance of sexual desire. The Hebrew term *mišgal* seems to have been applied both for the Arabic *al-ǧimāʿ*, sexual intercourse, coitus, as well as *al-bāh* or *al-šahwa al-bāhiyya*, sexual desire, libido.

Sciatica … the tongue and the foot become thick: Ms. Escorial reads *dāʾ al-fīl*, in my edition understood as elephantiasis, while Ms. Parma in its stead reads גיד הנשה, sciatica. According to Ms. Escorial the whole leg and the foot become enormous, while Ms. Parma, instead of leg, Ar. *al-sāq*, reads לשון, 'tongue.' It is most likely a corruption, as Ms. Escorial (§ 12:6) reads "… sciatica combined with heat in the leg; and for elephantiasis combined with heat of touch and darkening of complexion—this is a disease with which the whole leg and foot become enormous."

12:5 **In the case of this illness [i.e., sanguine fever]**: Ms. Parma does not mention sanguine fever. See 12:7 in the edition of Ms. Escorial.

Galen's preparation: This prescription and the instructions of its usage correspond to Galen in *Meth. Med. 11*.

74 Lane, *An Arabic-English Lexicon*, p. 465.
75 Kahl, *The Sanskrit, Syriac and Persian Sources in the Comprehensive Book of Rhazes*, p. 208.

> … the best of all the medications I know, and the one which is safer to use for hemorrhages from the meninges, is the one I shall speak of. Mix one part of frankincense with half a part of aloes, and then, when it comes to the time for use, mix in the white of an egg to such a degree that the whole has a honeylike consistency. Next, let this be taken up by the softest hairs of a hare, and then let it be applied in abundance to the vessel and to the whole wound. Bind externally with a linen cloth in an underbandage, making the first four or five turns on the hemorrhaging vein itself, and from that point, distribute it to the root of the vessel in those parts where it is possible to distribute to the root, which is almost all parts except for the meninges. Then, when you release it on the third day, if the medication is still adhering safely to the wound, apply another encircling bandage, moistening the tampon from the hairs, as you bound it initially. If the first tampon should fall off spontaneously, gently compress the root of the vessel with your finger until there is no further flow, then remove your finger carefully and apply another tampon.[76]

13:3 **Frankincense**: Ms. Escorial reads "one part of frankincense, and half a part of aloe." It is not certain to what Ms. Parma refers with כנדר שיאן.

Tip of a probe: Ms. Parma reads †*r'š hmwl*†. While Fellmann, in *Das Aqrābād̲īn al-Qalānisī*, presents the term *ḥamūl*, as suppositories or a tampon-like mass, and Galen (12:5 above) mentions a 'tampon' in his preparation, this interpretation seems less fitting given the various consistencies of the prescriptions in Qalānisī: powdery to thick liquids and pastes intended for vaginal or rectal insertion, not solid suppositories.[77] Consequently the term is better understood as *roš hamūl*, the tip of an applicator tool used to place the medicinal paste onto the wound. This interpretation aligns with the existing translation מכחול, meaning a probe or a stylus, which corresponds to the Arabic *mīl*, used for the application of medicinal substances and makeup.[78]

As previously mentioned: Ms. Escorial presents the instructions in Galen's remedy (Ms. Escorial § 13:3), while "as previously mentioned" is a part of the other prescription presented right after.

---

76 Galen, *Meth. Med. II*, V, 320K–321K (LCL: 517: 22–25).

77 Fellmann, *Das Aqrābād̲īn al-Qalānisī*, no. 3. 30, pp. 207–208.

78 Bos, *Novel Medical and General Hebrew Terminology from the 13th Century*, Volume 2, p. 60, and Volume 4, p. 99.

13:5 **Another prescription**: The measures differ between Ms. Parma and Ms. Escorial: See the prescription in Ms. Escorial (13:10):

chicken fat	
rose oil	5 *miṯqāls*
white wax	3 *miṯqāls*
tragacanth	
litharge	
ceruse	equal parts

Melt five *miṯqāls* of chicken fat and rose oil in three *miṯqāls* of white wax on fire. Remove from the fire, and add tragacanth, litharge, and ceruse. Use according to the need.

For additional prescriptions and more instructions, see chapter 13 in the edition of Ms. Escorial.

14:1 **Cupping**: For more on cupping vessels, see Bliquez, *The Tools of Asclepius*, p. 56 ff.

14:2 **The lateral parts of the neck**: Ms. Parma reads והצדעים, 'and the temples.' However, cupping the temples is not mentioned in Ms. Escorial, which in this passage reads 'the lateral parts of the neck.' Therefore, emendation to והצדדים.

14:9 **For women …**: While Ms. Escorial reads "for women whose facial complexion is fair and whose skin is white," Ms. Parma reads "for women who are fleshy and have a white complexion." For more, see commentary for § 14:9 in Ms. Escorial.

14:15 **Another treatise on cauterisation**: Possibly referring to al-Rāzī's treatise on cauterisation, *De sectionibus et cauteriis et ventosis*.[79]

… our book *BeMal'akat haYadayim*: Several Hebrew manuscripts in various locations and collections featuring the words מלאכת היד can be found by searching for instance at the website of the National Library of Israel. The name suggests that the treatise focuses on manual procedures.

---

79 *De sectionibus et cauteriis et ventosis*, by al-Rāzī, 13th century, MS 167/ff. 19^{v}–21^{r}. Western Medieval Manuscripts, MS. University of Edinburgh Library Heritage Collections.

Indices

1 Index of *materia medica*

Including foodstuffs and compound drugs. The items have been arranged according to the Hebrew alphabetical order, and include the Arabic terms spelled with Hebrew characters, as they occur in Ms. Parma, as well as their Arabic equivalents in Ms. Escorial. The references are given in an abbreviated form. The index of *materia medica* is followed by an abridged index of *materia medica*. See the *key to index of materia medica* for English-Hebrew-Arabic.

אגאס *aggas*: *iǧǧāṣ* إجاص plum: Cf. DTr I, no. 97. (p. 184): Prunus domestica and its varieties in the Rosaceae family. Cf. Galen, *Alim. Fac.*, II:31 (p. 94): According to Galen, plums are laxative due to their moisture and viscidity, and beneficial for moistening and cooling the stomach.

אספידאג' *isfīdāǧ* إسفيداج ceruse: Cf. Ibn Ǧanāḥ I, no. 76 (p. 278): ceruse, white lead.

אספינך *isfānāḫ* إسفاناخ spinach: Cf. Schmucker, *Firdaws*, no. 30 (p. 67): Spinacia oleracea L., spinach.

אתרוג *etrog*: *utruǧǧ* أترج citron: Cf. DTr I, no. 90 (p. 178): Citrus Limon [L.] Burm. (Citrus medica L.) et. al.

בנפסג *banafsaǧ* بنفسج violet: Cf. DTr IV, no. 110 (pp. 623–624): Viola odorata L., the leaves, flowers, seeds and roots of which were used as emetics and laxatives.

ברבריס *barbārīs* برباريس barberry, berberis: Cf. DTr I, no. 62 (pp. 145–146): *barbārīs* usually refers to Berberis vulgaris L., barberry. Dioscurides did not describe the barberry, which was unknown to the Greeks, but a rose plant, which most authors consider Crataegus oxyacantha L., hawthorn. The confusion may have arisen from the Arabs who understood barberry and hawthorn to be the same plant.

ג'לב *ǧullāb* جلاب julep, rose water syrup: Cf. Fellmann, *Qalānisī*, no. 3. 27. (p. 201): A syrup made of rose water, sugar, and perhaps other ingredients. It is used both as a cooling drink and as a purgative. For a simple julep one takes two parts of sugar mixed with six parts of rose water, boils it until half of it remains and removes the foam. Powdered saffron is added, and the drink may be dissolved with ice.

גליא *ġāliya* الغالية al-ġāliya: Cf. Fellmann, *Qalānisī*, no. 3. 22. (p. 196): A perfume blend that comes in various types, the basic components of which are musk and ambergris that are mixed with ben oil. Various other fragrances may be added.

גרעין *garʿin*: *bizr*, pl. *buzūr* بزر ج. بزور seed; spices: Cf. Ibn Ǧanāḥ I, no. 145 (p. 338): *Bizr*, seed; oil made of seeds. Cf. Dozy, *Supplément aux dictionnaires arabes*, p. 81: In plural it can also mean spices.

דבש *devaš*: *ʿasal* عسل honey: Cf. DTr II, no. 64 (p. 238): Mel commune, honey, praised as a medicine since the ancient times and used in electuaries, syrups, herbal and sour honeys, ointments, suppositories and enemas.

דרציני *dārṣīnī* دارصيني cinnamon: Cf. Ibn Ǧanāḥ I, no. 239 (p. 431): "*Dārṣīnī*, derived from the Persian *dār chīnī* ('Chinese wood'), is the common Arabic name of cinnamon (Cinnamomum verum J.Presl; Lauraceae […])".

הנדבא *hindibāʾ* هندباء endive: Cf. Ibn Ǧanāḥ I, no. 275 (pp. 460–461): endive, Cichorium endivia L. There are two types of *hindibāʾ*, *al-sarīs*, from the Greek σέρις, that grows in gardens, and another that grows in the wild that comes in two varieties. Like the Greek term σέρις, the Arabic *hindibāʾ* can also mean chicory (Cichorum intybus L.; Compositae). Cf. DTr II, no. 114 (p. 280): *hindibāʾ*, endive, that is *al-sarīs*, from the Greek σέρις. There are three varieties of *al-sarīs:* two wild, and one tame. The species are Cichorum intybus L., and Cichorum endivia L., endive, Compositae, and Lactuca serriola, of which endive is probably the latter.

ורד *vered*: *ward* ورد rose: Cf. DTr I, no. 68 (p. 155): Genus Rosa, numerous species of the Rosaceae family.

חבוש *ḥabbuš*: *safarǧal* سفرجل quince: Cf. DTr I, no. 87 (p. 176): Cydonia oblonga Mill., Rosaceae. Cf. Galen, *Alim. Fac.* II:23 (pp. 89–90): Galen, calling these Cydonian and Strouthian apples, mentions that quinces are more astringent than other apples, thus good for preserving. He refers to his own medication of the Strouthian apple, i.e., quince, containing quince juice, honey, white pepper, ginger, and vinegar, that he used to treat people with anorexia.

חזרת *ḥazeret*: *ḫass* خس lettuce: Either *ḫass barrī* (DTr IV, no. 18, p. 530) or *ḫass bustānī*, Lactuca sativa L. (DTr II, no. 119, p. 284).

חמץ *ḥomeṣ*: *ḫall* خل vinegar: Cf. Fellmann, *Qalānisī*, no. 3. 33. (pp. 210–211): Vinegar itself was regarded as a medicine, as it was thought to have a cooling effect. Vinegar also serves as a solubiliser. Cf. Fellmann, *Qalānisī*, no. 3. 84. (pp. 267–268): Alkaloids can be extracted from the drugs better with vinegar than with water, because they form a soluble compound with it. Thus, vinegar extracts are usually stronger than decoctions made with water. Although this chemical process naturally was unknown, the increased effect was most evidently noticed.

טבשיר *ṭabāšīr* طباشير tabasheer, bamboo chalk; Cf. Ibn Ǧanāḥ II, no. 904, (p. 1035): "'Tabasheer' is a white substance obtained from the nodal joints of bamboo (Bambusa bambos (L.) Voss)."

יין *yayin*: *nabīḏ* نبيذ wine: Cf. Nasrallah, pp. 468–470: wine made by using either dates, *dāḏī* (strong date wine), or grapes, or a combination of these. Cf.

Galen, *Alim. Fac.* III:39 (pp. 149–150): "The thick, red ones are the most useful of all wines for the production of blood, since they require the least change into it".

כאפור *kāfūr* كافور camphor: Cf. DTr III, no. 24 (p. 370): The white, translucent mass obtained from Cinnamomum camphora [L.], or Drybalanops aromatica, Dipterocarpaceae. Cf. Ibn Ǧanāḥ I, no. 211 (p. 398): "the bract (*qishr*) of the inflorescence of the date palm".

כזבור *kuzbura* كزبرة coriander: DTr III, no. 60 (p. 411): Coriandrum sativum L., used both medically and as a spice. The name originates from Akkadian. Cf. Nasrallah (p. 662): Both the seeds and the green herb have hot and moist properties. The seeds are thought to strengthen and delight the heart. Fresh coriander leaves improve digestion and induce sleep.

כיאר שנבר *ḫiyāršanbar* خيارشنبر cassia fistula: Cf. Ibn Ǧanāḥ II, no. 875 (p. 1010): "The loanword *khiyārshanbar* refers to purging cassia, also known as 'Indian laburnum', 'golden rain', or 'golden shower tree' (Cassia fistula L., Leguminosae). The Arabic term is derived from the Persian form *khiyār-chanbar* composed of *khiyār* ('cucumber') and *chanbar* ('circle, collar, necklace')."

כמתרא *kummaṯrā* كمثرى pear: Cf. DTr I, no. 91 (p. 179): Pyrus communis L., Rosaceae. The word comes originally from Akkadian.

כנדר *kundur* كندر frankincense: Cf. DTr I, no. 30 (p. 113): *al-kundur*, synonymous with *al-lubān* or *al-lūbān*, is frankincense, the dried gum resin of Boswellia species, particularly Boswellia Carteri Birdw., Burseraceae. It originates from Southern Arabia and Somalia, especially Šiḥr in Oman, as mentioned by Dioscorides.

כתירא *kaṯīrā'* كثيراء tragacanth: Cf. DTr III, no. 21 (p. 366): the gum resin that forms in the root and stem of several species of Astragalus gummifer Labill et. al.

לובן ביצים *loven beiṣim*: *bayāḍ al-bayḍ* بياض البيض egg white: in Ms. Escorial and Ms. Parma used in dressings to treat wounds.

מטבך *maṭbūḫ* مطبوخ decoction: Cf. Fellmann, *Qalānisī*, no. 3. 63. (pp. 245–246): decoctions are juices of drugs when cooked in water. Boiling on light to medium fire allows the powers of the drugs to release without being destroyed. The purpose of decoctions is to soften the nature and to purify it.

מיבא *mayba* ميبة mayba: Cf. Fellmann, *Qalānisī*, no. 3. 53 (p. 238): Mayba is a composite drink made from quince juice and wine. Quince juice is boiled with honey until the mixture defoams and thickens, and sugar and various spices are added.

מים *mayim*: *mā'* ماء water: Cf. Fellmann, *Qalānisī*, no. 3. 53. (p. 239): Water, *mā'*, usually refers to a drug extract that is made with water.

מלח *melaḥ*: *milḥ* ملح salt: Cf. Schmucker, *Firdaws*, no. 737: salt.

מורדסאנג' *murdāsanǧ* مرداسنج synonymous with *martak* مرتك: Cf. Ibn Ǧanāḥ II, no. 543 (p. 716): litharge, lead oxide.

מסך *misk* مسك musk: Cf. Ibn Ǧulǧul, *Dio.*, no. 33 (p. 51): Musk, the glandular secretion of the male musk deer (Moschus moschiferus L., Cervidae), obtained from the preputial sac near the navel of the animal.

מסתק *mastik*: *maṣṭakā* مصطكى mastic: Cf. Ibn Ǧanāḥ II, no. 562 (p. 733): mastic, resin of Pistacia lentiscus L. (Anacardiaceae).

משקה *mašqe*: *šarāb*, *ašriba* شراب ج. أشربة syrup, potion: Cf. Fellmann, *Qalānisī*, no. 3. 87. (p. 269): Syrups prepared of fruit and other juices, boiled with sugar and honey until they have a consistency similar to oxymel or apple syrup. When you squeeze fruit or vegetables, the resulting juice is 'press juice,' i.e., sap (*ʿuṣāra*). When the juice is thickened by boiling, or by leaving it in the sun, it is called 'thickened juice' (*rubb*), and when sugar is added and it is thickened, it is called syrup (*šarāb*). Syrup contains more sugar in relation to fruit.

משקה הבסר *mašqe ha-boser*: *ḥiṣrim* حصرم verjuice: Cf. Schmucker, *Firdaws*, no. 245 (p. 167): juice of unripe grapes. Cf. Liddell/Scott, p. 1229a: "An acidic juice obtained by pressing unripe grapes, or a juice of other unripe fruits". Lane (*An Arabic-English Lexicon*, p. 584) mentions that crude and sour grapes (ḥiṣrim), when rubbed on the body in the bath, either bruised or pulverised, strengthens and cools the body.

משקה הדבש *mašqe ha-devaš*: *šarāb al-ʿasal* شراب العسل melicratum: Cf. Riddle, *Dio. Pharm. Med.*, p. 144: "Very popular as a drink and as a medicine in antiquity was melicraton, or water mead (V. 9). This was a mixture of honey and water allowed to ferment. Among its usages was one for coughs."

סבסתן *sabistān* سبستان sebesten: Cf. Ibn Ǧanāḥ II, no. 666 (pp. 825–826): "*sabistān* is a common Arabic name 'sebesten fruits' produced by Cordia myxa L. ('Assyrian plum', Boraginaceae)."

סכנג'בין *sikanǧubīn* سكنجبين Oxymel, or sour honey: Cf. Fellmann, *Qalānisī*, no. 3. 84. (pp. 267–268): a potion composed of vinegar and honey. For pure oxymel one part of wine vinegar, two parts of fresh water, and three parts of *ṭabarzad* sugar are boiled until the liquid becomes consistent. This recipe could be used as a base, and altered by changing the honey to sugar, or the vinegar to quince juice and the like. Alkaloids can be extracted from the drugs better with vinegar than with water, because they form a soluble compound with it. Thus, vinegar extracts are usually stronger than decoctions made with water. Although this chemical process naturally was unknow, the increased effect was most evidently noticed. As for sugar and honey, that generally were considered interchangeable, they were credited for enhancing the moist properties. Thus, oxymel helped to combine the power of drugs with the medicinal effects of vinegar and sugar.

סכרי *sukkar* سكر sugar: Cf. DTr II, no. 65 (p. 238): Saccharum officinarum L., cane sugar, or sugar cane. It is said to have been brought from India to Egypt in the ancient times. Used both for its medicinal effects and for its taste.

סמי הריח *sammei ha-reaḥ*: *rayāḥīn* رياحين fragrant herbs: Cf. Schmucker, *Firdaws*, no. 332 (p. 209): plural of *rayḥān*, a generic name for fragrant herbs, such as basil. Cf. Nasrallah (p. 669): "All the aromatic herbs and plants such as the numerous varieties of mint, basil, and myrtle, are indispensable ingredients in cooking, for medicinal preparations, and in social gatherings where people sniff them for refreshment and pleasure."

סנבל *sunbul al-ṭīb* سنبل الطيب Indian nard: Cf. Schmucker, *Firdaws*, no. 403 (p. 248): Valeriana jatamansi Roxb. (Valerianaceae), Indian nard.

סנדל *ṣandal* صندل sandalwood: Cf. Schmucker, *Firdaws*, no. 461: white sandalwood, Santalum album L. (Santalaceae); red sandalwood, Pterocarpus santalinus L. (Papilionaceae). Cf. Dozy, *Supplément aux dictionnaires arabes*, pp. 358–359, on the sobriquet *maqāṣīrī*: white sandalwood, *sandalos cetrinos*, of yellowish colour. This yellow, pale species is called *santalum citrinum* in pharmacies, in Latin *santalum pallidum* or *santalum odoratum*. There are several kinds of sandal: the best is the yellow sandal, that has an aromatic smell, and it is called *maqāṣīrī*. *Maqāṣīrī* is yellow, *Ǧawrī* is white. Cf. DTr III, no. 38 (p. 385): ʿAbdallāh b. Ṣāliḥ says that even thyme, Thymus serpullum L., Labiatae is called *ṣandal*.

עדשים *ʿadašim*: *ʿadas* عدس lentils: Cf. DTr II, no. 91 (pp. 255–256): Lens culinaris Medik. Considered difficult to digest if consumed continuously, causing several issues. Cf. Galen, *Alim. Fac.*, I:18, p. 58: "Their juice, as stated previously, is the reverse of astringent. This is why if, after boiling them in water, one were to drink it seasoned with salt or fish sauce, and oil as well, the draught is aperient. But on boiling it twice, as described, the soup prepared from these lentils has the opposite property to the juice—drying up gastric fluxes and increasing the tone in the oesophagus, intestines and the stomach as a whole. This is why it is an appropriate food for those with gastric or dysenteric complaints."

ענאב *ʿunnāb* عناب jujube: Cf. Ibn Ǧanāḥ II, no. 736 (p. 542): Ziziphus jujuba Mill., also called Chinese date. Cf. Galen, *Alim. Fac.* II:32 (p. 95): Galen viewed jujube only as "poorly nutritious and difficult to concoct, and at the same time bad for the stomach".

ענב אלתעלב *ʿinab al-ṯaʿlab* عنب الثعلب nightshade: Cf. DTr IV, no. 63 (p. 573 f.): Several species of nightshade plants from the Solanaceae family, including e.g., Solanum nigrum L., Solanum villosum L., Solanum dulcamara L., Solanum alkekengi L., Atropa belladonna L. They have a soporific effect that can lead to death.

פירות *perot*: *fawākih* فواكه fruit: Cf. Galen, *Alim. Fac.* II, 7 (p. 76): "pears, apples, figs, peaches and pomegranates, and all such fruits that are useful to people as food".

פלפל ארוך *pilpel arok̲*: *dārfulful* دارفلفل long pepper: Cf. DTr III, no. 134 (p. 498): Piper longum L., Piperaceae. Cf. Dioscorides, *GHD*, Book II, no. 189 (p. 199): All types of pepper generally have warming, diuretic, digestive, and dissolving properties. Cf. Nasrallah (p. 648): long pepper is beneficial for treating cold-related illnesses, strengthening the stomach, and for aiding digestion.

פקוס *faqqūṣ*: melon: Cf. Lane, *An Arabic-English Lexicon*, p. 2427 *faqqūṣ*: "*A melon* (بِطِّيخَة) *before it has become ripe* (—) *now applied in Egypt to the cucumis sativus* (or *common cucumber*)."

צבר *ṣabir* صبر aloe: Cf. Ibn Ǧanāḥ II, no. 522 (pp. 696–697): "*Ṣabir* is the common Arabic name of aloe (Aloe vera (L.) Burm.f.; or Aloe ferox Mill.)."

צמג ערבי *ṣamġ ʿarabī* صمغ عربي gum Arabic: Cf. Schmucker, *Firdaws*, no. 460 (p. 282): gum from Acacia gummifera, A. spirocarpa, i.e., Mimosa gummifera, A. vera, i.e., Mimosa nilotica. Cf. Abdelkareem (p. 184): the fluid from Acacia seyal or Acacia senegal trees, used in traditional medicine for pain relief, as a glue, and several other ailments.

קישוא *qiššuʾ*: *qarʿ* قرع gourd, pumpkin: Cf. DTr II, no. 116 (p. 282): Three different plants from the cucurbitaceae family: Cucurbita maxima, Cucurbita pepo, Lagenaria vulgaris.

קיתא *qiṯṯāʾ* قثاء cucumber: Cf. Ibn Ǧulǧul, *Dio.*, no. 43 (p. 57): often treated as synonymous to *ḫiyār*, Cucumis sativus L. and Var. Cf. DTr IV, no. 139 (pp. 655–656): *al-qiṯṯāʾ al-barrī*, also known as *qiṯṯāʾ al-ḥimār*, i.e., Ecballium elaterium, squirting cucumber.

קרנפל *qaranful* قرنفل cloves: Cf. Ibn Ǧulǧul, *Dio.*, no. 19 (p. 34): cloves, "Syzygium aromaticum [L.] Merr. et L.M. Perry, Myrtaceae (Caryophyllus aromaticus L.)."

קרצה ר. אקרץ *qurṣ, aqrāṣ* قرص ج. أقراص pastille: Cf. Fellmann, *Qalānisī*, no. 3. 75 (p. 257): Drugs that are crushed and made in the form of pastilles. In singular also *qurṣa*.

ריבס *ribbas*: *rāwand ṣīnī* راوند صيني Chinese rhubarb: Cf. DTr III, 2 (p. 344): Chinese rhubarb, Rheum palmatum var. tanguticum, Polygonaceae, used as a laxative and astringent for gastrointestinal ailments. Cf. Schmucker, *Firdaws*, no. 321 (pp. 205–206): *rāwand ṣīnī* at times designates a separate species, at times a synonym for *rāwand*, for which it is representative as the most well-known species: Chinese rhubarb, usually called Rheum palmatum var. tanguticum, medicinal rhubarb, native to high Asia (Tibet and the Chinese provinces of Kansu and Shensi).

רג׳לא *riğla* رجلة purslane: Cf. Ibn Ğanāḥ II, no. 751 (pp. 892–893): common purslane, Portulaca oleracea L., Portulacaceae.

רמון *rimmon*: *rummān* رمان pomegranate: Cf. DTr I, no. 81 (p. 170): The fruit of Punica granatum L. et. al., Punicacaea. Cf. Dioscorides, *GHD*, Book I, 151 (p. 80): Dioscorides identifies three sorts of pomegranates: the sweet, that is the best for the stomach; a sharp one, that helps a burning stomach; and a species that in its taste resembles wine, that is of middle strength. They all are tasty and good for the stomach, yet do not nourish.

שמן *šemen*: *duhn* دهن oil: Cf. Fellmann, *Qalānisī*, no. 3. 13. (p. 183): pure oil, or medicinal oil.

שער ארנבת *seʿar arnevet*: *wabar al-arnab* وبر الأرنب hare's fur: in Ms. Escorial and Ms. Parma an ingredient in a dressing.

שעוה *šaʿava*: *šamʿ* شمع wax (Ibn Ğanāḥ II, no. 539, p. 713).

שעורים *seʿorim*: *šaʿīr* شعير barley: Cf. DTr II, no. 72 (p. 242): parent plant for barley is Hordeum vulgare L, and var., Gramineae.

תמר הינדי *tamr hindī* تمر هندي tamarind: Cf. Ibn Ğulğul, *Dio.*, no. 5 (p. 30): Tamarindus indica L., Leguminosae.

תפוח *tappuaḥ*: *tuffāḥ* تفاح apple: Cf. DTr I, no. 86 (p. 175): understood by most authors as Malus sylvestris [L.] Mill. (Pyrus Malus L.).

2 Abridged Index of *materia medica*

Hebrew	Arabic	Arabic Romanised	English
אגס	إجاص	*iğğāṣ*	plum
אקרץ	أقراص	*aqrāṣ*	pastilles
אספידאג׳	إسفيداج	*isfīdāğ*	ceruse, white lead
אספינך	إسفاناخ	*isfānāḫ*	spinach
אתרוג	أترج	*utruğğ*	citron
בנפסג	بنفسج	*banafsağ*	violet
ברבריס	برباريس	*barbārīs*	berberis, barberry
ג׳לב	جلاب	*ğullāb*	julep
גליא	الغالية	*al-ġāliyya*	*ġāliya*
גרעין	بزر	*bizr*	seed; spices
דבש	عسل	*ʿasal*	honey
דרציני	دارصيني	*dārṣīnī*	cinnamon
הנדבא	هندباء	*hindibāʾ*	endive
ורד	ورد	*ward*	rose

(*cont.*)

Hebrew	Arabic	Arabic Romanised	English
חבוש	سفرجل	*safarğal*	quince
חזרת	خس	*ḫass*	lettuce
חמץ	خل	*ḫall*	vinegar
טבשיר	طباشير	*ṭabāšīr*	bamboo chalk
יין	نبيذ	*nabīḏ*	wine
כאפור	كافور	*kāfūr*	camphor
כזבור	كزبرة	*kuzbura*	coriander
כיאר שנבר	خيارشنبر	*ḫiyāršanbar*	cassia fistula
כמתרא	كمثرى	*kummaṯrā*	pear
כנדר	كندر	*kundur*	frankincense
כתירא	كثيراء	*kaṯīrā*ʾ	tragacanth
לב	لب	*lubb*	pith
לובן ביצים	بياض البيض	*bayāḍ al-bayḍ*	egg white
מטבך	مطبوخ	*maṭbūḫ*	decoction
מיבא	ميبة	*mayba*	*mayba*
מים	ماء	*mā*ʾ	water
מלח	ملح	*milḥ*	salt
מרדסאנג׳	مرداسنج	*murdāsanğ*	litharge
מסך	مسك	*misk*	musk
מסתק	مصطكى	*maṣṭakā*	mastic
משקה	شراب	*šarāb*	syrup
משקה הבסר	حصرم	*ḥiṣrim*	verjuice
משקה הדבש	شراب العسل	*šarāb al-ʿasal*	melicratum
סבסתן	سبستان	*sabistān*	sebesten
סכנג׳בין	سكنجبين	*sikanğubīn*	oxymel
סכרי	سكر	*sukkar*	sugar
סמי הריח	رياحين	*rayāḥīn*	fragrant herbs
סנבל	سنبل الطيب	*sunbul al-ṭīb*	Indian nard
סנדל	صندل	*ṣandal*	sandalwood
עדשים	عدس	*ʿadas*	lentils
ענאב	عناب	*ʿunnāb*	jujube
ענב אלתעלב	عنب الثعلب	*ʿinab al-ṯaʿlab*	nightshade
פירות	فواكه	*fawākih*	fruit
פלפל ארוך	دارفلفل	*dārfulful*	long pepper
פקוס	فقوص	*faqqūṣ*	melon
צבר	صبر	*ṣabir*	aloe

(cont.)

Hebrew	Arabic	Arabic Romanised	English
צמג ערבי	صمغ عربي	*ṣamġ ʿarabī*	gum Arabic
קישוא	قرع	*qarʿ*	gourd
קרנפל	قرنفل	*qaranful*	cloves
קיתא	قثاء	*qiṯṯāʾ*	squirting cucumber
קרצה ר. אקרץ	قرص ج. أقراص	*qurṣ, aqrāṣ*	pastille
ריבס	راوند	*rāwand*	rhubarb
רג׳לא	رجلة	*riǧla*	purslane
רמון	رمان	*rummān*	pomegranate
שמן	دهن	*duhn*	oil
שער ארנבת	وبر الأرنب	*wabar al-arnab*	hare's fur
שעוה	شمع	*šamʿ*	wax
שעורים	شعير	*šaʿīr*	barley
תמר הינדי	تمر هندي	*tamr hindī*	tamarind
תפוח	تفاح	*tuffāḥ*	apple

3 Key to Index of *materia medica*

aloe	צבר	صبر
apple	תפוח	تفاح
melon	פקוס	فقوص
bamboo chalk	טבשיר	طباشير
barley	שעורים	شعير
berberis; barberry	ברבריס	برباريس
camphor	כאפור	كافور
cassia fistula	כיאר שנבר	خيارشنبر
ceruse, white lead	אספידאג	إسفيداج
cinnamon	דרציני	دارصيني
citron	אתרוג	أترج
cloves	קרנפל	قرنفل
coriander	כזבור	كزبرة
cucumber, squirting	קיתא	قثاء
decoction	מטבך	مطبوخ
egg white	לובן ביצים	بياض البيض

endive	הנדבא	هندباء
fragrant herbs	סמי הריח	رياحين
frankincense	כנדר	كندر
fruit	פירות	فواكه
gourd	קישוא	قرع
gum Arabic	צמג ערבי	صمغ عربي
hare's fur	שער ארנבת	وبر الأرنب
honey	דבש	عسل
Indian nard	סנבל	سنبل الطيب
jujube	ענאב	عناب
julep	ג׳לב	جلاب
lentils	עדשים	عدس
lettuce	חזרת	خس
litharge	מרדסאנג׳	مرداسنج
long pepper	פלפל ארוך	دارفلفل
mayba	מיבא	ميبة
mastic	מסתק	مصطكى
melicratum	משקה הדבש	شراب العسل
musk	מסך	مسك
nightshade	ענב אלתעלב	عنب الثعلب
oil	שמן	دهن
oxymel	סכנג׳בין	سكنجبين
pastille	קרצה	قرص
pear	כמתרא	كمثرى
pith	לב	لب
plum	אגס	إجاص
pomegranate	רמון	رمان
purslane	רג׳לא	رجلة
quince	חבוש	سفرجل
rhubarb, Chinese	ריבס	راوند صيني
rose	ורד	ورد
salt	מלח	ملح
sandalwood	סנדל	صندل
seed; spices	גרעין	بزر
sebesten	סבסתן	سبستان
spinach	אספינך	إسفاناخ
sugar	סכרי	سكر
syrup	משקה	شراب
tamarind	תמר הינדי	تمر هندي

tragacanth	כתירא	كثيراء
verjuice	משקה הבסר	حصرم
vinegar	חמץ	خل
violet	בנפסג	بنفسج
water	מים	ماء
wax	שעוה	شمع
wine	יין	نبيذ

4 Index of Foods and Dishes

אלסומקיא	السماقية	*al-summāqiyya*	*al-summāqiyya*
אלעדסיא	العدسية	*al-ʿadasiyya*	*al-ʿadasiyya*
אלרומאניאה	الرمانية	*al-rummāniyya*	*al-rummāniyya*
אלתפחיא		*al-tuffāḥiyya*	
בשול השעורים	ماء الشعير	*māʾ al-šaʿīr*	barley broth
בשר הגדיים	لحم جدي	*laḥm ğady*	goat meat
בשר הטלאים	لحم خروف	*laḥm ḫarūf*	mutton
דלעיה		*dullāʿiyya*	
הביצים הרכים	البيض النيمبرشت	*al-bayḍ al-nīmbarišt*	soft-cooked eggs
הצרמיא	حصرمية	*ḥiṣrimiyya*	*ḥiṣrimiyya*
לבות לחם לביבות הפת	لباب الخبز	*lubāb al- ḫubz*	breadcrumbs
מי הבשר	ماء اللحم	*māʾ al-laḥm*	meat broth
מרק התרנגולים	ماء الفروج	*māʾ al-farrūğ*	pullet broth
רג׳ליה		*riğliyya*	
תרנגול	فروج	*farrūğ*	pullet
תרנגולים עם חמץ	فراريج محمضات	*farārīğ muḥammaḍāt*	soured pullets
תרנגולים צלויים	فراريج مشوية	*farārīğ mašwiyya*	grilled pullets

5 Index of Weights and Measures

Presenting the weights and measures that occur in Ms. Parma with their equivalents in Ms. Escorial, and an estimated value based on Hinz.[1]

1 Hinz, Walther, Handbuch der Orientalistik, Abt. 1, Der Nahe und der Mittlere Osten, Erg. - Bd 1. H. 1, *Islamische Masse und Gewichte: umgerechnet ins metrische System*, Brill, Leiden, 1955.

dirham (3,125 g)	זוז	درهم	*dirham*
ounce, *ūqiyya* (33,85 g)	אוקיא	أوقية	*ūqiyya*
pound, *raṭl* (406,25 g)	ליטר	رطل ج. أرطال	*raṭl, arṭāl*
part	חלק ר. חלקים	جزء ج. أجزاء	*ǧuz', aǧzā'*

6 Index of Personal Names

7 Index of Places

8 Index of Works Cited

9 Index of Prescriptions

For a variety of prescriptions, see *index of prescriptions* in part 1. Below an index of prescriptions present in Ms. Parma.

10 Index of Some Medical Terms

Including Arabic terms spelled with Hebrew characters, as they occur in Ms. Parma, and the Arabic equivalents of the terms in Ms. Escorial.

eivar	איבר	عضو	part
admimut	אדמימות	حمرة	redness
ot	אות	دليل	indication
eiḵut	איכות	كيفية	method
iṣtomḵa	אצטומכא	معدة	stomach
al-akḥal	אלאכחל	الأكحل	median cubital vein
al-intišār	אלאנתשאר	الانتشار	al-intišār
al-usaylim	אלאסילם	الأسيلم	vena salvatella
al-ʿirq al-madīnī	אלערק אלמדיני	العرق المدني	Guinea worm
isṭenisut	אסטניסות	غثيان	nausea

ba’uš	באוש	نتن	bad smell
bawwāb	בואב	بواب	pylorus
bawāsīr	בואסיר	بواسير	haemorrhoids
buḥḥat al-ṣawt	אלבחוחה אלצות	بحة الصوت	hoarseness of voice
biqquʿa	בקוע	شقاق	fissures
beiṣim	ביצים	الأنثيان	testicles
al-ibṭī	אלבטאן	الإبطي	axillary veins
al-bāsilīq	אלבסליק	الباسليق	basilic vein

gubba	גבה	غدّة	gland
gavninut ha-kaved	גבנינות הכבד	حدبة الكبد	convex side of the liver

guf	גוף	بدن	body
gid	גיד	عرق	vein
gid ha-naše	גיד הנשה	عرق النسا	sciatic vein, sciatica
gid dofeq	גיד דופק	عرق ضارب	pulsatile veins
gid bilti dofeq	גיד בלתי דופק	عرق غير ضارب	non-pulsatile veins
gilgul ha-roš	גלגול הראש		dizziness
ḏabūliyya	דבוליא	ذبولية	marasmus
devequt	דבקות	لزوم	adhesion
dam	דם	دم	blood
dam ha-neḥirayim	דם הנחירים	رعاف	nosebleed; epistaxis
dummal	דמאל	دمل	boil
dofeq	דופק	نبض	pulse
defiqa	דפיקה	ضربان	throbbing
haggarat ha-zeraʿ ha-niqret al-iḥtilām	הגרת הזרע הנקראת אלאחתילאם	احتلام	nocturnal emission
hakkaʾa	הכאה	ضربة	blow
hanhaga	הנהגה	تدبير	regimen
heʿṣer ha-dam	העצר הדם	احتقان الدم	congestion of blood
haqqaza	הקזה	فصد	phlebotomy, blood-letting
haqqafa	הקפה	نوبة	paroxysm
haraqa	הרקה	استفراغ	evacuation
hattaḵa	התכה	تحليل	dissolution
veset	וסת	طمث	menstruation, menses
zeiʿa	זיעה	عرق	sweat
zukam	זכאם	زكام	rheum
zeroʿa	זרוע	ذراع	forearm
zeraʿ	זרע	–	semen
ḥabal al-ḏirāʿ	חבל אלדרע	حبل الذراع	vena cephalica pollicis
ḥikkuḵ	חכוך	حكة	itching
ḥabbura	חבורה	قرح	ulcer
ḥiǧāb	חג׳אב	حجاب	diaphragm
ḥiǧāma	חג׳אמה	حجامة	cupping

ḥulša	חולשה	ضعف	weakness
ḥulšat ha-re’ut ha-niqret al-ʿašāwa	חולשת הראות הנקרא אלעשאוא	عشاوة	visual impairment called nyctalopia
ḥaze	חזה	صدر	chest
ḥazarat ha-haqqaza	חזרת ההקזה	تثنية	additional removal of blood; epaphairesis
ḥoli	חלי	علّة	illness
ḥoli al-sulāq	חלי אלסלאק	سلاق	ptilosis
ḥoli al-sakta	חלי אלסכתה	سكتة	apoplexy
ḥoli ha-kefiya	חלי הכפייה	صرع	epilepsy
ḥoli malinḵuniya	חלי מלנכוניא	مالنخونيا	melancholy
ḥoli pittul ha-gidim ha-niqra al-dawālī	חלי פתול הגידים הנקרא אלדואלי	الدوالي	illness of twisted veins called varicose veins
ḥoli ha-ʿeinayim ha-niqra al-ramad	חלי העינים הנקרא אלרמאד	رمد	ophthalmia
ḥole	חולה	عليل	patient
ha-ḥelev ha-meḵase et ha-qerev	החלב המכסה את הקרב	ثرب	omentum
ḥamimut	חמימות	حار	heat
ḥamimut ṭivʿit	חמימות טבעית	الحار الغريزي	innate heat
ḥaniqot	חניקות	خوانيق	diphtheria
ṭevaʿ	טבע	طبيعة	Nature; natural constitution
ṭeḥol	טחול	طحال	spleen
ṭeḥorim	טחורים	بواسير	haemorrhoids
yeṣi’a	יציאה	إخراج	extraction
ke’ev	כאב	وجع	pain
ke’ev ha-ʿeinayim	כאב העינים	وجع العين	ophthalmalgia
ke’evei ha-peraqim	כאבי הפרקים	أوجاع المفاصل	arthritis
ke’ev roš	כאב ראש	صداع	headache
kaved	כבד	كبد	liver
ḵadar	כדר	خدر	numbness
koved	כובד	ثقل	heaviness
koaḥ	כוח	قوة	strength; faculty

koaḥ ḥiyuni	כוח חיוני	القوة الحيوانية	animal faculty
kosot ha-meṣiṣa	כוסות המציצה	محجمة ج. محاجم	cupping vessels
kaluf	כלוף	كلف	freckles
kammut	כמות	كمية	quantity

lev	לב	قلب	heart
labba	לבה	لبة	jugular fossa
leha'a	להאה	لهاة	uvula
leḥa	ליחה	خلط	humour
lesatot	לסתות	لثة	gums

ma'abiḍ al-rukba	מאבץ אלרכבא	مأبض الركبة	popliteal fossa
ma'aqin	מאקין	ماق	canthus internus, the inner corner of the eye
maġṣ	מגץ	مغص	gripes
moaḥ	מוח	دماغ	brain
mursa	מורסה	ورم	swelling; tumour
mursat ha-moaḥ ha-ḥama ha-niqret al-širsām	מורסת המוח החמה הנקראת אלשרסאם	شرسام	phrenitis
mursat ha-ṣela'ot	מורסת הצלעות	ذات الجنب	pleurisy
mezeg	מזג	مزاج	disposition
mazon	מזון	غذاء	nutriment
meḥiṣa	מחיצה	طبقة	tunic
min	מין	صنف	kind
meitar ha-zero'a	מיתר הזרוע		cord of the forearm
millui	מלוי	امتلاء	overfilling; plethos
millui kefi ha-ḥalalim	מלוי כפי החללים	امتلاء بحسب الأوعية	overfilling relating to vessels
millui kefi ha-koaḥ	מלוי כפי הכוח	امتلاء بحسب القوة	overfilling affecting the strength
minhag	מנהג	عادة	custom
ha-masak ha-niqra al-ḥiǧāb	המסך הנקרא אלחג׳אב	حجاب	diaphragm
me'ayim	מעים	أمعاء	intestines
mi'sam	מעצם	معصم	wrist
meṣaḥ	מצח	جبهة	forehead
miṣnefet	מצנפת	عصابة	bandage

miqve	מקוה	مثانة	bladder
maqom	מקום	موضع	site, spot
marpeq	מרפק	مرفق	elbow
mišgal	משגל	جماع	sexual intercourse
mešiḵa	משיכה	جذب	drawing
matuaḥ	מתוח	تمدد	expansion
nazla	נזלה	نزلة	catarrh
neḥir	נחיר	منخر	nostril
nuqrat ha-roš	נקרת הראש	نقرة الرأس	hollow of the neck
nefiḥa	נפיחה	التهاب	swelling; inflammation
nefila	נפילה	سقطة	fall
negaʿim	נגעים	بثور	pustules
nemiḵut ha-qol	נמיכות הקול	بحة الصوت	hoarseness of voice
sibba	סבה	سبب	cause
sibbuv ha-roš ha-niqra al-duwwār	סבוב הראש הנקרא אלדואר	دوار	vertigo
sabal	סבל	ريح السبل	[wind of] pannus
sakta	סכתה	سكتة	apoplexy
sulāq	סלאק	سلاق	ptilosis
silliyya	סליאה	سلية	phthisis
sammim	סמים	أدوية	drugs
saʿfa	סעפא	سعفة	cradle cap
ʿor	עור	جلد	skin
ʿaṭuf / ʿaluf	עטוף / עלוף	غشي	unconsciousness
ʿeṣev	עצב	عصب	nerve
ʿaṣal	עצל	عضل	muscle
ʿaṣela	עצלה	كسل	laziness
ʿaṣirat ha-veset	עצירת הוסת	احتباس الحيض	amenorrhea
ʿikkul	עכול	هضم	digestion
ʿippuš	עפוש	عفن	putrefaction
ʿaqev	עקב	كعب	ankle
ʿirq al-nasa	ערק אלניסא	عرق النسا	sciatica
paḥad	פחד	خيفة	fear
pi ha-isṭomḵa	פי האצטומכא	فم المعدة	orifice of the stomach

pi ha-ṭabbaʿat	פי הטבעת	مقعدة	anus
panim	פנים	وجه	face; kind
peʿula	פעולה	فعل	effect; activity
pereq	פרק	مفصل	joint
ṣedadim	צדדים	–	flanks; sides
ṣedaʿayim	צדעים	صدغان	temples
ṣaraʿat	צרעת	جذام	leprosy
al-ṣafin	צפאן	الصافن	saphenous vein
al-kāhil	קאהל	الكاهل	interscapular region
qaddaḥat	קדחת	حمى	fever
qol	קול	صوت	voice
qawlang	קולנג׳	قولنج	colic
qiʾ	קיא	قيء	vomiting
al-qīfāl	אלקיפאל	القيفال	cephalic vein
qulāʿ	קלע	قلاع	aphthae
qerum	קרום	غشاء	membrane
roš	ראש	رأس	head
rabw	רבו	ربو	asthma
ribbui	רבוי	كثرة	excess
reiʾa	ריאה	رئة	lungs
refuʾa	רפואה	علاج	treatment
rifion ha-daʿat	רפיון הדעת	بلادة الذهن	want of intellect
reḥem	רחם	رحم	uterus
razon	רזון	هزال	emaciation
ramad	רמד	رمد	ophthalmia
retiḥa	רתיחה	غليان	boiling
šidra	שדרה	صلب	spinal column
šilšul	שלשול	إسهال	diarrhoea
šilšul ha-dam	שלשול הדם	أختلاف الدم	bloody diarrhoea
šawṣa	שוצא	شوصة	pleuritis
šaqīqa	שקיקא	شقيقة	migraine
šarāsīf	שראסיף	شراسيف	false ribs
širyān	שרין	شريان	artery
seriṭa	שריטה	شرط	scarification
serifat ha-dam	שריפת הדם	احتراق الدم	combustion of blood

širsām	שרסאם	شرسام	phrenitis
šeten	שתן	بول	urine
toʿelet	תועלת	منفعة	benefit
hitpašṭut ha-eivarim	התפשטות האיברים	تمطٍ	stretching
tenuʿa	תנועה	حركة	movement
teʿura	תעורה	سهر	insomnia
taṯāʾub	תתאב	تثاؤب	yawning

Bibliography and Abbreviations

Abbott, Nabia, *Studies in Arabic Literary Papyri 2 Qur'anic Commentary and Tradition*, University of Chicago Press, Chicago, 1967

Abdelkareem: Abdelkareem A. Ahmed, 'Health Benefits of Gum Arabic and Medicinal Use' in *Gum Arabic: Structure, Properties, Application and Economics*. Elsevier 2018. Chapter 16, pp. 183–210 (Accessed online on June 15th, 2022)

Alam, Houshang, 'Cassia', in *Encyclopædia Iranica*, Vol. v, Fasc. 1, pp. 62–63, 1990, https://iranicaonline.org/articles/cassia-a-genus-of-shrubs-and-trees-of-the-family-leguminosae, accessed on June 22nd, 2022.

Albucasis, 936–1013.—*Albucasis On Surgery and Instruments / a definitive ed. of the Arabic text with Engl. transl. and comment. by M.S. Spink and G.L. Lewis*, London, 1973

Aristotle, *Problems*: Aristotle. *Problems, Volume 1: Books 1–19*. Edited and translated by Robert Mayhew. Loeb Classical Library 316. Cambridge, MA: Harvard University Press, 2011

Ashkenazi, Shmuel & Jarden, Dov, *Ozar rashe tevot: Thesaurus of Hebrew Abbreviations*, R. Mass, Jerusalem, 1978

Bakich, Michael E., *The Cambridge Guide to the Constellations* / Cambridge University Press, Cambridge, 1995

Bīrūnī, Risāla: Bīrūnī (973–1048), *Risāla li-l-Bīrūnī fī fihrist kutub Muḥammad ibn Zakariyyā' al-Rāzī*, ed. Paul Kraus, Paris, al-Qalam, 1936

Bliquez, Lawrence J., *The Tools of Asclepius: Surgical Instruments in Greek and Roman Times*. Leiden: Brill, 2015

Bos, Gerrit, *Novel Medical and General Hebrew Terminology from the 13th Century, Volume Two*, Brill, Leiden, 2018

Bos, Gerrit, *Novel Medical and General Hebrew Terminology from the 13th Century, Volume Four*, Brill, Leiden, 2019

Bos, Gerrit & Fischer, Klaus-Dietrich, *A Glimpse into Medical Practice among Jews around 1500*, Brill, Leiden, 2021

Brain, Peter, *Galen on Bloodletting: A Study of the Origins, Development and Validity of His Opinions, with a Translation of the Three Works*, Cambridge University Press, Cambridge, 1986

Clementi, Elisabetta M. & Misiti, Francesco, 'Potential Health Benefits of Rhubarb', in Watson, Ronald Ross. & Preedy, Victor R. (eds.) *Bioactive foods in promoting health [Electronic source] probiotics and prebiotics*, Academic Press, London, 2010, pp. 407–432

De Koning, *Trois Traités d'Anatomie Arabes*: Rhazes (ca. 854–ca. 925), *Trois traités d'anatomie arabes = Ṯalāṯ rasā'il arabiyya fī l-tašrīḥ*, [traduction de] Pieter de Koning, Inst. für Geschichte der Arabisch-Islamischen Wissenschaften an der Johann Wolfgang Goethe Univ., Frankfurt am Main, 1986[1903]

Derenbourg, Hartwig (reviewed and completed by Renaud), *Les manuscrits arabes de l'Escurial 2:2*, Paris, 1941

Dioscorides, *GHD*: Dioskorides Pedanius (40–90), *The Greek Herbal of Dioscorides*, edited and first printed A.D. 1933 by Robert T. Gunther, Classics of Medicine Library, New York, 1996

Dozy, Reinhart Pieter Anne. *Supplément aux dictionnaires arabes*, 2 éd., Brill, Leiden, 1927

DTr: Dioscurides Pedanius & Dietrich, Albert (ed.), *Dioscurides Triumphans: ein anonymer arabischer Kommentar (Ende 12. Jahrh. n. Chr.) zur Materia medica: arabischer Text nebst kommentierter deutscher Übersetzung*, Vandenhoeck & Ruprecht, Göttingen, 1988

El-Rouayheb, Khaled & Schmidtke, Sabine (eds.), *The Oxford Handbook of Islamic Philosophy*, Oxford University Press, New York, NY, 2017

Fellmann, *Qalānisī*: Fellmann, Irene, *Das Aqrābād̲īn al-Qalānisī: quellenkritische und begriffsanalytische Untersuchungen zur arabisch-pharmazeutischen Literatur*, In Kommission bei Steiner, Beirut, 1986

Fonahn, Adolf, *Arabic and Latin Anatomical Terminology: Chiefly from the Middle Ages*, Kristiania, 1922

Freimark, Peter, *Das Vorwort als literarische Form in der arabischen Literatur*. Diss. Münster, Westfalen, 1967

Gacek, Adam, *Handbuch der Orientalistik Abt. 1 Der Nahe und Mittlere Osten = The Near and Middle East. Vol. 98 Arabic manuscripts: Arabic Manuscripts: A Vademecum for Readers*, Brill, Leiden, 2009

Gacek, Adam, 'Taxonomy of Scribal Errors and Corrections in Arabic Manuscripts', in *Theoretical approaches to the transmission and edition of Oriental manuscripts: proceedings of a symposium held in Istanbul, March 28–30, 2001* / edited by Judith Pfeiffer, Manfred Kropp, 2007, pp. 217–235

Gacek, *The Arabic Manuscript Tradition*: Gacek, Adam, *Handbuch der Orientalistik Abt. 1 Der Nahe und Mittlere Osten = The Near and Middle East. Bd 58 The Arabic manuscrip[t] tradition: a glossary of technical terms and bibliography*, Brill, Leiden, 2001

Galen, *Alim. Fac.*: Galenos (129–199), *On the Properties of Foodstuffs = De alimentorum facultatibus*, introduction, translation, and commentary by Owen Powell; with a foreword by John Wilkins, Cambridge University Press, Cambridge, 2003

Galen, *Com. Hip. Ep.*: Galenos (129–199), *Commentary on Hippocrates' Epidemics book I, parts I–III* [Electronic source], edition of the Arabic version with English translation and notes by Uwe Vagelpohl, De Gruyter Akademie Forschung, Berlin, 2014

Galen, *Cur. Rat. Ven. Sect.*: Galen. De curandi ratione per venae sectionem—On Treatment by Venesection, in Brain, Peter, *Galen on Bloodletting: A Study of the Origins,*

Development and Validity of His Opinions, with a Translation of the Three Works, Cambridge University Press, Cambridge, 1986

Galen, De locis affectis: Galenos (129–199), *Galen On the Affected Parts: transl. from the Greek text with explanatory notes*, ed. Rudolph E. Siegel, Basel, 1976

Galen, *Dis.*: Galenos (129–199), *Galen on Diseases and Symptoms, translated, with introduction and notes*, by Ian Johnston, Cambridge University Press, Cambridge, 2006

Galen, Inst. Log.: Galen (129–199), *Galen's Institutio Logica, English Translation, Introduction, and Commentary by Kieffer, John Spangler* [Electronic source], The Johns Hopkins Press, Baltimore, 1964

Galen, *Meth. Med.*: Galen. *Method of Medicine, Volumes I–III: Books 1–14*. Edited and translated by Ian Johnston, G.H.R. Horsley. Loeb Classical Library 516, 517, 518. Cambridge, MA: Harvard University Press, 2011

Galen, *Meth. Med. G*: Galen. *On the Constitution of the Art of Medicine. The Art of Medicine. A Method of Medicine to Glaucon*. Edited and translated by Ian Johnston. Loeb Classical Library 523. Cambridge, MA: Harvard University Press, 2016

Galen, *Meth. Med. Hankinson*: Galenos (129–199)—*De Methodo Medendi (Kühn X 1–1021), On the Therapeutic Method: books I and II*, translated with an introduction and commentary by R.J. Hankinson, Clarendon Press, Oxford, 1991

Galen, *Nat. Fac.*: Galen. *On the Natural Faculties*. Translated by A.J. Brock. Loeb Classical Library 71. Cambridge, MA: Harvard University Press, 1916

Galen, *Opt. Med. Ex.*: Galenos (129–199), *On Examinations by which the Best Physicians are Recognized, edition of the Arabic version with English translation and commentary by Albert Z. Iskandar* = [Galeni De optimo medico cognoscendo libelli versionem Arabicam / primum edidit, in linguam Anglicam vertit, commentatus est Albert Z. Iskandar], Akademie-Vlg., Berlin, 1988

Galen, *PHP*: Galenos, *Galen on the Doctrines of Hippocrates and Plato, De Placitis Hippocratis et Platonis* (Kühn V 181–805), ed., tr. and comm. by Philip De Lacy, CMG V 4. 1. 2., Akademie-Vlg., Berlin, 1980

Galen, *Temp.*: Galenos, *On Temperaments. On Non-Uniform Distemperment. The Soul's Traits Depend on Bodily Temperament*. Edited and translated by Ian Johnston. Loeb Classical Library 546. Cambridge, MA: Harvard University Press, 2020

Galen, *UP*: Galenos (129–199), *De usu partium*, I–XVII (Kühn III 1–933) and Kühn IV 1–366, Helmreich (1907–1909), *On the Usefulness of the Parts of the Body*, Volumes 1 and 2, Translation from the Greek with an introduction and commentary by Margaret Tallmadge May, Ithaca, New York, 1996

Galen, Ven. Sect. Ad. Er.: Galen. Galeni de Venae Sectione adversus Erasistratum Liber—On Venesection against Erasistratus, in Brain, Peter, *Galen on Bloodletting: A Study of the Origins, Development and Validity of His Opinions, with a Translation of the Three Works*, Cambridge University Press, Cambridge, 1986

Galen, Ven. Sect. Ad. Er. Rom.: Galen. Galeni de Venae Sectione Adversus Erasistrateos Romae Degentes—On Venesection against the Erasistrateans at Rome, in Brain, Peter, *Galen on Bloodletting: A Study of the Origins, Development and Validity of His Opinions, with a Translation of the Three Works*, Cambridge University Press, Cambridge, 1986

Garrison, F.H., *The History of Bloodletting*, New York. A.R. Elliott Publishing Company, 1913

Gesenius, Wilhelm, *Gesenius' Hebrew and Chaldee Lexicon to the Old Testament Scriptures*, James Duncan, London, 1832

Goodman, L.E., '*The Greek Impact on Arabic Literature*', in Beeston, A.F.L. (red). *Arabic literature to the end of the Umayyad period*. Cambridge University Press, Cambridge, 1983, pp. 460–482

Grohmann, Adolf, *Arabische Paläographie T. 2 Das Schriftwesen: die Lapidarschrift*, Wien, 1971

Gutas, Dimitri, *Greek Thought, Arabic Culture: the Graeco-Arabic Translation Movement in Baghdad and Early 'Abbāsid Society* (*2nd–4th/8th–10th centuries*), London, Routledge, 1998

Hankinson: Hankinson, R.J., *Galen's Theory of Causation*. In ANRW II 37:2,1994

Hinz, *Islamische Masse und Gewichte*: Walther, *Handbuch der Orientalistik, Abt. 1, Der Nahe und der Mittlere Osten, Erg. -Bd 1. H. 1, Islamische Masse und Gewichte: umgerechnet ins metrische System*, Brill, Leiden, 1955

Hippocrates, *AWP; Epidemics I; Epidemics III; Nut.*: Hippocrates. *Ancient Medicine. Airs, Waters, Places. Epidemics 1 and 3. The Oath. Precepts. Nutriment*. Edited and translated by Paul Potter. Loeb Classical Library 147. Cambridge, MA: Harvard University Press, 2022

Hippocrates, *Critical Days*: Hippocrates. *Coan Prenotions. Anatomical and Minor Clinical Writings*. Edited and translated by Paul Potter. Loeb Classical Library 509. Cambridge, MA: Harvard University Press, 2010

Hippocrates, *De Alimento*: Hippocrates, (ca. 460–ca. 370 BC), *Kitāb Buqrāṭ fī l-aḫlāṭ and Kitāb al-ġiḏā' li-Buqrāṭ: On humours and On nutriment*, ed. and transl. with introd. notes and glossary by J.N. Mattock. Cambridge, 1971

Hippocrates, *Epidemics 2, 4–7*: Hippocrates. *Epidemics 2, 4–7*. Edited and translated by Wesley D. Smith. Loeb Classical Library 477. Cambridge, MA: Harvard University Press, 1994

Hippocrates, *Nat. Hom.; Regimen III; Dreams*: Hippocrates, Heracleitus. *Nature of Man. Regimen in Health. Humours. Aphorisms. Regimen 1–3. Dreams. Heracleitus: On the Universe*. Translated by W.H.S. Jones. Loeb Classical Library 150. Cambridge, MA: Harvard University Press, 1931

Hippocrates, *Places in Man*: Hippocrates. *Places in Man. Glands. Fleshes. Prorrhetic 1–2. Physician. Use of Liquids. Ulcers. Haemorrhoids and Fistulas*. Edited and translated by Paul Potter. Loeb Classical Library 482. Cambridge, MA: Harvard University Press, 1995

Hippocrates, *Reg. Ac.*: Hippocrates. *Prognostic. Regimen in Acute Diseases. The Sacred Disease. The Art. Breaths. Law. Decorum. Physician (Ch. 1). Dentition.* Translated by W.H.S. Jones. Loeb Classical Library 148. Cambridge, MA: Harvard University Press, 1923

Holmes, Brooke, 'Medicine', in *The Oxford Handbook of Hellenic Studies*, Graziosi, B., Vasunia, P. and Boys-Stones, G., Oxford University Press, Oxford, 2009

Hoyland, Robert G., *Seeing Islam as Others Saw It: a Survey and Evaluation of Christian, Jewish, and Zoroastrian Writings on Early Islam*, Darwin Press, Princeton, N.J., 1997

Ḥunayn ibn Isḥāq, *'Ašr maqālāt fī l-'ayn*: Ḥunayn ibn Isḥāq al-'Ibādī (809–873) (1996 [1928]). *'Ašr maqālāt fī l-'ayn* (*Ten Treatises on the Eye*), Frankfurt am Main: Institute for the History of Arabic-Islamic Science at the Johann Wolfgang Goethe University, 1996 [1928]

Ibn Abī Uṣaybi'a, *A Literary History of Medicine*: Aḥmad ibn al-Qāsim (d. 1269 or 1270), *A Literary History of Medicine: the 'Uyūn al-anbā' fī ṭabaqāt al-aṭibbā' of Ibn Abī Uṣaybi'ah Volume 3–2*, Annotated English translation / edited and translated by Emilie Savage-Smith, Simon Swain, Geert Jan van Gelder; with Ignacio Sánchez, N. Peter Joosse, Alasdair Watson, Bruce Inksetter and Franak Hilloowala, Brill, Leiden, 2020

Ibn Abī Uṣaybi'a, Ṭabaqāt: Ibn Abī Uṣaybi'a, Aḥmad ibn al-Qāsim (d. 1269 or 1270), *A Literary History of Medicine: the 'Uyūn al-anbā' fī ṭabaqāt al-aṭibbā'* of Ibn Abī Uṣaybi'ah Volume 2–2, Arabic edition / edited and translated by Emilie Savage-Smith, Simon Swain, Geert Jan van Gelder; with Ignacio Sánchez, N. Peter Joosse, Alasdair Watson, Bruce Inksetter and Franak Hilloowala, Brill, Leiden, 2020

Ibn Ǧanāḥ: Ibn Janāḥ, Abū al-Walīd Marwān, (ca. 990–ca. 1050), Marwān ibn Janāḥ: *On the Nomenclature of Medicinal Drugs* (*Kitāb al-talkhīṣ*)*: edition, translation and commentary, with special reference to the Ibero-Romance terminology*, edited by Gerrit Bos, Fabian Käs, Mailyn Lübke, Guido Mensching, Brill, Leiden, 2020

Ibn al-Ǧazzār, *Zād al-Musāfir*: McVaugh, Michael R., Bos, Gerrit & Käs, Fabian—*Ibn Al-Jazzār's Zād Al-Musāfir Wa-qūt Al-ḥāḍir. Provisions for the Traveller and Nourishment for the Sedentary: Books I and II*: Diseases of the Head and the Face, Brill, Boston, 2022

Ibn Ǧulǧul, *Dio.*: Ibn Ǧulǧul, Sulaymān ibn Ḥassān (976–1009), *Die Ergänzung Ibn-Ǧulǧul's zur Materia medica des Dioskurides:* arabischer Text nebst kommentierter deutscher Übersetzung, hrsg. von Albert Dietrich, Vandenhoeck und Ruprecht, Göttingen, 1993

Ibn Ǧulǧul, *Ṭabaqāt*: Ibn Ǧulǧul, Sulaymān ibn Ḥassān, 976–1009.—*Les generations des medecins et des sages. Ṭabaqāt al-atibbā' wa-l-ḥukamā'*. Ecrit composé en 377 H.

par Abu Dawud Sulaiman Ibn Hassan ibn Gulgul Al-Andalusi. Ed. critique par Fu'ad Sayyid.—1955

Ibn Māsawayh: Ibn Māsawaih, *Traité sur les substances simples aromatiques par Yohanna ben Massawaih*, ed. P. Sbath. Bulletin de l'Institut d'Égypte 19 (1937) 5–27, (https://archive.org/details/BIE-19-1936-1937) accessed online on June 15th, 2022

Ibn al-Nadīm, *Fihrist*: Ibn al-Nadīm, Muḥammad ibn Isḥāq (10th century), *The Fihrist of al-Nadīm: a tenth-century survey of Muslim culture* / Bayard Dodge ed. and transl., Columbia U.P., New York, 1970

Ibn Sīnā, *Risāla fī l-Qawlanǧ*: Ibn Sīnā, 'Risāla fī l-Qawlanǧ,' in *Kitāb al-qūlanǧ: Le livre de la colique, al-Rāzī; édition critique et traduction de Soubhi M. Hammami.* (pp. 157–175), Aleppo University, Institute for the History of Arabic Science, Aleppo, 1983

Iskandar, Albert Zaki, 'Ar-Rāzī, the Clinical Physician (Al-Rāzī aṭ-ṭabīb al-iklīnīkī)', in *Islamic Medical and Scientific Tradition: critical concepts in Islamic studies, Vol. I*, (ed. Peter E. Pormann). Routledge, Milton Park, Abingdon, 2011. (pp. 207–253)

Kahl, *The Dispensatory of Ibn al-Tilmīḏ*: Ibn al-Tilmīḏ, Hibat Allāh ibn Ṣā'id (1073 or 1074–1164 or 1165), *The Dispensatory of Ibn al-Tilmīḏ: Arabic text, English translation, study and glossaries*, by Oliver Kahl, Brill, Leiden, 2007

Kahl, *Sābūr ibn Sahl; The Small Dispensatory*: Kahl, Oliver, Sābūr ibn Sahl; *The Small Dispensatory. Translated from the Arabic, together with a study and glossaries*, Brill, 2003

Kahl, Oliver, *The Sanskrit, Syriac and Persian Sources in the Comprehensive Book of Rhazes*, Brill, Leiden, 2015

Al-Kindī, *Aqrābāḏīn*: Al-Kindī, Ya'qūb b. Isḥāq (d. ca. 873), *The Medical Formulary, or Aqrābādhīn of al-Kindī, translated, with a study of its materia medica by Martin Levey*, Wisconsin University Press, Milwaukee, 1966

Al-Khalidi, Rūḥī, *Al-Kīmiyā' 'ind al-'Arab*, Mu'assasat Hindāwī li-l-ta'līm wa-l-ṯaqāfa, Cairo, Egypt, 2013

Al-Kindī, Ya'qūb b. Isḥāq (d. ca. 873), *Kitāb kīmiyā al-'iṭr wat-taṣ'īdāt = Buch über die Chemie des Parfüms und die Destillationen*, transl. by K. Garbers, Leipzig, 1948

Käs, Mineralien: Käs, Fabian, *Die Mineralien in der arabischen Pharmakognosie: eine Konkordanz zur mineralischen Materia medica der klassischen arabischen Heilmittelkunde nebst überlieferungsgeschichtlichen Studien*, Harrassowitz Verlag, Wiesbaden, 2010

Lane, Edward William, *An Arabic-English Lexicon: derived from the best and the most copious Eastern sources*, Williams and Norgate, London, 1863–1893

Liddell, Henry George & Scott, Robert, *A Greek-English Lexicon, revised by Henry Stuart Jones*, Clarendon, Oxford, 1968

Liddell, Henry George & Scott, Robert, *An Intermediate Greek-English Lexicon: founded upon the seventh edition of Liddell and Scott's Greek-English lexicon*, Oxford University Press, Oxford, 2000[1889]

Maimonides, *Aphorisms 1–5*: Maimonides, Moses (1138–1204), *Medical Aphorisms, a parallel Arabic-English edition = Kitāb al-fuṣūl fī al-ṭibb Treatises 1–5, edited, translated, and annotated by Gerrit Bos*, Brigham Young University Press, Provo, Utah, 2004

Maimonides, *Aphorisms 10–15*: Maimonides, Moses (1138–1204), *Medical Aphorisms, a parallel Arabic-English edition = Kitāb al-fuṣūl fī al-ṭibb Treatises 10–15, edited, translated, and annotated by Gerrit Bos*, Brigham Young University Press, Provo, Utah, 2007

Maimonides, *Aphorisms 22–25*: Maimonides, Moses (1135–1204), *Medical Aphorisms, a parallel Arabic-English edition Treatises 22–25, edited, translated, and annotated by Gerrit Bos*, Brigham Young University Press, Provo, Utah, 2016

Maimonides, *Glossary*: Maimonides, Moses (1138–1204), *Glossary of Drug Names: translated from Max Meyerhof's French edition*, ed. by Fred Rosner, Philadelphia, 1979

Maimonides, *RH*: Bos, Gerrit, *Maimonides On the Regimen of Health*: *A New Parallel Arabic-English Translation by Gerrit Bos with Critical Editions of Medieval Hebrew Translations by Gerrit Bos and Latin Translations by Michael R. M* [Electronic source], Brill, 2019

Maimonides, *Rules*: Maimonides, Moses (1135–1204), *On Rules Regarding the Practical Part of the Medical Art = Kitāb qawānīn al-juz' al-ʿamalī min ṣināʿa al-ṭibb*: a parallel Arabic-English edition, edited by Gerrit Bos and Y. Tzvi Langermann, Brigham Young University Press, Provo, Utah, 2013

Martin, Richard C. (ed.), *Encyclopedia of Islam and the Muslim World*, Gale, 2004

Mattern, Susan P., *Prince of medicine: Galen in the Roman world*, Oxford University Press, NY, 2013

Minorsky: *Ḥudūd al-ʿālam = The Regions of the World: a Persian geography 372 A.H.–928 A.D.*, translated and explained by V. Minorsky, London, 1937

Montanari, Franco, *The Brill Dictionary of Ancient Greek*, Brill, Leiden, 2015

Nasr, Seyyed Hossein, *Islamic Philosophy from Its Origin to the Present: Philosophy in the Land of Prophecy*, State University of New York Press, Albany, 2006

Nasrallah, *Annals of the caliphs' kitchens*: Ibn Sayyār al-Warrāq, al-Muẓaffar ibn Naṣr, *Annals of the Caliphs' Kitchens: Ibn Sayyār al-Warrāq's tenth-century Baghdadi cookbook*, English translation with introduction and glossary by Nawal Nasrallah; Arabic text edited by Kaj Öhrnberg and Sahban Mroueh, Brill, Leiden, 2010

Netter, Frank H., *Atlas of Human Anatomy*, Seventh edition, Elsevier, Philadelphia, PA, 2018[2019]

Nutton, Vivian, *Ancient Medicine*, Routledge, London, 2004

Penn, Michael Philip, 'Monks, Manuscripts, and Muslims: Syriac Textual Changes in Reaction to the Rise of Islam', Hugoye: *Journal of Syriac Studies*, Vol. 12.2, 235–257. Beth Mardutho: The Syriac Institute and Gorgias Press, 2009

Perho, Irmeli, *The Prophet's Medicine: a Creation of the Muslim Tradionalist Scholars*, Finnish Oriental Society, Diss. Helsinki, University of Helsinki, 1995

Pormann, Peter E., 'Translations of Medical and Occult Texts into Arabic and Syriac and their Contexts after 80/700' in Brentjes, Sonja, *Routledge Handbook on the Sciences in Islamicate Societies: Practices From the 2nd/8th to the 13th/19th Centuries*, Taylor & Francis, London, 2022

Pormann, Peter E., *The Cambridge Companion to Hippocrates*, Cabridge University Press, 2018

Pormann, Peter E. & Savage-Smith, Emilie, *Medieval Islamic Medicine*, Edinburgh University Press, Edinburgh, 2007

Qusṭā ibn Lūqā, *Al-adwiya al-mushila*: Qusṭā ibn Lūqā (ca. 820–ca. 912), *On Purgative Drugs and Purgation = Kitāb Qusṭā ibn Lūqā fī al-adwiya al-mushila wa-l-ʿilāǧ bi-l-ishāl*, edition, translation and commentary by Lena Ambjörn, Institute for the History of Arabic-Islamic Science at the Johann Wolfgang Goethe University, Frankfurt am Main, 2004

Qusṭā ibn Lūqā, *Kitāb fi l-Faṣd*, Un inedito scritto medico di Qusṭā ibn Lūqā sulla flebotomia, ed. tr. Celentano and Marra; in: *Atti della V settimana di studi Sangue e antropologia. Riti e culto*, Rome, 1984, pp. 273–460

Qusṭā ibn Lūqā, *Numbness*: Qusṭā ibn Lūqā (ca. 820–ca. 912), *Qusṭā ibn Lūqā On Numbness: a book on numbness, its kinds, causes and treatment according to the opinion of Galen and Hippocrates*, edition, translation and commentary by Lena Ambjörn, Diss. Lund University, Stockholm, 2000

Qusṭā ibn Lūqā, *Safar al-Ḥaǧǧ*: Qusṭā ibn Lūqā (ca. 820–ca. 912), *Qusṭā ibn Lūqā's Medical Regime for the Pilgrims to Mecca: The Risāla fī tadbīr safar al-ḥajj*, edited with translation and commentary by Gerrit Bos, Brill, Leiden, 1992

Al-Rāzī, *Asrār*: Al-Rāzī, Abū Bakr Muḥammad ibn Zakarīyāʾ (865?–925?), *The Alchemy of Al-Razi: a translation of the "Book of Secrets"*, edition and translation by Gail Marlow Taylor, Createspace, North Charleston, 2014

Al-Rāzī, *De. Cur. Puer.* Bos, Gerrit & McVaugh, Michael, Al-Razi, *On the Treatment of Small Children (De curis puerorum)*, Brill, 2015

Al-Rāzī, *Faṣd Alukah*: *Maqāla anšaʾahā Muḥammad ibn Zakariyyāʾ al-Rāzī fī l-Faṣd*, https://www.alukah.net/culture/0/5123/ مقالة-أنشأها-محمد-بن-زكريا-الرازي-في-22% 22%الفصد/#_ftn1

Al-Rāzī, *Ḥāwī II*: Rhazes (854–ca. 925), *Kitāb al-Ḥāwī fī l-Ṭibb al-ǧuzʾ 2. Fī amrāḍ al-ʿayn.* al-Ṭabʿah 1. Hyderabad-Deccan, 1955

Al-Rāzī, *Ḥāwī XI*: Rhazes (ca. 854–ca. 925), *Kitāb al-Ḥāwī fī l-Ṭibb al-ǧuzʾ 11. Fī amrāḍ al-ḥayyāt wa-l-dīdān fī l-baṭn wa-l-bawāsīr wa-ḥadab wa-l-niqris wa-l-dawālī wa-dāʾ al-fīl* ... al-Ṭabʿah 1, Hyderabad-Dekkan, 1962

Al-Rāzī, *Kitāb al-Iklīl*: Kahl, Oliver & Sharp Cockrell, Henrietta, *The Book of the Crown (Kitāb al-Iklīl) of Pseudo-Rhazes*, Islamic Philosophy, Theology and Science, Texts and Studies, Volume: 123., Brill, 2023

Al-Rāzī, *al-Kitāb al-Manṣūrī fī l-Ṭibb*: Abū Bakr Muḥammad ibn Zakariyyāʾ al-Rāzī, *al-Kitāb al-Manṣūrī fī l-Ṭibb*, šarḥ wa-taḥqīq wa-taʿlīq: al-Duktūr Ḥāzim al-Bakrī al-Ṣadīqī, Maʿhad al-Maḫṭūṭāt al-ʿArabiyya (al-Munaẓẓama al-ʿArabiyya li-l-Tarbiya wa-l-Ṯaqāfa wa-l-ʿUlūm), al-Kuwayt, al-ṭabʿa al-ūlā 1408 H.—1987 M.

Al-Rāzī, *Kitāb al-Qawlanǧ*: Rhazes (ca. 854–ca. 925), *Kitāb al-qūlanǧ: Le livre de la colique*, édition critique et traduction de Soubhi M. Hammami, Institute for the History of Arabic Science, Aleppo, 1983

Al-Rāzī, *Naqras*: Rhazes (ca. 854–ca. 925), *Maqālah fī al-naqras, Treatise on Gout, li-Abī Bakr al-Rāzī*, Maktabat al-Iskandariyyah, al-Iskandariyyah, 2003

Al-Rāzī, Muḥammad Ibn-Zakarīyā, 865–925. *On Phlebotomy* / Abū Bakr Muḥammad ibn Zakariyyāʾ al-Rāzī; edition, translation and commentary by Juhan Björn, Joint Faculties of Humanities and Theology, Centre for Languages and Literature, Lund University, Diss. Lund, 2023

Al-Rāzī, *Spiritual Physick*: Rhazes (ca. 854–ca. 925), *The "Spiritual Physick" of Rhazes*, translated from the Arabic by Arthur J. Arberry, J. Murray, London, 1950

Richler, Benjamin & Beit-Arié, Malachi (eds.), *Hebrew Manuscripts in the Biblioteca Palatina in Parma: a Catalogue*, Hebrew University of Jerusalem, Jewish National and University Library, Jerusalem, 2001

Riddle, *Dio. Pharm. Med.*: Riddle, John M., *Dioscorides on Pharmacy and Medicine*, Univ. of Texas Press, Austin, 1985

Rufus, *Melancholy*: Rufus Ephesius, *On Melancholy*, edited by Peter E. Pormann, Mohr Siebeck, Tubingen, 2008

Rufus, *Quaestiones medicinales*: Rufus Ephesius, *Die Fragen des Arztes an den Kranken*, herausgegeben, übersetzt und erläutert von Hans Gärtner = *Rufi Ephesii Quaestiones medicinales*, Akademie-Vlg., Berlin, 1962

Saif, *Islamicate Occult Sciences in Theory and Practice*: *Islamicate Occult Sciences in Theory and Practice*, edited by Liana Saif, Francesca Leoni, Matthew Melvin-Koushki, Farouk Yayha. Brill, Leiden, 2020

Samir, *Actes du premier Congrès international d'études arabes chrétiennes*, Congrès international d'études arabes chrétiennes, (*Goslar, septembre 1980*), éd. par Khalil Samir, Pont. institutum studiorum Orientalium, Roma, 1982

Savage-Smith, Emilie, 'Were the Four Humours Fundamental to Medieval Islamic Medical Practice?' in: *The Body in Balance: Humoral Theory in Practice*, ed. by Elisabeth Hsu and Peregrine Horden. [Epistemologies of Healing, vol. 6], Berghahn Books, Oxford, 2013, pp. 89–106

Scheper, Karin, *The Technique of Islamic Bookbinding: Methods, Materials and Regional Varieties*, Second Revised Edition. Brill, Leiden/Boston, 2019

Schmucker, *Firdaws*: Schmucker, Werner, *Die pflanzliche und mineralische materia medica im Firdaus al-Ḥikma des ʿAlī ibn Sahl Rabbān aṭ-Ṭabarī*, Diss., Bonn, 1969

Sezgin, Fuat, *Geschichte des arabischen Schrifttums, Bd 3, Medizin, Pharmazie, Zoologie, Tierheilkunde bis ca. 436 H*, Brill, Leiden, 1970

Siegel, Rudolph E., *Galen's System of Physiology and Medicine: an analysis of his doctrines and observations on bloodflow, respiration, humors and internal diseases*, Basel, 1968

Stroumsa, Sarah, *Freethinkers of Medieval Islam*: Ibn al-Rāwandī, Abū Bakr al-Rāzī and their impact on Islamic thought, Brill, Boston, Mass., 1999

Swain, Simon, '*Social Stress and Political Pressure: On Melancholy in Context*', in: Pormann, Peter E., (ed.) *On melancholy / Rufus of Ephesus*. Sapere (No. 12). Tübingen: Mohr Siebeck, 2008, pp. 113–138

Al-Ṭabarī, *Amrāḍ al-ʿayn*: al-Ṭabarī. Aḥmad ibn Muḥammad, *Amrāḍ al-ʿayn wa ʿilāǧātuhā min kitābay al-muʿālaǧāt al-Buqrāṭiyya wa Firdaws al-Ḥikma*, Mu'assasat al-Furqān, London, 1998

Tang, Weici & Eisenbrand, Gerhard, *Chinese Drugs of Plant Origin: chemistry, pharmacology, and use in traditional and modern medicine*, Springer-Vlg., Berlin, 1992

Temkin, Owsei, *Galenism: Rise and Decline of a Medical Philosophy*, Ithaca, 1973

Ullmann, Manfred, *Islamic Medicine*, Edinburgh Univ. Press, Edinburgh, 1978

Ullmann, *Die Medizin im Islam*: Ullmann, Manfred, *Handbuch der Orientalistik. Abt. 1, Der Nahe und der Mittlere Osten*, Erg. -Bd 6. Abschnitt 1, *Die Medizin im Islam*. Leiden: Brill, 1970

Ullmann, Manfred, *Wörterbuch zu den griechisch-arabischen Übersetzungen des 9. Jahrhunderts*, Harrassowitz, Wiesbaden, 2002–2007

Waines, David, 'Dietetics in Medieval Islamic Culture', in *Islamic Medical and Scientific Tradition: critical concepts in Islamic studies, Vol. II*, (ed. Peter E. Pormann). Routledge, Milton Park, Abingdon, 2011 (pp. 99–115)

Wehr, Hans, *A Dictionary of Modern Written Arabic* (*Arabic-English*). 4th ed. considerably enl. and amended by the author. Student ed., Spoken Languages Services, Urbana, Ill., 1994

Young, M.J.L., Latham, J.D. & Serjeant, R.B. (eds.), *Religion, Learning and Science in the Abbasid Period*, Cambridge Univ. Press, Cambridge, 1990.

Index of Arabic Terms

Index of Hebrew Terms

Index of General Terms

www.ingramcontent.com/pod-product-compliance
Ingram Content Group UK Ltd.
Pitfield, Milton Keynes, MK11 3LW, UK
UKHW020846290926
15470UKWH00004B/1582

9 789004 762275